Efficiency in Kinesiology: Innovative Approaches in Enhancing Motor Skills for Athletic Performance 2.0

Efficiency in Kinesiology: Innovative Approaches in Enhancing Motor Skills for Athletic Performance 2.0

Editor

Diego Minciacchi

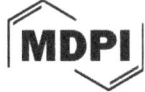

Basel • Beijing • Wuhan • Barcelona • Belgrade • Novi Sad • Cluj • Manchester

Editor
Diego Minciacchi
Experimental and Clinical
Medicine
University of Florence
Florence
Italy

Editorial Office
MDPI AG
Grosspeteranlage 5
4052 Basel, Switzerland

This is a reprint of articles from the Special Issue published online in the open access journal *Journal of Functional Morphology and Kinesiology* (ISSN 2411-5142) (available at: www.mdpi.com/journal/jfmk/special_issues/U53IMNF269).

For citation purposes, cite each article independently as indicated on the article page online and as indicated below:

Lastname, A.A.; Lastname, B.B. Article Title. *Journal Name* **Year**, *Volume Number*, Page Range.

ISBN 978-3-7258-2060-3 (Hbk)
ISBN 978-3-7258-2059-7 (PDF)
doi.org/10.3390/books978-3-7258-2059-7

© 2024 by the authors. Articles in this book are Open Access and distributed under the Creative Commons Attribution (CC BY) license. The book as a whole is distributed by MDPI under the terms and conditions of the Creative Commons Attribution-NonCommercial-NoDerivs (CC BY-NC-ND) license.

Contents

Vincenzo Sorgente and Diego Minciacchi
Efficiency in Kinesiology: Innovative Approaches in Enhancing Motor Skills for Athletic Performance 2.0
Reprinted from: *J. Funct. Morphol. Kinesiol.* **2024**, *9*, 137, doi:10.3390/jfmk9030137 1

Jatin P. Ambegaonkar, Matthew Jordan, Kelley R. Wiese and Shane V. Caswell
Kinesiophobia in Injured Athletes: A Systematic Review
Reprinted from: *J. Funct. Morphol. Kinesiol.* **2024**, *9*, 78, doi:10.3390/jfmk9020078 5

Andreas Hegdahl Gundersen, Hallvard Nygaard Falch, Andrea Bao Fredriksen and Roland van den Tillaar
The Effect of Sex and Different Repetition Maximums on Kinematics and Surface Electromyography in the Last Repetition of the Barbell Back Squat
Reprinted from: *J. Funct. Morphol. Kinesiol.* **2024**, *9*, 75, doi:10.3390/jfmk9020075 19

Nor Fazila Abd Malek, Ali Md Nadzalan, Kevin Tan, Abdul Muiz Nor Azmi, Rajkumar Krishnan Vasanthi, Ratko Pavlović, et al.
The Acute Effect of Dynamic vs. Proprioceptive Neuromuscular Facilitation Stretching on Sprint and Jump Performance
Reprinted from: *J. Funct. Morphol. Kinesiol.* **2024**, *9*, 42, doi:10.3390/jfmk9010042 32

Alessandro Cudicio and Valeria Agosti
Beyond Belief: Exploring the Alignment of Self-Efficacy, Self-Prediction, Self-Perception, and Actual Performance Measurement in a Squat Jump Performance—A Pilot Study
Reprinted from: *J. Funct. Morphol. Kinesiol.* **2024**, *9*, 16, doi:10.3390/jfmk9010016 43

Israel Caraballo, Luka Pezelj and Juan José Ramos-Álvarez
Analysis of the Performance and Sailing Variables of the Optimist Class in a Variety of Wind Conditions
Reprinted from: *J. Funct. Morphol. Kinesiol.* **2024**, *9*, 18, doi:10.3390/jfmk9010018 56

Renata Jirovska, Anthony D. Kay, Themistoklis Tsatalas, Alex J. Van Enis, Christos Kokkotis, Giannis Giakas and Minas A. Mina
The Influence of Unstable Load and Traditional Free-Weight Back Squat Exercise on Subsequent Countermovement Jump Performance
Reprinted from: *J. Funct. Morphol. Kinesiol.* **2023**, *8*, 167, doi:10.3390/jfmk8040167 64

Giorgos Anastasiou, Marios Hadjicharalambous, Gerasimos Terzis and Nikolaos Zaras
Reactive Strength Index, Rate of Torque Development, and Performance in Well-Trained Weightlifters: A Pilot Study
Reprinted from: *J. Funct. Morphol. Kinesiol.* **2023**, *8*, 161, doi:10.3390/jfmk8040161 76

Athanasios Mandroukas, Ioannis Metaxas, Yiannis Michailidis and Thomas Metaxas
Muscle Strength and Joint Range of Motion of the Spine and Lower Extremities in Female Prepubertal Elite Rhythmic and Artistic Gymnasts
Reprinted from: *J. Funct. Morphol. Kinesiol.* **2023**, *8*, 153, doi:10.3390/jfmk8040153 87

Nikolaos Manouras, Christos Batatolis, Panagiotis Ioakimidis, Konstantina Karatrantou and Vassilis Gerodimos
The Reliability of Linear Speed with and without Ball Possession of Pubertal Soccer Players
Reprinted from: *J. Funct. Morphol. Kinesiol.* **2023**, *8*, 147, doi:10.3390/jfmk8040147 102

S. Howard Wittels, Eric Renaghan, Michael Joseph Wishon, Harrison L. Wittels, Stephanie Chong, Eva Danielle Wittels, et al.
A Novel Metric "Exercise Cardiac Load" Proposed to Track and Predict the Deterioration of the Autonomic Nervous System in Division I Football Athletes
Reprinted from: *J. Funct. Morphol. Kinesiol.* **2023**, *8*, 143, doi:10.3390/jfmk8040143 . . . . **114**

Paul T. Donahue, Ayden K. McInnis, Madelyn K. Williams and Josey White
Examination of Countermovement Jump Performance Changes in Collegiate Female Volleyball in Fatigued Conditions
Reprinted from: *J. Funct. Morphol. Kinesiol.* **2023**, *8*, 137, doi:10.3390/jfmk8030137 . . . . **125**

Eric Renaghan, Harrison L. Wittels, Luis A. Feigenbaum, Michael Joseph Wishon, Stephanie Chong, Eva Danielle Wittels, et al.
Exercise Cardiac Load and Autonomic Nervous System Recovery during In-Season Training: The Impact on Speed Deterioration in American Football Athletes
Reprinted from: *J. Funct. Morphol. Kinesiol.* **2023**, *8*, 134, doi:10.3390/jfmk8030134 . . . . **134**

Lea R. Stenerson, Bridget F. Melton, Helen W. Bland and Greg A. Ryan
Running-Related Overuse Injuries and Their Relationship with Run and Resistance Training Characteristics in Adult Recreational Runners: A Cross-Sectional Study
Reprinted from: *J. Funct. Morphol. Kinesiol.* **2023**, *8*, 128, doi:10.3390/jfmk8030128 . . . . **144**

Pasquale J. Succi, Brian Benitez, Minyoung Kwak and Haley C. Bergstrom
Analysis of Individual $\dot{V}O_{2max}$ Responses during a Cardiopulmonary Exercise Test and the Verification Phase in Physically Active Women
Reprinted from: *J. Funct. Morphol. Kinesiol.* **2023**, *8*, 124, doi:10.3390/jfmk8030124 . . . . **155**

George Giatsis, Vassilios Panoutsakopoulos, Christina Frese and Iraklis A. Kollias
Vertical Jump Kinetic Parameters on Sand and Rigid Surfaces in Young Female Volleyball Players with a Combined Background in Indoor and Beach Volleyball
Reprinted from: *J. Funct. Morphol. Kinesiol.* **2023**, *8*, 115, doi:10.3390/jfmk8030115 . . . . **167**

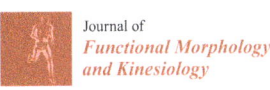

Editorial

Efficiency in Kinesiology: Innovative Approaches in Enhancing Motor Skills for Athletic Performance 2.0

Vincenzo Sorgente * and Diego Minciacchi

Kinesiology and Motor Control (Ki.Mo.Co.) Laboratory, Department of Experimental and Clinical Medicine, Physiological Sciences Section, University of Florence, 50134 Florence, Italy; diego.minciacchi@unifi.it
* Correspondence: vincenzo.sorgente@unifi.it

Citation: Sorgente, V.; Minciacchi, D. Efficiency in Kinesiology: Innovative Approaches in Enhancing Motor Skills for Athletic Performance 2.0. *J. Funct. Morphol. Kinesiol.* **2024**, *9*, 137. https://doi.org/10.3390/jfmk9030137

Received: 29 July 2024
Revised: 6 August 2024
Accepted: 12 August 2024
Published: 14 August 2024

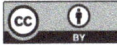

Copyright: © 2024 by the authors. Licensee MDPI, Basel, Switzerland. This article is an open access article distributed under the terms and conditions of the Creative Commons Attribution (CC BY) license (https://creativecommons.org/licenses/by/4.0/).

1. Introduction

The second edition of the Special Issue titled "Efficiency in Kinesiology: Innovative approaches in enhancing motor skills for Athletic Performance" has been effectively concluded, significantly enriching the discourse on "efficiency in kinesiology" by presenting a diverse array of innovative research findings and methodologies aimed at optimizing athletic performance and motor-skill development (https://www.mdpi.com/2411-5142/8/3/111, accessed on 28 July 2024).

Research from the last few decades has established a solid foundation for enhancing athletic performance through various biomotor and technical training and monitoring methodologies [1–4]. However, the ever-expanding field of sports science incessantly proposes new methodologies and technologies, as well as their applications, aimed at evaluating, improving, and predicting motor performance. These innovations attract attention from academics, practitioners, and the general public alike. Yet, the adoption of new approaches often outpaces the scientific validation process, resulting in a clash between popular methods that may lack robust scientific support and validated techniques which may fail to gain traction in practical settings.

Given the dynamic nature of sports science and the relentless pursuit of improved competitive performance, the development and dissemination of novel scientific approaches is crucial for both trainers and researchers. A comprehensive understanding of the advantages and limitations of these methods is essential to effectively evaluate, predict, and model athletic performance across various levels, from amateur to elite.

The present Special Issue addresses the critical gaps in our knowledge by exploring innovative approaches to enhancing motor skills and athletic performance. A broad palette of experimental experiences cover a wide range of sports including weightlifting, volleyball, sailing, soccer, running, American football, and gymnastics. Each of these sporting activities present unique challenges, requiring specific training and performance evaluation methodologies.

By examining multifaceted approaches, this latest collection aims to provide a deeper understanding on how to optimize athletic training and performance. A total of fifteen manuscripts were accepted for publication and inclusion in this Special Issue.

2. Overview of Published Articles

This collection of studies presents a comprehensive examination of several aspects of athletic performance and biomechanics across different sports and activities, highlighting their critical role in enhancing athletic achievements. The main components of the findings in this new issue of Efficiency in Kinesiology are described below.

Female volleyball players showed notable adaptations in their jump mechanics when transitioning from rigid surfaces to sand, leveraging the stretch-shortening cycle for better performance, underscoring the importance of surface-specific training [5]. Additionally, in physically active women, reliability in VO2max measurements was high, although individual variations necessitate personalized assessments, emphasizing the need for individualized training protocols [6]. In the realm of running-related injuries, they were shown to be more prevalent among those with higher running volumes and performance-driven motives, indicating the necessity for tailored injury prevention strategies to ensure athletes' long-term health and performance sustainability [7]. Moreover, high exercise cardiac loads were found to detrimentally impact running speed and autonomic nervous system recovery in collegiate football players, stressing the significance of balanced training and recovery protocols to maintain optimal performance [8]. Furthermore, the cardiac loads of exercise proved to be a reliable predictor of autonomic nervous system deterioration, aiding in the prevention of overtraining and highlighting the value of monitoring physiological loads [9]. Sport-specific training significantly enhanced jump performance in female volleyball players [10], while fitness tests for linear speed were validated as being reliable for monitoring pubertal soccer players, supporting their use in evaluating and improving athletic performance [11]. In rhythmic and artistic gymnastics, specialized training contributed to a superior range of motion in joints and muscle strength in prepubertal athletes, showcasing the benefits of early targeted training on neuromuscular development [12]. The reactive strength index from drop jumps emerged as a strong predictor of weightlifting performance [13], although unstable load back squats did not significantly improve countermovement jump performance, indicating the need for further research in resistance training methodologies [14]. In addition, self-efficacy was closely linked to squat jump performance, reflecting the importance of psychological factors in athletic achievements and suggesting potential areas for intervention [15]. In sailing, performance variables like velocity and maneuvers made were influenced by wind conditions, with notable gender differences in maneuver frequency, emphasizing the need for context-specific performance analysis [16]. Dynamic stretching and proprioceptive neuromuscular facilitation were both effective in enhancing vertical jump height and sprint performance, highlighting effective warm-up techniques [17]. The "sticking region" in squats revealed biomechanical variations based on sex and repetitions, crucial for optimizing training regimens. Finally, the isometric peak torque and rate of torque development provided valuable insights into the neuromuscular fitness of weightlifters, underscoring their predictive power for performance outcomes and the importance of monitoring these metrics for improved training results [18]. The only systematic review of this Special Issue is dedicated to kinesiophobia, a condition marked by an intense fear of physical movement following an injury, presenting a significant barrier to rehabilitation. Central to understanding this condition is the Tampa Scale of Kinesiophobia, a tool to assess the degree of fear and its impact on daily life. These mental factors not only amplify the fear of movement, but also perpetuate a cycle of inactivity and psychological distress. By addressing these underlying issues, particularly through measures that reduce anxiety, bolster self-confidence, and challenge avoidance behaviors, more effective strategies for managing kinesiophobia and promoting physical recovery can be developed [19].

These findings collectively highlight the intricate interplay of biomechanics, training, psychological factors, and environmental conditions in shaping athletic performance, stressing the significance of a holistic approach to athletic development.

3. Conclusions

Grounded in the research reported above, several potential directions for future study can establish a proficient and novel framework for the enhancement of athletic performance. In light of this new editorial, we propose the following directions to continue advancing the field of sports science.

First, the application of emerging technologies, such as wearable sensors and machine learning, is a promising avenue to enhance performance evaluation and prediction models. Wearable sensors can provide real-time data on various performance metrics, while machine learning algorithms can analyze these data to offer insights and predict future performance trends.

Additionally, conducting long-term studies to assess the chronic effects of various training methodologies and their transferability to real-world sports settings is crucial. Longitudinal research can reveal the long-term benefits or drawbacks of specific training regimens, helping to fine-tune practices for sustained athlete development.

Furthermore, developing personalized training regimens based on individual biomechanical, physiological, and psycho-cognitive profiles to optimize performance and reduce injury risk remains essential [20–24]. Personalized programs can adapt to changes in an athlete's condition over time, ensuring continuous optimization and safety.

Moreover, another key direction is encouraging collaboration between sports scientists, coaches, psychologists, and engineers to create holistic training programs that address all facets of athletic performance. Cross-disciplinary efforts can lead to comprehensive training solutions that incorporate physical conditioning, mental resilience, and advanced technological support.

Finally, it is also vital to investigate the impact of early specialization versus diversified training in young athletes to determine the best practices for long-term athletic development. Understanding the balance between specialized and varied training in youths can guide practices that maximize potential and minimize burnout- or overuse-related injuries.

By addressing these areas, future research can provide valuable insights and practical applications, ultimately enhancing the effectiveness of training programs and improving athletic performance across all levels. In particular, it may be worthwhile to promote umbrella reviews to enhance the breadth and depth of scholarly understanding.

In conclusion, we wish to gratefully acknowledge the essential contributions from all of the authors, reviewers, and editors toward this Special Issue. Given the great success of this Special Issue, we have launched a third edition. We believe that this topic has the potential to propel sports science forward by connecting cutting-edge scientific research with practical on-field training methods and experiences.

Author Contributions: Conceptualization, methodology, formal analysis, writing—original draft preparation review and editing, V.S. and D.M. All authors have read and agreed to the published version of the manuscript.

Conflicts of Interest: The authors declare no conflicts of interest.

References

1. Hughes, W.; Healy, R.; Lyons, M.; Nevill, A.; Higginbotham, C.; Lane, A.; Beattie, K. The effect of different strength training modalities on sprint performance in female team-sport athletes: A systematic review and meta-analysis. *Sports Med.* **2023**, *53*, 993–1015. [CrossRef] [PubMed]
2. Meyers, M.C. Enhancing sport performance: Merging sports science with coaching. *Int. J. Sports Sci. Coach.* **2006**, *1*, 89–100. [CrossRef]
3. Booth, M.A.; Orr, R. Effects of plyometric training on sports performance. *Strength Cond. J.* **2016**, *38*, 30–37. [CrossRef]
4. Harries, S.K.; Lubans, D.R.; Callister, R. Resistance training to improve power and sports performance in adolescent athletes: A systematic review and meta-analysis. *J. Sci. Med. Sport* **2012**, *15*, 532–540. [CrossRef]
5. Giatsis, G.; Panoutsakopoulos, V.; Frese, C.; Kollias, I. Vertical Jump Kinetic Parameters on Sand and Rigid Surfaces in Young Female Volleyball Players with a Combined Background in Indoor and Beach Volleyball. *J. Funct. Morphol. Kinesiol.* **2023**, *8*, 115. [CrossRef] [PubMed]
6. Succi, P.; Benitez, B.; Kwak, M.; Bergstrom, H. Analysis of Individual VO_{2max} Responses during a Cardiopulmonary Exercise Test and the Verification Phase in Physically Active Women. *J. Funct. Morphol. Kinesiol.* **2023**, *8*, 124. [CrossRef]
7. Stenerson, L.; Melton, B.; Bland, H.; Ryan, G. Running-Related Overuse Injuries and Their Relationship with Run and Resistance Training Characteristics in Adult Recreational Runners: A Cross-Sectional Study. *J. Funct. Morphol. Kinesiol.* **2023**, *8*, 128. [CrossRef]
8. Renaghan, E.; Wittels, H.; Feigenbaum, L.; Wishon, M.; Chong, S.; Wittels, E.; Hendricks, S.; Hecocks, D.; Bellamy, K.; Girardi, J.; et al. Exercise Cardiac Load and Autonomic Nervous System Recovery during In-Season Training: The Impact on Speed Deterioration in American Football Athletes. *J. Funct. Morphol. Kinesiol.* **2023**, *8*, 134. [CrossRef]
9. Wittels, S.; Renaghan, E.; Wishon, M.; Wittels, H.; Chong, S.; Wittels, E.; Hendricks, S.; Hecocks, D.; Bellamy, K.; Girardi, J.; et al. A Novel Metric "Exercise Cardiac Load" Proposed to Track and Predict the Deterioration of the Autonomic Nervous System in Division I Football Athletes. *J. Funct. Morphol. Kinesiol.* **2023**, *8*, 143. [CrossRef]

10. Donahue, P.; McInnis, A.; Williams, M.; White, J. Examination of Countermovement Jump Performance Changes in Collegiate Female Volleyball in Fatigued Conditions. *J. Funct. Morphol. Kinesiol.* **2023**, *8*, 137. [CrossRef]
11. Manouras, N.; Batatolis, C.; Ioakimidis, P.; Karatrantou, K.; Gerodimos, V. The Reliability of Linear Speed with and without Ball Possession of Pubertal Soccer Players. *J. Funct. Morphol. Kinesiol.* **2023**, *8*, 147. [CrossRef] [PubMed]
12. Mandroukas, A.; Metaxas, I.; Michailidis, Y.; Metaxas, T. Muscle Strength and Joint Range of Motion of the Spine and Lower Extremities in Female Prepubertal Elite Rhythmic and Artistic Gymnasts. *J. Funct. Morphol. Kinesiol.* **2023**, *8*, 153. [CrossRef] [PubMed]
13. Anastasiou, G.; Hadjicharalambous, M.; Terzis, G.; Zaras, N. Reactive Strength Index, Rate of Torque Development, and Performance in Well-Trained Weightlifters: A Pilot Study. *J. Funct. Morphol. Kinesiol.* **2023**, *8*, 161. [CrossRef] [PubMed]
14. Jirovska, R.; Kay, A.; Tsatalas, T.; Van Enis, A.; Kokkotis, C.; Giakas, G.; Mina, M. The Influence of Unstable Load and Traditional Free-Weight Back Squat Exercise on Subsequent Countermovement Jump Performance. *J. Funct. Morphol. Kinesiol.* **2023**, *8*, 167. [CrossRef] [PubMed]
15. Cudicio, A.; Agosti, V. Beyond Belief: Exploring the Alignment of Self-Efficacy, Self-Prediction, Self-Perception, and Actual Performance Measurement in a Squat Jump Performance—A Pilot Study. *J. Funct. Morphol. Kinesiol.* **2024**, *9*, 16. [CrossRef] [PubMed]
16. Caraballo, I.; Pezelj, L.; Ramos-Álvarez, J. Analysis of the Performance and Sailing Variables of the Optimist Class in a Variety of Wind Conditions. *J. Funct. Morphol. Kinesiol.* **2024**, *9*, 18. [CrossRef] [PubMed]
17. Malek, N.; Nadzalan, A.; Tan, K.; Nor Azmi, A.; Krishnan Vasanthi, R.; Pavlović, R.; Badau, D.; Badau, A. The Acute Effect of Dynamic vs. Proprioceptive Neuromuscular Facilitation Stretching on Sprint and Jump Performance. *J. Funct. Morphol. Kinesiol.* **2024**, *9*, 42. [CrossRef] [PubMed]
18. Hegdahl Gundersen, A.; Nygaard Falch, H.; Bao Fredriksen, A.; Tillaar, R. The Effect of Sex and Different Repetition Maximums on Kinematics and Surface Electromyography in the Last Repetition of the Barbell Back Squat. *J. Funct. Morphol. Kinesiol.* **2024**, *9*, 75. [CrossRef]
19. Ambegaonkar, J.; Jordan, M.; Wiese, K.; Caswell, S. Kinesiophobia in Injured Athletes: A Systematic Review. *J. Funct. Morphol. Kinesiol.* **2024**, *9*, 78. [CrossRef]
20. Shieh, S.F.; Lu, F.J.; Gill, D.L.; Yu, C.H.; Tseng, S.P.; Savardelavar, M. Influence of mental energy on volleyball competition performance: A field test. *PeerJ* **2023**, *11*, e15109. [CrossRef]
21. Singh, A.; Kaur Arora, M.; Boruah, B. The role of the six factors model of athletic mental energy in mediating athletes' well-being in competitive sports. *Sci. Rep.* **2024**, *14*, 2974. [CrossRef] [PubMed]
22. Kaufman, K.A.; Glass, C.R.; Arnkoff, D.B. Evaluation of Mindful Sport Performance Enhancement (MSPE): A new approach to promote flow in athletes. *J. Clin. Sport Psychol.* **2009**, *3*, 334–356. [CrossRef]
23. Carraça, B.; Serpa, S.; Guerrero, J.P.; Rosado, A. Enhance sport performance of elite athletes: The mindfulness-based interventions. *Cuad. Psicol. Deporte* **2018**, *18*, 79–109.
24. Stone, M.J.; Knight, C.J.; Hall, R.; Shearer, C.; Nicholas, R.; Shearer, D.A. The psychology of athletic tapering in sport: A scoping review. *Sports Med.* **2023**, *53*, 777–801. [CrossRef]

Disclaimer/Publisher's Note: The statements, opinions and data contained in all publications are solely those of the individual author(s) and contributor(s) and not of MDPI and/or the editor(s). MDPI and/or the editor(s) disclaim responsibility for any injury to people or property resulting from any ideas, methods, instructions or products referred to in the content.

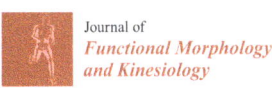

Journal of
Functional Morphology and Kinesiology

Review

Kinesiophobia in Injured Athletes: A Systematic Review

Jatin P. Ambegaonkar *, Matthew Jordan, Kelley R. Wiese and Shane V. Caswell

Sports Medicine Assessment Research & Testing (SMART) Laboratory, George Mason University, Manassas, VA 20110, USA; mjorda@gmu.edu (M.J.); kwiese2@gmu.edu (K.R.W.); scaswell@gmu.edu (S.V.C.)
* Correspondence: jambegao@gmu.edu; Tel.: +1-703-993-2123

Abstract: Athletes have a high risk of injury. Kinesiophobia is a condition in which an individual experiences a fear of physical movement and activity after an injury occurs. Our purpose was to systematically review the literature about Kinesiophobia in athletes. A systematic review was conducted in February 2023 using PubMed, CINAHL, SPORTDiscus, Web of Science, Cochrane Library, and Medline. Studies were included if they were peer-reviewed, in English, within the last 20 years and included athletes who had been injured and tracked Kinesiophobia. Articles were checked for quality via the modified Downs and Black checklist. Fourteen studies were included in the review and had an average "fair" quality score. Authors examined Kinesiophobia in injured athletes with mostly lower-extremity injuries. Kinesiophobia was associated with lower physical and mental outcomes. Kinesiophobia exists in athletes and can affect both physical and mental factors. The Tampa Scale of Kinesiophobia (TSK) was the most common tool used to examine Kinesiophobia. Common mental factors associated with Kinesiophobia include anxiety, low confidence, and fear avoidance.

Keywords: Tampa Scale of Kinesiophobia; fear of reinjury; fear of movement

Citation: Ambegaonkar, J.P.; Jordan, M.; Wiese, K.R.; Caswell, S.V. Kinesiophobia in Injured Athletes: A Systematic Review. *J. Funct. Morphol. Kinesiol.* **2024**, *9*, 78. https://doi.org/10.3390/jfmk9020078

Academic Editor: Diego Minciacchi

Received: 25 March 2024
Revised: 12 April 2024
Accepted: 18 April 2024
Published: 19 April 2024

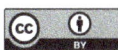

Copyright: © 2024 by the authors. Licensee MDPI, Basel, Switzerland. This article is an open access article distributed under the terms and conditions of the Creative Commons Attribution (CC BY) license (https://creativecommons.org/licenses/by/4.0/).

1. Introduction

Approximately 8.6 million sports-related injuries occur every year [1]. Sports-related injury can result not only in physical disability, but may also have psychological impacts [2,3]. Kinesiophobia is a psychological concept that affects the athletic population and can have a negative impact on rehabilitation progression and return to sport [3]. Kinesiophobia is defined as an irrational and debilitating fear of physical movement and activity resulting from feeling vulnerable to painful injury or reinjury [4]. This fear consequently affects the athlete both physically (e.g., decreased muscular strength, impaired proprioception, and decreased range of motion) [5–8] and psychologically (e.g., anxiety, depression, and decreased health-related quality of life) [7–10]. Fear of movement tends to increase pain-related fear and can be associated with safety-seeking behaviors, such as the avoidance of certain movements [7].

Authors have previously used the terms Kinesiophobia, fear of movement, and fear of reinjury interchangeably in previous literature [3,4,11]. For the purpose of this article, fear of movement and fear of injury are separately, operationally defined in regard to Kinesiophobia. Previous authors have described a fear of movement as occurring at the early stage post-injury in which the patient is hesitant to perform a basic movement, such as walking [3]. Fear of reinjury is commonly used during the later stages of rehabilitation where the patient is hesitant to participate in functional athletic movements (e.g., cutting) [3]. Fear of reinjury can be triggered in settings in which the athlete was initially injured [3].

Athletes who are experiencing Kinesiophobia are likely to experience reduced physical function, affecting their ability to progress through rehabilitation programs and their quality of life [9]. In some cases, Kinesiophobia is reported to negatively affect functional outcomes because patients may be hesitant to complete triggering rehabilitation exercises, delaying the recovery process and leading to decreased strength and range of motion [6]. However,

Kinesiophobia may be overlooked because practitioners may not be aware of the concept or they may assume the athlete is eager to return to play [4].

The fear avoidance model [7] explains how and why injuries can result in Kinesiophobia and other factors, such as chronic pain. When an athlete suffers an injury and experiences pain, they either have high or low catastrophization, which determines their fear levels [7]. Low fear levels allow the athlete to interpret the pain as non-threatening, promoting normal recovery [7]. However, if an athlete perceives the pain as threatening, likely causing a fear of movement, it can lead to Kinesiophobia [7]. Kinesiophobia can present in many individuals either post-injury or following surgery, but the length of time in which Kinesiophobia persists varies across individuals [11–16]. Irrespective of its onset, Kinesiophobia complicates a full return to participation in sport [11,15,16]. Prior authors note that less than 50% of athletes return to pre-injury activity levels [14,15,17]. Furthermore, fear of movement and/or fear of reinjury can delay the Return-to-Play (RTP) process and may negatively impact rehabilitation outcomes. For example, a fear of movement may lead to decreased muscular strength, increased postural sway, and impaired proprioception, perpetuating chronic conditions that hinder an athlete's athletic ability [5,8].

Overall, despite the existence of Kinesiophobia and the negative outcomes associated with Kinesiophobia, relatively limited literature exists describing the presence of Kinesiophobia in athletes and current practices to address Kinesiophobia. This gap in the literature is problematic because clinicians may not know how to properly rehabilitate and return athletes who have a fear of movement or reinjury. Additionally, an awareness of Kinesiophobia allows the healthcare team to implement objective Kinesiophobia measures into rehabilitation protocols and ensure the athlete possesses the confidence and psychological readiness to return to play. Thus, the purpose of this study was to systematically review the current literature examining Kinesiophobia in injured athletes.

2. Materials and Methods

2.1. Search Strategy and Study Selection

This review was conducted in accordance with the Preferred Reporting Items for Systematic Reviews and Meta-Analyses (PRISMA) guidelines [18]. Six electronic databases were systematically searched through 25 February 2023, including PubMed, CINAHL, SPORTDiscus, Web of Science, Cochrane Library, and Medline. Articles were included if they were published within the last 20 years to ensure the evidence was current and relevant. The inclusion criteria and exclusion criteria that were applied to this review can be seen in Table 1, and the search strategy and terms used can be found in Table 2.

Table 1. Inclusion and exclusion criteria in studies examining Kinesiophobia in injured athletes.

Inclusion Criteria	Exclusion Criteria
Athletes who have been injured	Reviews
Track Kinesiophobia	Case studies
Peer-reviewed	Conference proceedings
English articles	
Published within last 20 years	

Table 2. Search strategy and search terms used to examine Kinesiophobia in injured athletes.

Step	Search Terms	Boolean Operator	PubMed	CINAHL Plus	Sport Discus	Web of Science	Cochrane Library	MedLine
1	Kinesiopho *		140	925	439	1459	874	1446
2	Injur *		108,825	368,476	169,496	952,027	71,764	1,417,231
3	athlet *		9353	80,516	397,997	95,466	11,813	111,143
4	Reinjur *		172	1477	579	943	259	1207
5	Fear *		10,450	51,694	10,568	156,481	11,475	122,033

Table 2. Cont.

Step	Search Terms	Boolean Operator	PubMed	CINAHL Plus	Sport Discus	Web of Science	Cochrane Library	MedLine
6	Moveme *		54,609	96,129	85,431	732,726	39,633	637,703
7	1, 2	AND	7	44	42	47	10	66
8	7, 4	AND	2	12	9	10	4	13
9	5, 6	AND	341	1474	685	5980	915	3695
10	7, 9	AND	2	18	17	17	2	0
11	1, 2, 4,	AND, OR	32	216	0	379	144	338
12	11, 5, 6	AND, OR	23	152	0	312	89	235
13	11, 9	AND	14	99	0	229	49	146
14	1, 5, 6,	AND, OR	439	2144	973	6885	1590	4697
15	1, 4, 5	AND, OR	157	1062	495	1555	907	1555
16	14, 3	AND	13	981	504	1522	887	1508
17	15, 3	AND	16	1002	471	1506	880	1504
18	1, 3, 2, 4, 9	AND, OR	13	18	17	19	2	20

The asterisk sign indicates a truncation of the word and allows a wildcard search for all the variable endings of the root word.

2.2. Data Extraction

A two-part screening process was implemented following the initial search. First, two investigators screened article titles and abstracts to determine whether they were relevant to the scope of the review. Following, the full text of the articles was examined to determine inclusion and exclusion eligibility. A third expert reviewer resolved any disagreement or discrepancy to determine article inclusion and exclusion.

2.3. Methodological Rigor and Study Quality Assessment

The modified Downs and Black (mDB) checklist appraisal tool was used to assess the methodological rigor and study quality for the chosen articles [19]. This appraisal tool was designed to assess both randomized and non-randomized studies [19]. The mDB checklist consisted of 27 questions, separated into 5 categories (reporting, external validity, internal validity—bias, internal validity—confounding, and power), including how to score each question [19].

3. Results

3.1. Study Selection

During the initial literature search, 41 studies were screened. A total of 14 studies fit the inclusion criteria and are included in this review. The overall purpose of the included articles was to examine the presence of Kinesiophobia in injured athletes or use Kinesiophobia as a patient-reported outcome measure to examine the change over time (see Figure 1 depicting the PRISMA flowchart).

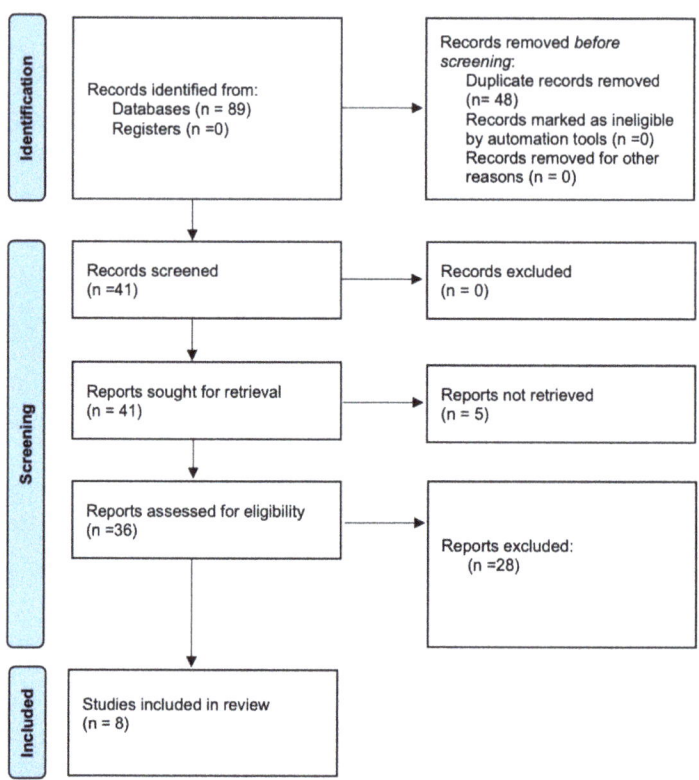

Figure 1. PRISMA flowchart of studies about Kinesiophobia in injured athletes.

3.2. Methodological Rigor and Study Quality Assessment

About half of the studies in this review were of higher quality (>71.4%). The highest scores on the MDB checklist were 27/28 and 20/28 [11,16,20–23] (see Table 3). All included studies directly stated the objective/aim, characteristics of participants, outcome measures, and main findings. Only two of the included studies described the intervention of interest [20,21]. Most of the studies did not have a treatment or placebo and were rather simply observing measures over time. Only one study [20] reported possible adverse events. Most studies reported participants lost to follow-up. External validity was determined to be overall good quality, with 11/14 studies scoring 3/3 within the category. Scores for internal validity—bias were mixed, due to subjects and researchers not being blinded in most studies. Internal validity—confounding results were mixed as well, due to the questions about randomization not being applicable to most of the included study designs. All but two studies [24,25] scored 1/1 for the power category. The lowest scores on the mDB checklist were 13/28 and 14/28 [24,25].

Table 3. Methodological rigor of studies examining Kinesiophobia in injured athletes using the modified Downs and Black (mDB) criteria.

Study	Reporting	External Validity	Internal Validity—Bias	Internal Validity—Confounding	Power	Total	%
Alshahrani 22 [5]	6	3	5	1	1	16	57.1
Bagheri 21 [25]	10	3	7	6	1	27	96.4
Fukano 20 [21]	7	1	5	1	0	14	50.0
Hart 19 [26]	7	0	5	2	1	15	53.6
Houston 14 [22]	8	3	5	3	1	20	71.4
Huang 19 [27]	7	3	3	4	1	18	64.3
Jedvaj 21 [24]	7	3	4	3	1	18	64.3
Kvist 04 [28]	6	3	5	3	1	18	64.3
Ohji 22 [29]	6	1	4	2	0	13	46.4
Paterno 18 [11]	7	3	5	4	1	20	71.4
Reinking 22 [20]	7	3	5	4	1	20	71.4
Slagers 21 [30]	7	3	5	4	1	20	71.4
Theunissen 19 [16]	7	3	5	4	1	20	71.4
Watanabe 23 [23]	6	3	4	2	1	16	57.1

3.3. Participant Characteristics

Participant characteristics are presented in Table 4. The researchers examined Kinesiophobia in both males (n = 561) and females (n = 423). The level of sport participation varied in the 14 studies included in the review. In one study, the authors examined adolescent athletes [20], three examined high-school and/or collegiate athletes [21–23], one examined professional athletes [24], two examined recreational athletes [5,25], and seven examined a combination of levels [11,16,26–30], such as recreational and collegiate athletes. The athletes played diverse sports, including running [25], football and lacrosse [21], alpine skiing [24], and various college sports, including baseball, basketball, futsal, gymnastics, lacrosse, soccer, softball, table tennis, tennis, and track and field [23]. Most studies examined athletes who had anterior cruciate ligament or other knee injuries [16,24–29], or ankle injuries [5,21,23,30].

Table 4. Participant characteristics in studies examining Kinesiophobia in injured athletes.

Study	Year	Training Level	Injury	Mean Age (y)	Sport	Female (n)	Male (n)	Total (n)
Alshahrani [5]	2022	Recreational	Functional Ankle Instability	23	Not Reported	21	34	55
Bagheri [25]	2021	Recreational	Patellofemoral Pain	28.35	Running	33	0	33
Fukano [21]	2020	Collegiate	Functional Ankle Instability	19.45	Football and Lacrosse	105	79	89
Hart [26]	2019	Athletes (Various Levels)	Anterior Cruciate Ligament	31	Not Reported	42	76	118
Houston [22]	2014	High School and Collegiate	Acute Musculoskeletal Injury (Inability to Fully Participate in Sport for at Least 2 Days)	17.9	Not Reported	11	11	22
Huang [27]	2019	Athletes (Various Levels)	Anterior Cruciate Ligament	32.4	Not Reported	81	141	222
Jedvaj [24]	2021	Professional	Knee Injury	24	Alpine skiing	22	11	33
Kvist [28]	2004	Athletes (Various levels)	Anterior Cruciate Ligament	27	Not Reported	28	34	62

Table 4. Cont.

Study	Year	Training Level	Injury	Mean Age (y)	Sport	Female (n)	Male (n)	Total (n)
Ohji [29]	2022	Athletes (Various Levels)	Anterior Cruciate Ligament	20	Not Reported	13	18	31
Paterno [11]	2018	Athletes (Various Levels)	Anterior Cruciate Ligament	16.2	Not Reported	Not Reported	Not Reported	40
Reinking [20]	2022	Adolescent	Concussion	15.85	Not Reported	24	25	49
Slagers [30]	2021	Athletes (Various Levels)	Achilles Tendon Rupture	42.6	Not Reported	16	34	50
Theunissen [16]	2013	Athletes (Various Levels)	Anterior Cruciate Ligament	30.5	Not Reported	43	59	102
Watanabe [23]	2023	Collegiate	Chronic Ankle Instability	20.5	Badminton, Baseball, Basketball, Futsal, Gymnastics, Lacrosse, Soccer, Softball, Table Tennis, Tennis, and Track and Field	5	37	42

3.4. Objective Measures of Kinesiophobia

The authors used several tests (see Table 5) and objective physical measures to assess Kinesiophobia (see Table 6) including joint-position sense [5], postural control [5], strength [11,29], joint laxity [21,29], muscle activity [29], and performance-based functions [11,16,20,26,29,30]. We found that authors commonly use performance-based functions, often via horizontal hops tests for distance (single leg or double leg), side to side hops, heel raises, and/or by examining peak vertical ground reaction forces. For example, Alshahrani et al. [5] examined how Kinesiophobia might affect ankle joint-position sense and found a significant positive correlation with ankle joint-position sense errors both in dorsiflexion and plantarflexion, as well as with postural control. Ohji et al. examined peak vertical ground reaction force and found no significant correlations between the vertical ground reaction force and TSK-11 scores. However, they found that vastus medialis muscle activity, while landing from a jump, was positively correlated with TSK-11 scores [29]. Finally, Paterno et al. found that patients who had higher TSK-11 scores were more likely to have a quadricep muscle strength symmetry and a hop limb symmetry lower than 90% [11]. Kinesiophobia had a high correlation with a fear of reinjury [11,21,22,28–30], fear of movement [5,21,23,26], and confidence levels [16,23,24,26,30] in lower limb movement. Other objective outcome measures previously used to assess Kinesiophobia include activity level [11], injury tracking [11], and reliability and validity of the TSK [27].

3.5. Subjective Measures of Kinesiophobia

Kinesiophobia can be measured subjectively using several surveys (see Table 5), including the Athlete Fear Avoidance Questionnaire (AFAQ) [21], the Reinjury Anxiety Inventory (RIAI) [22], the Tampa Scale of Kinesiophobia (TSK) [5,20–22,24–28,30], the TSK-11 [11,22,23,29], and the TSK-17 [16]. The TSK-17 is the standard scale, consisting of a 17-item checklist that has statements regarding fear of movement, reinjury, and fear-avoidance in which participants use a 4-point Likert scale to rate how much they agree or disagree with each statement [31]. The TSK-11 is a shortened version the TSK-17, consisting of 11 items rather than 17, and is used more commonly [31].

Table 5. Tests used to assess Kinesiophobia in injured athletes.

Study	Year	Test
Alshahrani [5]	2022	TSK
Bagheri [25]	2021	TSK
Fukano [21]	2020	AFAQ
Hart [26]	2019	TSK
Houston [22]	2014	TSK-11
Huang [27]	2019	TSK
Jedvaj [24]	2021	TSK
Kvist [28]	2004	TSK
Ohji [29]	2022	TSK-11
Paterno [11]	2018	TSK-11
Reinking [20]	2022	TSK
Slagers [30]	2021	TSK
Theunissen [16]	2019	TSK-17
Watanabe [23]	2023	TSK-11

TSK = Tampa Scale of Kinesiophobia; AFAQ = Athlete Fear Avoidance Questionnaire.

Table 6. Physical measures analyzed examining studies about Kinesiophobia in injured athletes.

Outcome Measure	Study	Specific Measure; Units
Ankle joint-position sense	Alashahrani 22 [5]	Dual digital inclinometer, degrees
Postural control	Alashahrani 22 [5]	Stabilometric force platform, mm squared
Knee symptoms and function	Bagheri 21 [25]	KOOS-ADLs and KOOS sports activities scale, 0–100
Joint laxity	Fukano 20 [21]	Ankle arthrometer, degrees
	Ohji 22 [29]	KT-1000, degrees
Functional instability	Fukano 20 [21]	Identification of functional ankle instability score, score
Performance-based function	Hart 19 [26]	Hops for distance, cm; side to side hops in 30 s, number; cross-over hop for distance, cm
	Ohji 22 [29]	SL hop distance, cm; SL jump landing: peak vertical ground reaction force, N; time to peak force; s
	Paterno 18 [11]	SL hop for distance, cm; triple hop for distance, cm; triple cross-over hop for distance, cm; 6 m timed hop, cm; limb symmetry index, %
	Slagers 21 [30]	SL heel-raise test for endurance; number; SL hop test for distance; cm, limb symmetry index, %
	Reinking 22 [20]	Reaction time, ms
	Theuniessen 19 [16]	IKDC-2000 score, 0–100
Strength	Ohji 22 [29]	Biodex system 4 (peak torque) measured isokinetic knee strength, N
	Paterno 18 [11]	Biodex isokinetic dynamometer-measured isometric quadricep femoris strength (peak torque), N
Muscle activity	Ohji 22 [29]	sEMG, Root Mean Square Activation (%maximum voluntary isometric contraction)

KOOS = Knee Injury and Osteoarthritis Outcome Score, ADL = Activities of Daily Living, SL = Single Leg; sEMG = Surface Electromyography.

Nine of the 14 articles only assessed a single measurement of Kinesiophobia using a survey [5,11,21,23,24,26–29]. The other five articles implemented a repeated measures design in which participants completed a survey multiple times (two to three) to examine the change in subjective Kinesiophobia levels over time [16,20,22,25,30]. Pain was also examined in several studies as an outcome measure, usually via a visual analog scale or patient-reported outcome measure questionnaires [16,23,25,26,29,30].

Ten studies examined how Kinesiophobia affected athletes psychologically, specifically at the time of RTP and beyond [11,16,20–24,26,28,30]. Researchers assessed many different psychological outcome measures, including Kinesiophobia [5,16,20,23,29,30], fear of movement/reinjury [21,22,24–26,28], patient reported fear [11,21,22], coping strategies [25], confidence [26], and anxiety [22] (see Table 7). Houston et. al, Reinking et al., Slagers et al., and Theunissen et al. examined how psychological symptoms of Kinesiophobia changed over time [16,20,22,30]. Overall, these four studies found that, as the athlete's physical symptoms improved over time during rehabilitation, Kinesiophobia and a fear of reinjury decreased for the majority of participants [16,20,22,30]. Individuals with mild to moderate musculoskeletal injuries experienced a significant improvement in TSK-11 and RIAI scores 3 weeks post-injury [22]. However, in individuals with an Achilles tendon rupture that were still psychologically impacted by Kinesiophobia 6 months post-injury, the presence of symptoms determined the amount of physical activity they were willing to complete [30]. In contrast, post-operative ACL reconstruction (ACLR) surgery patients were found to have a decreased level of Kinesiophobia 12 months following surgery, with the number of ACLR patients reporting high levels of Kinesiophobia decreasing by about 61% (92 to 36 patients) [16].

Table 7. Psychological measures analyzed in studies examining Kinesiophobia in injured athletes.

Outcome Measures	Study	Specific Measure
Kinesiophobia/fear of movement or reinjury	Alashahrani 22 [5]	TSK score in the range of 17–68
	Ohji 22 [29]	TSK-11 score
	Reinking 22 [20]	TSK-17 score in the range of 17–68
	Slagers 21 [30]	TSK score in the range of 17–68
	Theuniessen 19 [16]	TSK-17 score in the range of 17–68
	Watanabe 23 [23]	TSK-11 score
	Bagheri 21 [25]	TSK score
	Fukano 20 [21]	TSK-17 score in the range of 17–80
	Hart 19 [26]	TSK score in the range of 17–68
	Houston 14 [22]	TSK-11 score
	Jedvaj 21 [24]	TSK-17 score
	Kvist 04 [28]	TSK score
Coping strategies	Bagheri 21 [25]	Coping strategies questionnaire—27 items, categorized into 6 domains scored separately
Injury-related fear avoidance	Fukano 20 [21]	AFAQ score in the range of 10–50
	Houston 14 [22]	Fear Avoidance Beliefs Questionnaire
Knee confidence	Hart 19 [26]	(VAS) 0–10 and KOOS quality-of-life subscale
Psychological readiness to return to sport	Hart 19 [26]	ACL Return-to-Sport after Injury Scale, 0–100
Reinjury anxiety	Houston 14 [22]	Reinjury anxiety inventory, 28 items
Patient-reported fear	Paterno 18 [11]	TSK-11 score in the range of 11–44

TSK = Tampa Scale of Kinesiophobia; AFAQ = Athlete Fear Avoidance Questionnaire; VAS = Visual Analog Scale; KOOS = Knee Injury and Osteoarthritis Outcome Score; ACL = Anterior Cruciate Ligament.

Huang et al. examined the validity and reliability of the TSK, specifically the Japanese TSK (TSK-J), in patients with ACLR, and found good reliability but low validity and responsiveness [27]. They suggested that the TSK-J may not the best way to assess psychological factors in patients with ACL injuries [27]. Other patient-reported outcome measures include the visual analog scale (VAS) [32] for pain and the disablement in the physically active scale (DPAS) [8]. The VAS is used to track patients' pain progression or compare pain severity between patients with similar conditions [32]. The VAS can be administered using numerical rating scales, graphic rating scales, or curvilinear scales, and patients mark the point on the line that they feel represents their perception of pain [32]. While the VAS does not explicitly measure Kinesiophobia or fear, it may be a good tool to use in combination with the TSK for clinicians to track pain alongside fear levels. The DPAS is a tool that measures the level of disablement in physically active populations [8]. It consists of 16 items that assesses both physical health and mental health [8]. Higher scores indicate greater levels of disablement [8].

3.6. Other Measures of Kinesiophobia

Researchers in six studies assessed a one-time measurement of Kinesiophobia and used those scores, along with other outcome measures, to assess for correlations between outcome variables [11,21,23,24,26,28]. Fukano et al. compared TSK and AFAQ scores in individuals with functional ankle instability (FAI) to individuals who had sprained their ankle previously, but were not diagnosed with functional ankle instability (NFI) [21]. Individuals with FAI had higher TSK scores compared to those without functional ankle instability [21]. As a result, the authors concluded that the presence of an FAI could be associated with a higher level of fear of movement and reinjury [21].

Similarly, Watanabe et al. concluded that even a perceived instability with FAI patients may be related to Kinesiophobia [23]. Kvist et al. reported a weak negative correlation between the TSK and present pain, but patients who did not return to their pre-injury activity levels following ACLR had more fear of pain or reinjury [28]. This trend of patients not returning to their pre-injury activity levels was also observed by Paterno et al. and Hart et al. [11,26]. Psychological readiness to RTP and knee confidence are two factors that can determine whether an ACLR athlete is psychologically ready to return to sport or even perform specific movements, and could contribute to an athlete's ability to return to their to pre-injury activity levels [26].

Bagheri et al. conducted a randomized controlled trial on female recreational runners with patellofemoral pain syndrome (PFPS) to compare treatments of only exercise versus a combination of exercise and mindfulness [25]. The group that completed the mindfulness training, consisting of breathing, meditation, yoga, and stress reduction, reported a decreased fear of movement following the intervention [25].

4. Discussion

4.1. Primary Findings

The primary findings of this systematic review reveal that Kinesiophobia exists in athletes both physically and psychologically. The TSK is the most common tool in the literature to assess subjective accounts of Kinesiophobia. Psychological factors associated with Kinesiophobia include anxiety, confidence, and fear avoidance.

4.2. Methodological Rigor and Study Quality Assessment

The average score of the studies was 65%, or 18 points, which is a "fair" score [19]. Reporting items within the studies were described in most of the studies, and external validity was present in all but three studies. Still, given the relatively low sample sizes of studies in this review, we believe that additional longitudinal examinations are needed to examine the associations of Kinesiophobia with return-from-injury timelines in injured athletes. The articles in this review include cross-sectional, prospective cohort, and a randomized controlled trial. This finding indicates that there is an increasing interest in the area with researchers examining Kinesiophobia in injured athletes using multiple types of study designs.

4.3. Characteristics of Included Studies and Participant Demographics

The range of ages of athletes included in the studies was 15~42 years old. Across the studies, both male and female athletes were examined across many different levels of sport. Only one of the studies suggested that females had a higher chance of reporting higher TSK-11 scores [23], but there were only five females included in that particular study compared to 37 males. This ratio of females to males in this study made it difficult to make conclusive statements on the differences in Kinesiophobia levels between sexes. The majority of the researchers examined Kinesiophobia in athletes with lower-extremity injuries. Specifically, several authors examined Kinesiophobia in athletes with knee injuries, with anterior cruciate ligament (ACL) injury being the most common knee injury, supporting the idea that ACL injury and reconstuction are extensively associated with Kinesiophobia [16]. Several authors also examined Kinesiophobia in athletes with ankle instability, which is understandable given that a lateral ankle sprain is the most prevalent lower-extremity musculoskeletal injury in physically active individuals [33].

4.4. Tests Used to Assess Kinesiophobia

The TSK survey was most consistently used to measure Kinesiophobia. Although Huang et al. [27] indicate that the Japanese version of the TSK (TSK-J) may not the best way to assess psychological factors for patients with ACL injuries, most other researchers indicate the TSK as a means to objectively measure Kinesiophobia. We found that the TSK is the most popular measurement tool to assess Kinesiophobia because it is based on the fear avoidance model and has been found to be valid and reliable [27,34]. The TSK-11 is suggested for use with athletes because of its high reliability and satisfactory validity [31], but it is also a condensed version of the TSK. Thus, it does not take as much time for completion, increasing compliance. The shortened TSK-11 is also beneficial when athletes are completing it multiple times.

Other surveys, like the AFAQ, measure injury-related fear avoidance and can be taken alongside the TSK to provide a comprehensive understanding of any mental barriers an athlete is facing pertaining to fear of movement or reinjury [21]. Similar to the VAS, the DPAS may be a useful tool to incorporate alongside the TSK as the scale does not measure fear levels directly. By using these three surveys in conjunction with one another, clinicians can understand how the athlete perceives their fear, ability, and pain.

4.5. Physical Measures to Assess Kinesiophobia

Kinesiophobia was found to have negative impacts on strength and postural control [5,11,29]. Based on this information, there is a chance that an athlete who has high levels of Kinesiophobia will have resulting functional deficits. This idea can be tied to the fear avoidance model, where a high catastrophization of pain leading to high anxiety of pain perpetuates a cycle of a fear of movement [7]. This fear causes an avoidance of movement, which can inhibit the muscles, tendons, and ligaments around the area, thus leading to muscle atrophy, fibrosis, and functional impairment [5]. As a result, altered motor patterns occur, and can lead to decreased strength and postural control in the affected area [5].

Kinesiophobia is also associated with diminished performance-based function [11,16,20,26,29]. Performance-based function, or how well an athlete can perform an advanced set of movements, is related to the functional demands of their sport. Performance-based function aligns with Kinesiophobia more commonly as an athlete is closer to returning to a sport [3]. High Kinesiophobia and fear of reinjury levels can cause an athlete to reduce their exposure to physical activities, especially those in which they can possibly reinjure themselves, leading to a perception of limited function or an actual decrease in performance-based function [3]. This finding supports the importance for clinicians to track Kinesiophobia in their athletes to help address it, so that performance and functional levels do not continue to decrease. If Kinesiophobia is left unaddressed, everyday functional activities could be affected [9].

4.6. Limitations and Future Recommendations

We acknowledge some study limitations. First, despite using a comprehensive search strategy, we recognize that some relevant studies may have been excluded. For example, we did not find studies assessing Kinesiophobia for athletes with upper-extremity injuries, with only one study examining musculoskeletal injuries irrespective of location [22]. Additionally, there was an inconsistency in athlete level in the reviewed articles. Future researchers should assess athletes across levels (e.g., high school, collegiate, and professional) to understand how Kinesiophobia affects athletes at various levels when returning to play.

We also note the need for additional research to examine how Kinesiophobia affects athletes across several sports, since a majority of the included studies (11) did not report which sport was assessed. The information is needed because Kinesiophobia levels may vary across sports and athletic activities that involve contact with other players (e.g., soccer and wrestling) versus non-contact sports (e.g., tennis, and track and field). Therefore, the results of this review cannot be directly generalized to all types of athletes across levels and types of sport.

Future researchers should also examine treatment options for Kinesiophobia to identify the options that are most effective for addressing Kinesiophobia in athletes. It is important to note that none of the included articles described how effective repeated use over time was when using the TSK. Furthermore, only one study stated the minimal clinically important difference with the TSK, which was reported as a score of 4 [16]. However, this was only in regards to patients with low back pain [16]. Therefore, future researchers should examine minimal clinically important difference values with the TSK as well. This work can allow clinicians the opportunity to document meaningful objective measurements during the return-to-play process.

4.7. Clinical Implications and Applications

The primary clinical implication of the current study is that clinicians should be aware of the potential presence of Kinesiophobia in athletes post-injury. It is important for practitioners to monitor Kinesiophobia scores throughout the rehabilitation process to monitor both psychological and physical recovery in athletes to prevent a decrease in quality of life during the return-to-play process.

Furthermore, it is important to educate athletes, coaches, and the multidisciplinary healthcare team caring for the athletes about Kinesiophobia. This education could reduce the athletes' anxiety [3], and if all stakeholders (athletes, parents, coaches, and healthcare practitioners) are educated about Kinesiophobia and the anticipated symptoms, then everyone supporting the athlete through recovery may be able to recognize and address early signs of Kinesiophobia that could hinder the injury recovery process. If coaches know how to recognize Kinesiophobia-related signs that are diminishing an athlete's performance, they can communicate that to the athletic trainers and healthcare team. The healthcare team can then work with the athlete to overcome his/her fear. Likewise, if athletes are able to recognize and articulate their symptoms of Kinesiophobia, they can communicate their mental and physical barriers that may be inhibiting their optimal performance. Overall, once practitioners are equipped to recognize the signs of Kinesiophobia, they can integrate appropriate techniques into treatment strategies to proactively assess and address Kinesiophobia.

Practitioners can use the TSK as a means to objectively measure Kinesiophobia. The TSK is currently the only tool that specifically aims to measure Kinesiophobia [31]. The current review findings indicate that the TSK-11 is the preferred form of the TSK to use because it has high reliability and high validity compared to other versions [31]. The shortened TSK-11 also allows multiple administrations to objectively measure psychological Kinesiophobia feelings throughout the rehabilitation process.

In addition, the whole sports medicine team (e.g., athletic trainers, physical therapists, physicians, coaches, and others) can create a plan to address Kinesiophobia. This plan can include mindfulness or relaxation techniques that could reduce tension and anxiety [3,25]. The team can also work with the athlete to set goals, which provides the athlete with direction and the ability to visualize the progress that is made during rehabilitation [3]. Graded exposure may also be an effective technique to gradually expose the athlete to fearful movements to decrease Kinesiophobia levels [3]. Furthermore, appropriate social support may enhance the athlete's coping strategies [3]. Implementing education, recognition, assessment, and appropriate plans for athletes with Kinesiophobia will support athletes in overcoming their fears.

Overall, Kinesiophobia levels should be considered as an essential return-to-play criteria similar to pain, range of motion, and strength measurements. The current review provides evidence that there is an increasing amount of interest in the topic of Kinesiophobia in injured athletes, evidenced by the finding that, in the final included articles, almost all (13 of 14) of them were conducted within the last 10 years. Clinicians should implement proper education, recognition, assessment, and plan to help athletes with Kinesiophobia to overcome the condition. This education about Kinesiophobia can help clinicians, coaches, and athletes become aware of the condition so they know how to identify who may have Kinesiophobia, ultimately helping athletes become less fearful and gain confidence when recovering from an injury.

5. Conclusions

The current findings indicate that Kinesiophobia exists in athletes and can affect both physical and mental factors. The Tampa Scale of Kinesiophobia is the most common survey tool used to measure Kinesiophobia. Common psychological factors associated with Kinesiophobia include anxiety, confidence, and fear avoidance.

Author Contributions: Conceptualization, J.P.A. and M.J.; methodology, J.P.A., K.R.W. and M.J.; software, J.P.A., K.R.W. and M.J.; validation, J.P.A., K.R.W. and M.J.; formal analysis, J.P.A., M.J., K.R.W. and S.V.C.; investigation, J.P.A., K.R.W. and M.J.; resources, J.P.A., M.J., K.R.W. and S.V.C.; data curation, J.P.A., K.R.W. and M.J.; writing—original draft preparation, J.P.A. and M.J.; writing—review and editing, J.P.A., M.J., K.R.W. and S.V.C.; visualization, J.P.A. and M.J.; supervision, J.P.A.; project administration, J.P.A. All authors have read and agreed to the published version of the manuscript.

Funding: This research received no external funding.

Institutional Review Board Statement: Not applicable.

Informed Consent Statement: Not applicable.

Data Availability Statement: The data that support the findings of this study are available from the corresponding author, J.P.A., upon reasonable request.

Conflicts of Interest: The authors declare no conflicts of interest.

References

1. Sheu, Y.; Chen, L.; Hedegaard, H. Sports- and Recreation-Related Injury Episodes in the United States, 2011–2014. *Natl. Health Stat. Rep.* **2016**, *99*, 1–12.
2. Haraldsdottir, K.; Watson, A.M. Psychosocial Impacts of Sports-Related Injuries in Adolescent Athletes. *Curr. Sports Med. Rep.* **2021**, *20*, 104. [CrossRef]
3. Hsu, C.-J.; Meierbachtol, A.; George, S.Z.; Chmielewski, T.L. Fear of Reinjury in Athletes. *Sports Health* **2017**, *9*, 162–167. [CrossRef]
4. Stiller-Ostrowski, J.; Granquist, M.D.; Flett, R. Kinesiophobia. *Athl. Train. Sports Health Care* **2014**, *6*, 248–251. [CrossRef]
5. Alshahrani, M.S.; Reddy, R.S. Relationship between Kinesiophobia and Ankle Joint Position Sense and Postural Control in Individuals with Chronic Ankle Instability—A Cross-Sectional Study. *Int. J. Environ. Res. Public Health* **2022**, *19*, 2792. [CrossRef]
6. Brown, O.S.; Hu, L.; Demetriou, C.; Smith, T.O.; Hing, C.B. The Effects of Kinesiophobia on Outcome Following Total Knee Replacement: A Systematic Review. *Arch. Orthop. Trauma Surg.* **2020**, *140*, 2057–2070. [CrossRef]
7. Castanho, B.; Cordeiro, N.; Pinheira, V. The-Influence-of-Kinesiophobia-on-Clinical-Practice-in-Physical-Therapy-an-Integrative-Literature-Review. *Int. J. Med. Res. Health Sci.* **2021**, *10*, 78–94.
8. Hoch, J.M.; Druvenga, B.; Ferguson, B.A.; Houston, M.N.; Hoch, M.C. Patient-Reported Outcomes in Male and Female Collegiate Soccer Players during an Athletic Season. *J. Athl. Train.* **2015**, *50*, 930–936. [CrossRef]

9. Cross, S.J.; Gill, D.L.; Brown, P.K.; Reifsteck, E.J. Prior Injury, Health-Related Quality of Life, Disablement, and Physical Activity in Former Women's Soccer Players. *J. Athl. Train.* **2021**, *57*, 92–98. [CrossRef]
10. Wright, S.; Snyder Valier, A. Health-Related Quality of Life in Former Division II Collegiate Athletes Using the Disablement of the Physically Active Scale. *Athl. Train. Sports Health Care* **2021**, *13*, 85–92. [CrossRef]
11. Paterno, M.V.; Flynn, K.; Thomas, S.; Schmitt, L.C. Self-Reported Fear Predicts Functional Performance and Second ACL Injury after ACL Reconstruction and Return to Sport: A Pilot Study. *Sports Health* **2018**, *10*, 228–233. [CrossRef] [PubMed]
12. Vascellari, A.; Ramponi, C.; Venturin, D.; Ben, G.; Coletti, N. The Relationship between Kinesiophobia and Return to Sport after Shoulder Surgery for Recurrent Anterior Instability. *Joints* **2021**, *7*, 148–154. [CrossRef]
13. Raizah, A.; Alhefzi, A.; Alshubruqi, A.A.M.; Hoban, M.A.M.A.; Ahmad, I.; Ahmad, F. Perceived Kinesiophobia and Its Association with Return to Sports Activity Following Anterior Cruciate Ligament Reconstruction Surgery: A Cross-Sectional Study. *Int. J. Environ. Res. Public Health* **2022**, *19*, 10776. [CrossRef]
14. Ardern, C.L.; Taylor, N.F.; Feller, J.A.; Whitehead, T.S.; Webster, K.E. Psychological Responses Matter in Returning to Preinjury Level of Sport after Anterior Cruciate Ligament Reconstruction Surgery. *Am. J. Sports Med.* **2013**, *41*, 1549–1558. [CrossRef] [PubMed]
15. Randsborg, P.-H.; Cepeda, N.; Adamec, D.; Rodeo, S.A.; Ranawat, A.; Pearle, A.D. Patient-Reported Outcome, Return to Sport, and Revision Rates 7–9 Years after Anterior Cruciate Ligament Reconstruction: Results from a Cohort of 2042 Patients. *Am. J. Sports Med.* **2022**, *50*, 423–432. [CrossRef] [PubMed]
16. Theunissen, W.W.E.S.; van der Steen, M.C.; Liu, W.Y.; Janssen, R.P.A. Timing of Anterior Cruciate Ligament Reconstruction and Preoperative Pain Are Important Predictors for Postoperative Kinesiophobia. *Knee Surg. Sports Traumatol. Arthrosc. Off. J. ESSKA* **2020**, *28*, 2502–2510. [CrossRef] [PubMed]
17. Ardern, C.L.; Österberg, A.; Tagesson, S.; Gauffin, H.; Webster, K.E.; Kvist, J. The Impact of Psychological Readiness to Return to Sport and Recreational Activities after Anterior Cruciate Ligament Reconstruction. *Br. J. Sports Med.* **2014**, *48*, 1613–1619. [CrossRef]
18. Page, M.; McKenzie, J.; Bossuyt, P.; Boutron, I.; Hoffmann, T.; Mulrow, C. The PRISMA 2020 Statement: An Updated Guideline for Reporting Systematic Reviews. *BMJ* **2021**, *1*, 71. [CrossRef]
19. Downs, S.H.; Black, N. The Feasibility of Creating a Checklist for the Assessment of the Methodological Quality Both of Randomised and Non-Randomised Studies of Health Care Interventions. *J. Epidemiol. Community Health* **1998**, *52*, 377–384. [CrossRef]
20. Reinking, S.; Seehusen, C.N.; Walker, G.A.; Wilson, J.C.; Howell, D.R. Transitory Kinesiophobia after Sport-Related Concussion and Its Correlation with Reaction Time. *J. Sci. Med. Sport* **2022**, *25*, 20–24. [CrossRef]
21. Fukano, M.; Mineta, S.; Hirose, N. Fear Avoidance Beliefs in College Athletes with a History of Ankle Sprain. *Int. J. Sports Med.* **2020**, *41*, 128–133. [CrossRef] [PubMed]
22. Houston, M.N.; Cross, K.M.; Saliba, S.A.; Hertel, J. Injury-Related Fear in Acutely Injured Interscholastic and Intercollegiate Athletes. *Athl. Train. Sports Health Care J. Pract. Clin.* **2014**, *6*, 15–23. [CrossRef]
23. Watanabe, K.; Koshino, Y.; Kawahara, D.; Akimoto, M.; Mishina, M.; Nakagawa, K.; Ishida, T.; Kasahara, S.; Samukawa, M.; Tohyama, H. Kinesiophobia, Self-Reported Ankle Function, and Sex Are Associated with Perceived Ankle Instability in College Club Sports Athletes with Chronic Ankle Instability. *Phys. Ther. Sport Off. J. Assoc. Chart. Physiother. Sports Med.* **2023**, *61*, 45–50. [CrossRef] [PubMed]
24. Jedvaj, H.; Kiseljak, D.; Olivera, P. Kinesiophobia in Skiers with Knee Injuries. *Pol. J. Sport Tour.* **2021**, *28*, 24–29. [CrossRef]
25. Bagheri, S.; Naderi, A.; Mirali, S.; Calmeiro, L.; Brewer, B.W. Adding Mindfulness Practice to Exercise Therapy for Female Recreational Runners with Patellofemoral Pain: A Randomized Controlled Trial. *J. Athl. Train.* **2021**, *56*, 902–911. [CrossRef] [PubMed]
26. Hart, H.F.; Culvenor, A.G.; Guermazi, A.; Crossley, K.M. Worse Knee Confidence, Fear of Movement, Psychological Readiness to Return-to-Sport and Pain Are Associated with Worse Function after ACL Reconstruction. *Phys. Ther. Sport* **2020**, *41*, 1–8. [CrossRef] [PubMed]
27. Huang, H.; Nagao, M.; Arita, H.; Shiozawa, J.; Nishio, H.; Kobayashi, Y.; Kaneko, H.; Nagayama, M.; Saita, Y.; Ishijima, M.; et al. Reproducibility, Responsiveness and Validation of the Tampa Scale for Kinesiophobia in Patients with ACL Injuries. *Health Qual. Life Outcomes* **2019**, *17*, 150. [CrossRef] [PubMed]
28. Kvist, J.; Ek, A.; Sporrstedt, K.; Good, L. Fear of Re-Injury: A Hindrance for Returning to Sports after Anterior Cruciate Ligament Reconstruction. *Knee Surg. Sports Traumatol. Arthrosc.* **2005**, *13*, 393–397. [CrossRef] [PubMed]
29. Ohji, S.; Aizawa, J.; Hirohata, K.; Ohmi, T.; Mitomo, S.; Koga, H.; Yagishita, K. Association between Landing Biomechanics, Knee Pain, and Kinesiophobia in Athletes Following Anterior Cruciate Ligament Reconstruction: A Cross-Sectional Study. *PM&R* **2023**, *15*, 552–562. [CrossRef]
30. Slagers, A.J.; Dams, O.C.; van Zalinge, S.D.; Geertzen, J.H.; Zwerver, J.; Reininga, I.H.; van den Akker-Scheek, I. Psychological Factors Change during the Rehabilitation of an Achilles Tendon Rupture: A Multicenter Prospective Cohort Study. *Phys. Ther.* **2021**, *101*, pzab226. [CrossRef]
31. Miller, R.; Kori, S.; Todd, D. The Tampa Scale: A Measure of Kinesiophobia. *Clin. J. Pain* **1991**, *7*, 51–52. [CrossRef]
32. Delgado, D.A.; Lambert, B.S.; Boutris, N.; McCulloch, P.C.; Robbins, A.B.; Moreno, M.R.; Harris, J.D. Validation of Digital Visual Analog Scale Pain Scoring With a Traditional Paper-Based Visual Analog Scale in Adults. *J. Am. Acad. Orthop. Surg. Glob. Res. Rev.* **2018**, *2*, e088. [CrossRef] [PubMed]

33. Gribble, P.A.; Bleakley, C.M.; Caulfield, B.M.; Docherty, C.L.; Fourchet, F.; Fong, D.T.-P.; Hertel, J.; Hiller, C.E.; Kaminski, T.W.; McKeon, P.O.; et al. Evidence Review for the 2016 International Ankle Consortium Consensus Statement on the Prevalence, Impact and Long-Term Consequences of Lateral Ankle Sprains. *Br. J. Sports Med.* **2016**, *50*, 1496–1505. [CrossRef] [PubMed]
34. Shastri, M.; Nagarajan, M.; Maheshwari, S. Reliability and Validity of Kannada Version of Tampa Scale of Kinesiophobia (TSK-KA-11)-a Validation Study. *Indian J. Physiother. Occup. Ther.* **2022**, *16*, 15–19. [CrossRef]

Disclaimer/Publisher's Note: The statements, opinions and data contained in all publications are solely those of the individual author(s) and contributor(s) and not of MDPI and/or the editor(s). MDPI and/or the editor(s) disclaim responsibility for any injury to people or property resulting from any ideas, methods, instructions or products referred to in the content.

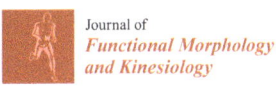

Article

The Effect of Sex and Different Repetition Maximums on Kinematics and Surface Electromyography in the Last Repetition of the Barbell Back Squat

Andreas Hegdahl Gundersen, Hallvard Nygaard Falch, Andrea Bao Fredriksen and Roland van den Tillaar *

Department of Sports Sciences, Nord University, 7600 Levanger, Norway;
andreasgundersen78@gmail.com (A.H.G.); falch7@hotmail.com (H.N.F.); andreabaof@hotmail.com (A.B.F.)
* Correspondence: roland.v.tillaar@nord.no

Abstract: During the ascent phase of a maximal barbell back squat after an initial acceleration, a deceleration region occurs as the result of different biomechanical factors. This is known as the sticking region. However, whether this region is similar in the last repetition of different repetition maximums and if sex has an impact on biomechanics of this region are not known. Therefore, this study investigated the effect of sex (men/women) and repetition maximum (1-, 3-, 6-, and 10RM) on kinematics and surface electromyography around the sticking region. Twenty-six resistance-trained individuals comprising 13 men (body mass: 82.2 ± 8.7; age: 23.6 ± 1.9; height: 181.1 ± 6.5) and 13 women (body mass: 63.6 ± 6.6; age: 23.9 ± 4.5; height: 166.0 ± 4.5) participated in the study. The main findings were that women, in comparison to men, displayed larger trunk lean and lower hip extension angles in the sticking region, possibly due to different hip/knee extensor strength ratios. Moreover, an inverse relationship was discovered between repetition range and timing from V_0 to V_{max2}, in which lower repetition ranges (1- and 3RM) were shorter in V_{max2} compared to higher ranges (6- and 10RM). It was concluded that this occurrence is due to more moments of inertia in lower repetition ranges. Our findings suggest that both sex and repetition range might induce different requirements during the squat ascent.

Keywords: resistance; angular velocity; strength; sticking region

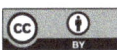

1. Introduction

The barbell back squat (squat) is a multi-joint resistance exercise incorporated into training programmes by a wide variety of cohorts, with the aim of enhancing everything from rehabilitation and health benefits to performance in sports, through increasing power, strength, and hypertrophy in the lower extremities [1]. Several studies have investigated biomechanical limiting factors in the squat among strength-trained individuals [2–8]. Several of those studies have separated the squat ascent into three regions: pre-sticking region (bottom position: V_0—first peak velocity: V_{max1}), sticking region (V_{max1}—minimum velocity: V_{min}), and post-sticking region (V_{min}—second peak velocity: V_{max2}) [5–7]. Larsen, et al. [9] observed that as loads increased, the sticking region occurred at lower barbell heights with lower hip and knee extension angles. The authors speculated that the lower sticking region observed with increased barbell load resulted in a disadvantageous internal moment arm position for the hip and knee extensors, as the gluteus maximus and vasti muscles have been reported to decrease their internal moment arm with increased flexion angles [10,11]. Moreover, two studies also reported a greater forward trunk lean when sets were taken within 80% of one repetition maximum (1RM), creating a larger moment arm and therefore increased rotational work at the hip [4,9].

The measurement of 1RM is a popular way of testing maximal strength among multiple different athletic cohorts because maximum external barbell load lifted for one repetition is representative of an athlete's ability to exert force [12]. Strength and hypertrophic responses are known to occur at multiple different repetition intervals [13]. The current consensus is that strength adaptions are maximised when training with heavier loads and lower per-set repetitions, while hypertrophic adaptions transpire on a larger spectrum of per-set repetitions but require proximity to muscular failure [13]. Therefore, training both strength and hypertrophic specifically should result in a sticking region in the final repetitions, as the literature suggests a sticking region to occur in lifts corresponding to >80% of 1RM [5,6]. However, none of the aforementioned studies have compared biomechanics around the sticking region directly between different RMs in the squat. In bench press, in the last repetition of 1-, 3-, 6-, and 10RM, kinematics and surface electromyography (sEMG) were compared [14], finding mostly similar sEMG and joint kinematics between the conditions, but higher barbell velocity across two events in 10RM compared to 1RM. The extension of these findings to the squat is currently unknown, as the squat engages larger muscle groups, which is known to impose heightened metabolic demands [15]. However, based upon Henneman's size principle, muscular excitation should remain similar across different RMs considering their proximity to failure is equal, as the principle relates the basis for size-ordered activation of motor units [16].

Biomechanical variations may be complicated further when accounting for differences between the sexes. Men are found to produce more force per unit of mass, which is on a populational average due to more muscle mass and less fat mass, thus expressing greater absolute and relative strength [17–19]. Additionally, greater sex differences in lean upper body mass compared to lean lower body mass were found [17–19]. When normalised for body mass, studies consistently find men to generate greater knee extensor torque than women during maximal effort contractions [20–23], which also seems to apply for the hip extensors [24–26]. In addition, women possess a knee/hip strength ratio close to 1, suggesting equal strength in knee and hip extensors [24]. Conversely, men had a ratio <1, which implies the hip extensors to be stronger relative to the knee extensors [24]. Furthermore, women have been shown to possess heightened strength endurance capacities at given relative loads [17,27,28]. This occurrence is postulated to arise from an augmented proportion of type 1 muscle fibres [17], better reliance on fat oxidation [27], lower oxygen demands attributable to lower muscle mass [27], and reduced work per repetition due to shorter limbs [29]. The precise mechanistic underpinnings of the observed disparities in strength endurance remain uncertain, with speculation that such variations may be reliant upon the specific strength task performed, as sEMG has been found to be similar between the sexes when normalised for strength [30]. Although several mechanisms could cause exercise form breakdown [9], similar sEMG and kinematics when comparing men and women in squats of different RM could indicate similar requirements for lifting through the sticking region and completing the squat ascent.

Therefore, the purpose of this study was to investigate the impact of four repetition maximums (1-, 3-, 6-, and 10RM) and sex on kinematics and sEMG amplitude of the last repetition in the squat. When viewed synergistically, this could provide insight on form breakdown as sets of different loads reach maximum. Such information could offer useful inputs in terms of training specificity when individualising training programs for strength and/or hypertrophy in the squat. Based on Larsen, Kristiansen, Nygaard Falch, Estifanos Haugen, Fimland and van den Tillaar [9], the Henneman's size principle, and Nimphius, et al. [30], it was hypothesised that no difference in sEMG would occur between neither RM nor sex [16]. Lastly, no kinematic differences were hypothesised between sexes, but based on Larsen, Kristiansen, Nygaard Falch, Estifanos Haugen, Fimland and van den Tillaar [9], the timing of different events was expected to be longer in the higher load (1- and 3RM) sets compared to lower load (6- and 10RM) sets.

2. Materials and Methods

2.1. Participants

A total of 26 recreationally strength-trained participants comprising both men ($n = 13$) and women ($n = 13$) volunteered to partake in the study (Table 1). Inclusion criteria stipulated that participants had to manage a squat equivalent to 1.2 × body mass (men) and 1 × body mass (women), adhering to the technique requirements established by the International Powerlifting Federation, which requires the femur to be parallel to the floor at bottom position. Additionally, participants had to declare absence of any injury or illness which could impede maximum effort. Furthermore, participants were instructed not to engage in any lower limb exercise and refrain from alcohol >48 h prior to testing. The risk and benefits of participation were explained both in writing and orally, and written consent had to be signed before participation. The study was approved by the local ethics committee and the Norwegian Centre for Research Data (project no. 701688), in conjunction with the latest alteration of the Helsinki Declaration.

Table 1. Mean age (years), height (cm), and body mass (kg) for men and women.

Sex	Age (Years)	Height (cm)	Body Mass (kg)
Men	23.6 ± 1.9	181.1 ± 6.5	82.2 ± 8.7
Women	23.9 ± 4.5	166.0 ± 4.5	63.6 ± 6.6

2.2. Procedure

To investigate the potential impact of sex and RM (1-, 3-, 6-, and 10RM) on kinematics and sEMG amplitude around the sticking region in the final repetition, a randomised mixed repeated-measures design was assessed.

The familiarisation test mirrored the same test protocol as the experimental test, serving to establish the appropriate load for each repetition range, whereas kinematic and sEMG data were collected solely during the experimental test session. To enhance ecological validity and reliability, stance width was standardised to the personal preference of each participant. The use of lifting aids (e.g., knee sleeves, lifting belt) was prohibited, with the exception of lifting shoes. Both sessions commenced with a standardised warm-up protocol squatting at incrementally higher percentages of estimated 1RM (40-, 60, 70, and 80%), before squatting 1-, 3-, 6-, and 10RM in a randomised order (Figure 1) decided by an online randomiser (https://www.random.org, accessed on 26 March 2024). The subjects were not restricted in lifting tempo and used their self-selected tempo, but were not allowed to remain at lockout for longer than 2 s. To minimise the risk of fatigue-induced performance, each participant was required to rest for a minimum of five minutes between each set for both test sessions. The familiarisation test started by acquiring the participant's preferred stance width and body height using a measuring tape, before body mass was measured with a standing scale (Sochnle Professional 7830, standing scale). Squatting depth at the bottom of the descending phase was defined in accordance with the technique regulations set by the International Powerlifting Federation, which necessitates the trochanter major to be inferior to the patella. To ensure reliability, appropriate squatting depth was monitored using a three-dimensional motion capture system.

For analysis, the squat ascent was separated into four events (bottom position: V_0, first peak velocity: V_{max1}, minimum velocity: V_{min}, and second peak velocity: V_{max2}), which divided the ascent into three different phases (V_0–V_{max1}: pre-sticking region, V_{max1}–V_{min}: sticking region, and V_{min}–V_{max2}: post-sticking region, Figure 1) [6].

sEMG data were recorded and analysed using Musclelab v.10.200.90.5095 (Ergotest Technology, Langesund, Norway). Electrodes sampling at 1000 Hz (Zynex Neurodiagnostics, Lone Tree, CO, USA) were lubricated and affixed lengthwise in the presumed direction of the underlying muscle fibre to the dominant side of 10 different muscles (erector spinae iliocostalis, gluteus maximus, gluteus medius, semitendinosus, bicep femoris, vastus lateralis, vastus medialis, rectus femoris, gastrocnemius, and soleus). The placement of the different electrodes was conducted according to SENIAM recommendations [31]. Prior to attachment, each participant underwent appropriate shaving and cleansing with alcohol to reduce interference from hair and dead skin. The root mean square of the unprocessed sEMG signal during the three regions (pre-sticking, sticking, and post-sticking) was computed by a hardware circuit network (frequency response 20–500 Hz, with a moving average filter of 100 ms width, securing an overall error rate of ±0.5%). sEMG was normalised by each individual peak sEMG amplitude during one of the regions of the last repetition of a repetition maximum and defined as 100%. A linear encoder sampling at 200 Hz (ET-Enc-02, Ergotest Technology AS, Langesund, Norway) was attached to the barbell and used to synchronise sEMG data and kinematics data to events and regions.

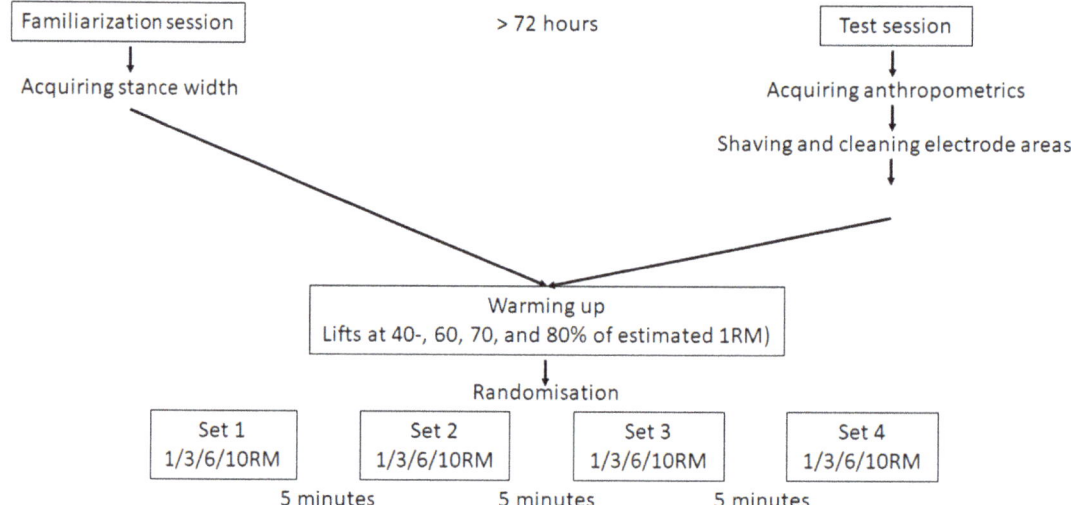

Figure 1. Test protocol.

Eight three-dimensional motion capture cameras (Qualisys, Gothenburg, Sweden) operating at a frequency of 500 Hz were used to track reflective markers for events V_0, V_{max1}, V_{min}, and V_{max2}. The reflective markers (14 mm) were placed on anatomical landmarks on both sides of the body (acromion, pelvis, iliac crest, posterior superior iliac spine, trochanter major, the medial and lateral condyle of the knee, medial and lateral malleolus, sternum, tuber calcanei, and 1st and 5th proximal phalanx), creating a three-dimensional measurement of each participant. This facilitated the determination of sagittal-plane kinematics for the hip, knee, and ankle joints, which in an erect standing position were defined as 180° for hip and knee, 90° for the ankle, and 0° for the trunk. Timing of the different events and peak joint angular velocities was calculated during the ascending phase. All kinematic data were transported via C3D files to Visual3D (C-motion, Germantown, MD, USA) for segment building and subsequent analysis. All joint angles were defined as the proximal segment relative to the distal segment, except the trunk angle which was defined as the trunk relative to the laboratory floor.

2.3. Statistical Analysis

Data were expressed as means and standard deviations (SD) per sex and normality of data were assessed and confirmed using the Shapiro–Wilk test. Differences in anthropometrics and lifted load at the different repetition maximums between the sexes were assessed with independent sample t-tests. To compare sex differences in joint kinematics, peak/minimum angular velocity, and timing across different repetition ranges (1-, 3-, 6-, and 10RM), a 2 (sex: men/women; independent measures) by 4 (event: V_0, V_{max1}, V_{min}, and V_{max2}; repeated measures) analysis of variance (ANOVA) was assessed. To compare sEMG amplitude between sexes, a mixed 2 (sex: men/women) by 4 (repetition range: 1-, 3-, 6-, and 10RM) by 3 (region: pre-sticking, sticking, and post-sticking) with repeated measures was assessed to compare each muscle. Post hoc comparison with a Holm–Bonferroni correction was conducted when significant differences were observed. The assumption of sphericity was controlled with Mauchly´s test of sphericity. If the assumption of sphericity was violated, the Greenhouse–Geisser adjusted p-value was reported. The level of significance was set at $p < 0.05$. Data are reported as means ± standard deviations. Effect size was evaluated as eta partial squared (η_p^2), whereby 0.01 to 0.06 η_p^2 constitutes a small effect, 0.06 to 0.14 was defined as a medium effect, and $0.14 > \eta_p^2$ was defined as a large effect [32]. The statistical analysis was conducted in IBM SPSS Statistics 27.0 (IBM, Armonk, NY, USA).

3. Results

Women were significantly lighter, shorter, and had a lower absolute and relative strength across all repetition ranges (Tables 1 and 2).

Table 2. Mean weights (kg) lifted for the different repetition ranges and mean relative strength for men and women.

Sex	1RM (kg)	3RM (kg)	6RM (kg)	10RM (kg)	Relative Strength
Men	100.3 ± 26.9	90.2 ± 25.0	81.8 ± 22.4	74.4 ± 21.4	1.3 ± 0.2
Women	77.8 ± 11.9	69.1 ± 11.3	62.5 ± 8.2	56.6 ± 8.2	1.2 ± 0.1

Significant sex differences were observed in hip extension angles at V_{min} and V_{max2}, and in trunk lean at V_{max1}, V_{min}, and V_{max2} ($F \geq 5.834$; $p \leq 0.026$; $\eta^2 \geq 0.235$). Post hoc testing revealed that the hip extension angle in men was significantly greater across all repetition ranges in V_{min} and V_{max2} when compared to women. Trunk lean angle in women was significantly higher across all repetition ranges at V_{max1} and V_{min} in comparison to men (Figure 2A). No significant sex differences were found in knee extension angle and ankle plantar flexion angle ($F \leq 2.355$; $p \geq 0.14$; $\eta^2 \leq 0.101$, Figure 2C,D).

A significant effect of repetition ranges (men and women together) was observed in both knee extension angle and ankle plantar flexion angle at V_{min} ($F \geq 3.689$; $p \leq 0.041$; $\eta^2 \geq 0.154$). Post hoc tests revealed that the knee extension angle and ankle plantar flexion were significantly greater in 6RM compared to 1RM at V_{min} (Figure 2C,D). No significant effect of repetition ranges was found in hip extension angle and trunk lean angle ($F \leq 1.614$; $p \geq 0.196$; $\eta^2 \leq 0.078$, Figure 2A,B). Furthermore, a significant interaction between repetition range and sex was observed in the knee extension angle at V_{max2} ($F \geq 5.415$; $p \leq 0.021$; $\eta^2 \geq 0.253$, Figure 2C).

A significant effect of repetition range on peak knee angular velocity was found ($F = 3.38$; $p = 0.025$; $\eta^2 = 0.158$). The post hoc test revealed the peak knee angular velocity to be significantly higher in 3- and 6RM compared to 10RM (Figure 3). No other significant effect of repetition range on peak angular velocity was observed in any of the other joints ($F \leq 2.044$; $p \geq 0.119$; $\eta^2 \leq 0.107$). Moreover, no significant differences between sexes ($F \leq 0.37$; $p \geq 0.08$; $\eta^2 \leq 0.13$, Figure 3) or interaction effects for peak angular velocity were discovered ($F \leq 1.41$; $p \geq 0.247$; $\eta^2 \leq 0.06$, Figure 3).

A significant effect of repetition range was found on the timing of V_{max2} ($F = 9.243$; $p < 0.001$; $\eta^2 = 0.327$), in which the timing of V_{max2} in 10RM was significantly shorter compared to 1- and 3RM. In addition, the timing of V_{max2} in 6RM was shorter in comparison to 1RM. No significant effects of repetition range were observed in the timing of V_{max1} and V_{min} ($F \leq 3.176$; $p \geq 0.07$; $\eta^2 \leq 0.137$). Lastly, no significant sex differences were discovered ($F \leq 1.085$; $p \geq 0.311$; $\eta^2 \leq 0.054$, Figure 4).

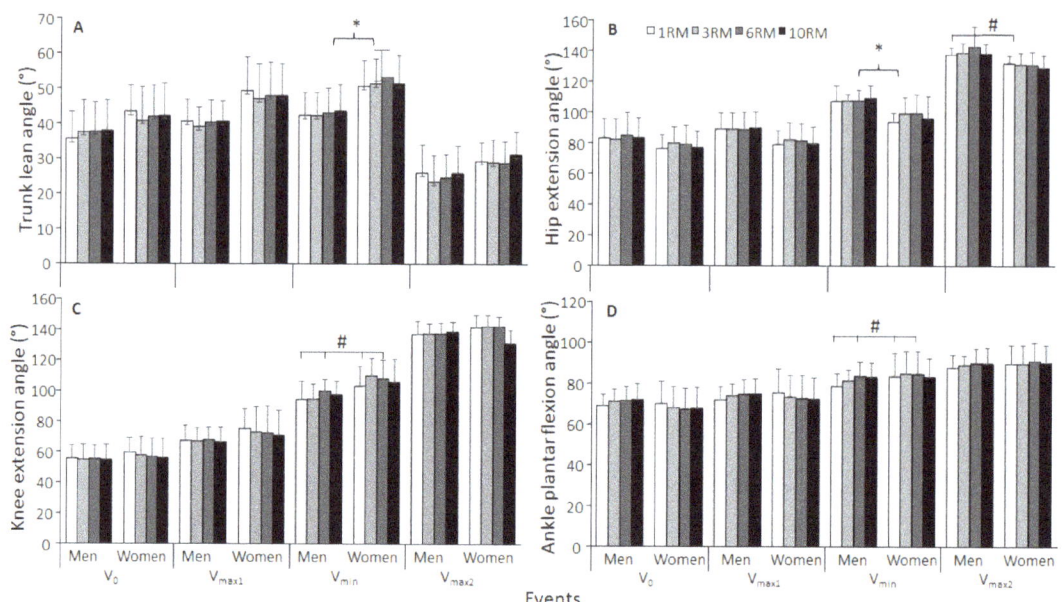

Figure 2. Mean ± SD (**A**) trunk, (**B**) hip, (**C**) knee, and (**D**) ankle angle at the different events of the last repetition during 1-, 3-, 6-, and 10RM barbell back squat. * Significantly different joint angles between sexes for all repetition ranges ($p < 0.05$). # Significantly different joint angles between two repetition ranges for both sexes ($p < 0.05$).

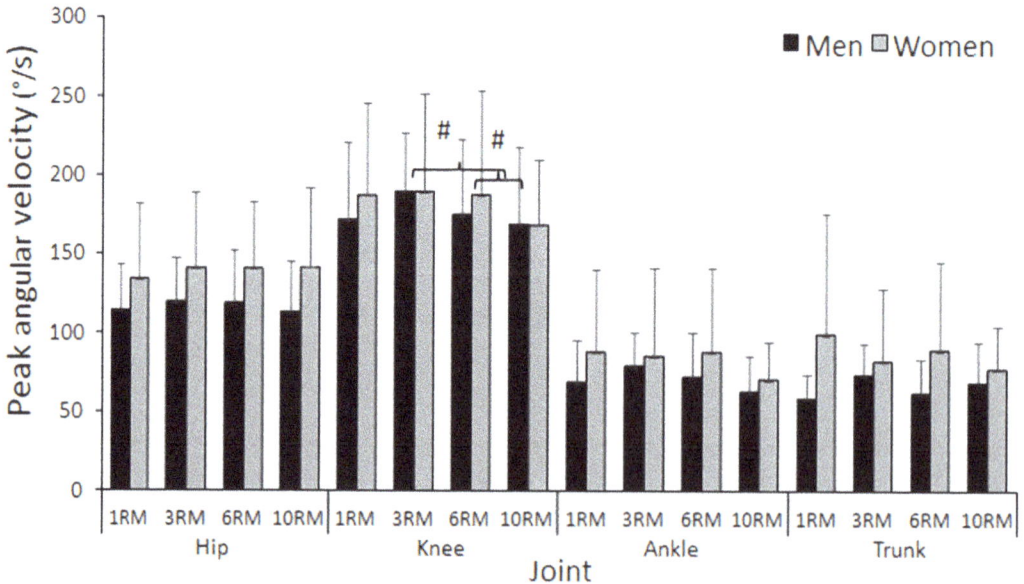

Figure 3. Mean ± SD peak angular velocity at the different events of the last repetition during 1-, 3-, 6-, and 10RM barbell back squat. # Significantly different peak angular velocity between these two repetition ranges for this joint ($p < 0.05$).

A significant effect of repetition range was observed in sEMG amplitude for the vastus medialis, vastus lateralis, soleus, and gastrocnemius in the post-sticking region, and for the vastus lateralis in the sticking region (F ≥ 4.019; $p \leq 0.011$; $\eta^2 \geq 0.041$, Figure 5D). Post hoc analysis revealed significantly higher sEMG amplitude when comparing 1RM with 10RM at the post-sticking region in the vastus medialis, vastus lateralis, soleus, and gastrocnemius. Additionally, the vastus lateralis showed higher sEMG amplitude when comparing 3RM with 6- and 10RM in the sticking region, and when comparing 3RM with 10RM at the post-sticking region. No significant effect of repetition range was observed in any of the other muscles (F ≤ 2.484; $p \geq 0.071$; $\eta^2 \leq 0.020$, Figure 5). Also, a significant effect of region was discovered in all muscles (F ≥ 6.382; $p \leq 0.012$; $\eta^2 \geq 0.148$), except at the erector spinae (F = 2.676; $p = 0.083$; $\eta^2 = 0024$, Figure 5B). In addition, significant interactions between sex and repetition range were found in the vastus lateralis and gluteus medius (F ≥ 3.168; $p \leq 0.049$; $\eta^2 \geq 0.023$, Figure 5B,E). Moreover, significant interactions between sex and region were discovered at the soleus (F ≥ 3.980; $p \leq 0.0027$; $\eta^2 \geq 0.030$, Figure 5I). Lastly, a significant interaction between region, repetition range, and sex was observed for both the gluteus medius and gluteus maximus (F ≥ 2.341; $p \leq 0.036$; $\eta^2 \geq 0.005$, Figure 5E,F). No significant interactions were found in any of the other muscles (F ≤ 2.748; $p \geq 0.078$; $\eta^2 \leq 0.020$, Figure 5).

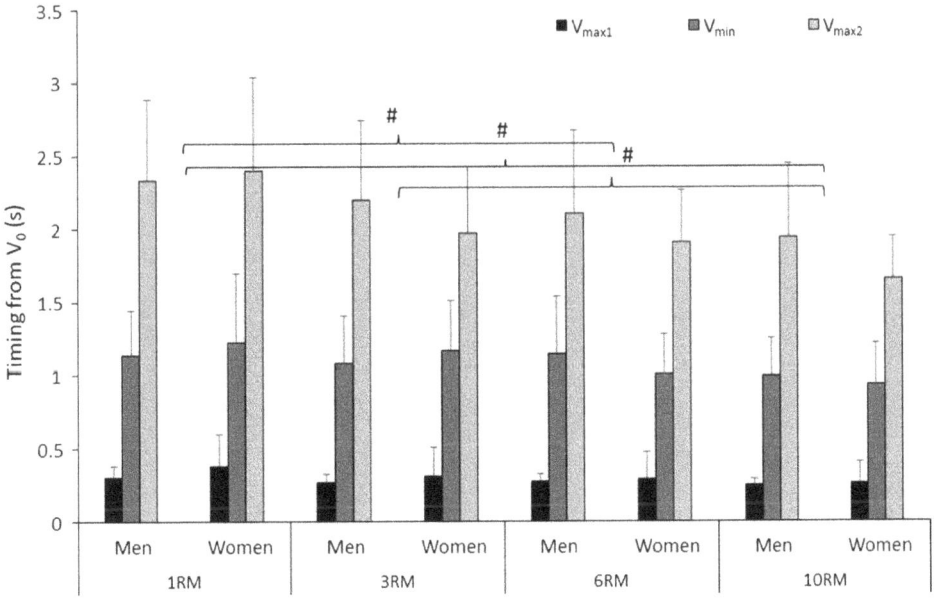

Figure 4. Mean ± SD of the timing from V_0 to the different events at the last repetition during 1-, 3-, 6-, and 10RM barbell back squat. # Significantly different timing of V_{max2} between these two repetition ranges for both sexes ($p < 0.05$).

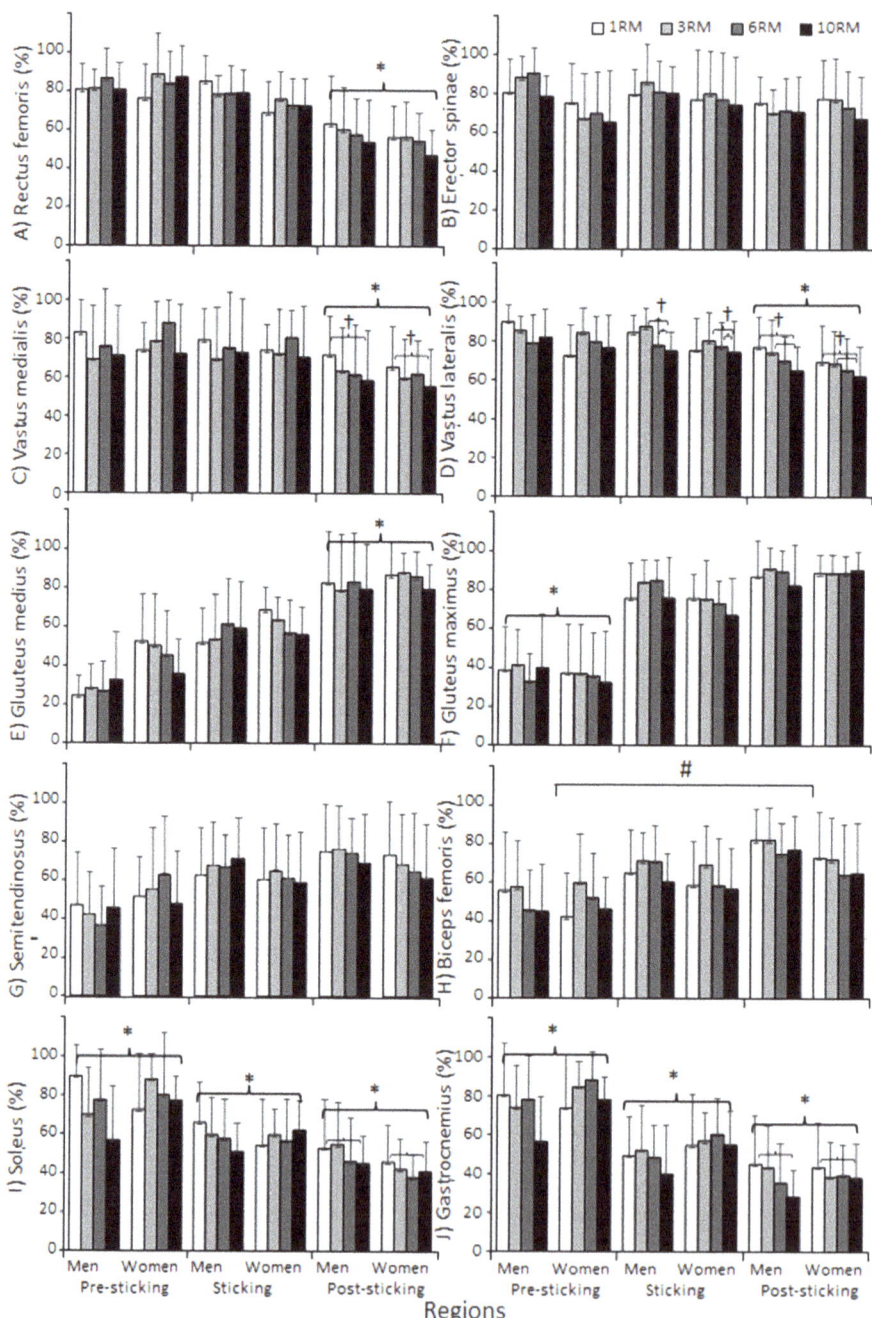

Figure 5. Mean ± SD of sEMG of the different muscles (**A–J**) during the different phases of the last repetition during 1-, 3-, 6-, and 10RM barbell back squat. * Significantly different sEMG for all repetition ranges for this region with all other regions ($p < 0.05$). # Significantly different sEMG for both men and women between these two regions for all repetition ranges ($p < 0.05$). † Significantly different sEMG between these two repetition ranges for this region ($p < 0.05$).

4. Discussion

The aim of this study was to investigate the effect of different RM ranges (1-, 3-, 6-, and 10RM) and sex on kinematics and sEMG amplitude around the sticking region in the final repetition of the squat. The main findings were that in all repetition ranges, women displayed a larger trunk lean and lower hip extension angle in the sticking region when compared to men. Furthermore, an inverse relationship between repetition range and timing from V_0 to V_{max2} was found, such that timing was shorter at 6- and 10RM compared to 1RM, and shorter at 10RM compared to 3RM. Lastly, the lower repetition range (1- and 3RM) displayed higher sEMG amplitude than the higher repetition range (6- and 10RM).

An inverse relationship between repetition range and timing from V_0 to V_{max2} was discovered, in that such timing was shorter for the higher repetition range (6- and 10RM) compared to the lower repetition range (1- and 3RM). From a biomechanical perspective, this was expected, as per-set repetitions and barbell load are inversely related; hence, lower per-set repetition ranges should be influenced by more moments of inertia, resulting in a slower ascent phase. This was in accordance with what was reported in bench press activity: significantly higher peak barbell velocities in the sticking region of 10RM compared to 1RM [14]. Conveniently, we observed a difference in timing to V_{max2}, which is the event subsequent to the sticking region. As such, when seen together with the findings from Larsen, Haugen and van den Tillaar [14], a tendency of velocity discrepancy between loads might exist in the sticking region. This is logical, as more inertia adds torque to the already heightened rotational work at the hip during the sticking region [3], which slows down the hip extension to keep the net hip moment similar.

Women displayed a larger trunk lean and lower hip extension angle in the sticking region in all repetition ranges when compared to men, which indicates technique differences between the sexes (Figures 2 and 6).

When normalised for body mass, studies consistently find men to generate greater knee and hip extensor torque than women during maximal effort contractions [20–26]. Stearns, Keim and Powers [24] found that the hip extensors of men were 44% stronger than the hip extensors of women, whereas the knee extensors of men were only 28% stronger than those of women (24). Additionally, women were found to possess a hip/knee extensor strength ratio close to 1, indicating parity in strength across knee and hip extensors. Conversely, men demonstrated a ratio <1, signifying a relative strength dominance in hip extensors compared to the knee extensors [24]. As reported by Larsen, Kristiansen and van den Tillaar [7], the knee moment contribution decreases in the sticking region, while hip moment arm and hip moment contribution increase. Also, the gluteus maximus has been found to be at a mechanical disadvantage to exert force in the sticking region [33]. Thus, when hip moment contribution increases in the sticking region, hip extensors have been viewed as a bottleneck in maximal squats [3]. Accordingly, the biomechanical requirements of the sticking region might disproportionally increase difficulty for lifters with weaker hip extensors relative to knee extensors. Therefore, as the hip joint is responsible for extending the hip, and thereby the trunk, slower extension of the hips in the sticking region could explain why the women of this study squat with increased hip extension angles and trunk lean in the sticking region. Even with higher peak angular hip and trunk extension velocities (Figure 2) of women (no significant moderate effect size), due to lower angles during the sticking region compared to men, these could only partly compensate for this later in the lift, as shown by similar trunk lean at V_{max2} (Figure 2A). The hip extension angle is still significantly higher in men, probably because the peak hip extension occurs at around V_{max2} [34]. However, more research regarding kinematic discrepancies between the sexes in maximal squats must be conducted in order to draw more concise conclusions.

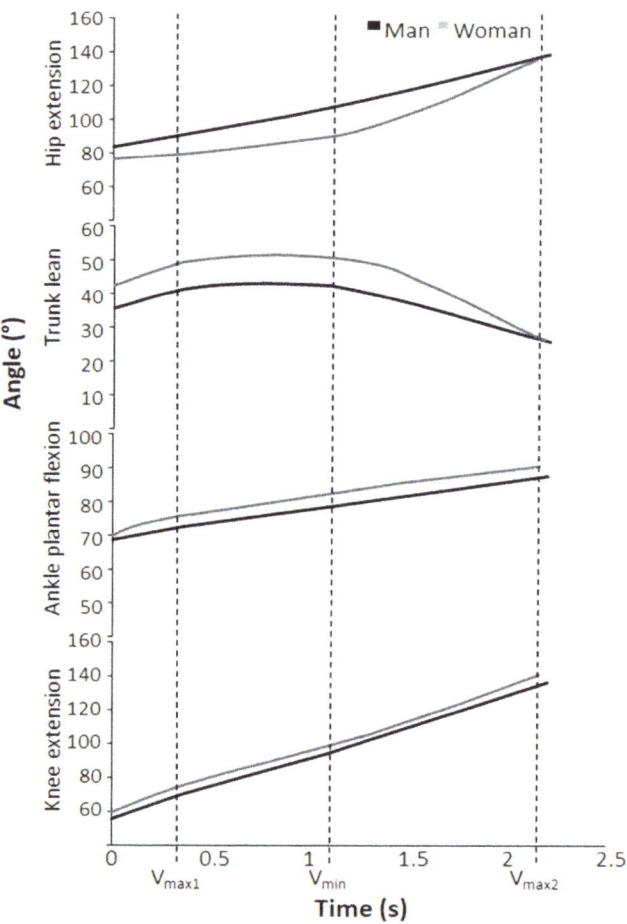

Figure 6. Two examples of joint angles over time during squats for a representative man and woman.

There were no significant sEMG findings supporting these kinematic sex differences, as both hip and knee extensors showed similar sEMG. However, the study used a mixed design, so sEMG was normalised, with each individual's peak sEMG amplitude defined as 100%. As such, comparing peak values between groups is not possible. Consequently, comparable sEMG only indicates that the timing of excitation is similar between sexes in the different regions.

It was hypothesised, likewise, that no differences would be found in sEMG activity between the repetition ranges, as the recruitment of motor units is size ordered. Hence, the highest threshold motor units would be recruited when the sets reached failure, creating similar sEMG amplitudes [16]. However, knee extensors (medial and lateral vastus) and plantar flexors displayed a lower sEMG amplitude at the post-sticking region in 10RM compared to 1 RM, with the vastus lateralis also reporting a lower sEMG amplitude in 6- and 10RM compared to 3RM at the sticking and post-sticking regions. Using a fatigue-inducing protocol, Tesch, et al. [35] found a parallel reduction in sEMG amplitude and maximum force in the knee extensors as the accumulation of lactic acid increased, possibly due to changes in action potential in the most acid-labile motor units. Exercise on multiple large muscle groups is known to increase acute metabolic demands [15], such that when combined with longer work duration in 10RM (>15 s) compared to 1 RM (<5 s), this may have caused higher threshold motor units to fail due to acidosis, which, in turn, reduced sEMG amplitude in 10RM. Additionally, previous research has observed reduced knee flexion and increased hip flexion as a high-repetition squat nears failure, making the lift increasingly hip dominant [36]. As such, knee extensors and ankle plantar flexors may have experienced heightened ATP depletion during initial repetitions in 10RM conditions [37], as the squat can be performed with a more knee-dominant technique when perceived effort is low (which also augments ankle dorsal flexion) [38]. Hence, recruitment of motor units and therefore sEMG amplitude in 10RM may be modulated by locally fatiguing factors, including ATP depletion and decreased oxidation associated with longer set duration [39–41].

This study has limitations that should be addressed. Firstly, despite the participants engaging in sets with varying loads, the consideration of body mass above the knees was omitted, which holds significance because it contributes to the absolute weight lifted. Secondly, bar placement was not standardised among participants, so we cannot exclude the possible influence of high-bar vs. low-bar technique. Thirdly, lifting tempo was not controlled for, which could influence the results. However, to avoid extra constraints on the subjects, which would make this study less ecological, it was decided that the lifting tempo and barbell placement between subjects was not standardised.

5. Conclusions

This study revealed notable variations in squatting technique between the sexes across all RMs (1-, 3-, 6-, and 10RM), with women exhibiting greater trunk lean and reduced hip extension angles compared to men in and around the sticking region, possibly due to differences in hip/knee extensor strength ratios. Additionally, an inverse relationship between timing to V_{max2} and repetition range was discovered, where timing was lower for lower repetition ranges (1–3RM) compared to higher repetition ranges (6–10RM), which might occur as heavier loads are influenced by more moments of inertia. Therefore, based upon the principle of specificity, sex and repetition range might induce different requirements during the ascent phase when squatting to volitional failure.

Author Contributions: Conceptualization: A.H.G. and R.v.d.T.; methodology: A.H.G. and R.v.d.T.; software: A.B.F. and A.H.G.; validation: R.v.d.T.; formal analysis: A.H.G., A.B.F. and R.v.d.T.; investigation: A.B.F. and H.N.F.; resources: A.H.G., A.B.F., H.N.F. and R.v.d.T.; data curation: A.B.F.; writing—original draft preparation: A.H.G.; writing—review and editing: A.H.G., H.N.F., A.B.F. and R.v.d.T.; visualization: A.H.G. and R.v.d.T.; project administration: R.v.d.T. All authors have read and agreed to the published version of the manuscript.

Funding: This research received no external funding.

Institutional Review Board Statement: The study was conducted according to the guidelines of the Declaration of Helsinki, and approved by the Norwegian Centre for Research Data (project no. 701688).

Informed Consent Statement: Informed consent was obtained from all subjects involved in the study.

Data Availability Statement: The data presented in this study are available on request from the corresponding author. The data are not publicly available due to national laws of the Norwegian government on privacy.

Conflicts of Interest: The authors declare no conflicts of interest.

References

1. McKean, M.R.; Dunn, P.K.; Burkett, B.J. Quantifying the movement and the influence of load in the back squat exercise. *J. Strength Cond. Res.* **2010**, *24*, 1671–1679. [CrossRef] [PubMed]
2. Escamilla, R.F.; Fleisig, G.; Lowry, T.M.; Barrentine, S.W.; Andrews, J.R. A three-dimensional biomechanical analysis of the squat during varying stance widths. *Med. Sci. Sports Exerc.* **2001**, *33*, 984–998. [CrossRef] [PubMed]
3. Maddox, E.U.; Bennett, H.J. Effects of external load on sagittal and frontal plane lower extremity biomechanics during back squats. *J. Biomech. Eng.* **2021**, *143*, 051006. [CrossRef]
4. Maddox, E.U.; Sievert, Z.A.; Bennett, H.J. Modified vector coding analysis of trunk and lower extremity kinematics during maximum and sub-maximum back squats. *J. Biomech.* **2020**, *106*, 109830. [CrossRef] [PubMed]

5. van den Tillaar, R. Effect of descent velocity upon muscle activation and performance in two-legged free weight back squats. *Sports* **2019**, *7*, 15. [CrossRef]
6. van den Tillaar, R.; Andersen, V.; Saeterbakken, A.H. The existence of a sticking region in free weight squats. *J. Hum. Kinet.* **2014**, *42*, 63–71. [CrossRef] [PubMed]
7. Larsen, S.; Kristiansen, E.; van den Tillaar, R. New insights about the sticking region in back squats: An analysis of kinematics, kinetics, and myoelectric activity. *Front. Sports Act. Living* **2021**, *3*, 691459. [CrossRef] [PubMed]
8. Myer, G.D.; Kushner, A.M.; Brent, J.L.; Schoenfeld, B.J.; Hugentobler, J.; Lloyd, R.S.; Vermeil, A.; Chu, D.A.; Harbin, J.; McGill, S.M. The back squat: A proposed assessment of functional deficits and technical factors that limit performance. *Strength Cond. J.* **2014**, *36*, 4. [CrossRef]
9. Larsen, S.; Kristiansen, E.; Nygaard Falch, H.; Estifanos Haugen, M.; Fimland, M.S.; van den Tillaar, R. Effects of barbell load on kinematics, kinetics, and myoelectric activity in back squats. *Sports Biomech.* **2022**; *online ahead of print*.
10. Németh, G.; Ohlsén, H. In vivo moment arm lengths for hip extensor muscles at different angles of hip flexion. *J. Biomech.* **1985**, *18*, 129–140. [CrossRef]
11. Visser, J.; Hoogkamer, J.; Bobbert, M.; Huijing, P. Length and moment arm of human leg muscles as a function of knee and hip-joint angles. *Eur. J. Appl. Physiol. Occup. Physiol.* **1990**, *61*, 453–460. [CrossRef]
12. Stone, M.; Stone, M.; Lamont, H. Explosive exercise. *Natl. Strength Cond. Assoc. J.* **1993**, *15*, 7–15. [CrossRef]
13. Schoenfeld, B.J.; Grgic, J.; Van Every, D.W.; Plotkin, D.L. Loading recommendations for muscle strength, hypertrophy, and local endurance: A re-examination of the repetition continuum. *Sports* **2021**, *9*, 32. [CrossRef] [PubMed]
14. Larsen, S.; Haugen, M.; van den Tillaar, R. Comparison of kinematics and electromyographic activity in the last repetition during different repetition maximums in the bench press exercise. *Int. J. Environ. Res. Public Health* **2022**, *19*, 14238. [CrossRef] [PubMed]
15. Kraemer, W.J.; Ratamess, N.A. Fundamentals of resistance training: Progression and exercise prescription. *Med. Sci. Sports Exerc.* **2004**, *36*, 674–688. [CrossRef] [PubMed]
16. Gordon, T.; Thomas, C.K.; Munson, J.B.; Stein, R.B. The resilience of the size principle in the organization of motor unit properties in normal and reinnervated adult skeletal muscles. *Can. J. Physiol. Pharmacol.* **2004**, *82*, 645–661. [CrossRef] [PubMed]
17. Miller, A.E.J.; MacDougall, J.; Tarnopolsky, M.; Sale, D. Gender differences in strength and muscle fiber characteristics. *Eur. J. Appl. Physiol. Occup. Physiol.* **1993**, *66*, 254–262. [CrossRef] [PubMed]
18. Janssen, I.; Heymsfield, S.B.; Wang, Z.; Ross, R. Skeletal muscle mass and distribution in 468 men and women aged 18–88 yr. *J. Appl. Physiol.* **2000**, *89*, 81–88. [CrossRef] [PubMed]
19. Monteiro, E.R.; Brown, A.F.; Bigio, L.; Palma, A.; dos Santos, L.G.; Cavanaugh, M.T.; Behm, D.G.; Corrêa Neto, V. Male relative muscle strength exceeds females for bench press and back squat. *J. Exerc. Physiol. Online* **2016**, *19*, 79–86.
20. Häkkinen, K.; Kraemer, W.; Newton, R. Muscle activation and force production during bilateral and unilateral concentric and isometric contractions of the knee extensors in men and women at different ages. *Electromyogr. Clin. Neurophysiol.* **1997**, *37*, 131–142.
21. Shultz, S.J.; Nguyen, A.-D.; Leonard, M.D.; Schmitz, R.J. Thigh strength and activation as predictors of knee biomechanics during a drop jump task. *Med. Sci. Sports Exerc.* **2009**, *41*, 857. [CrossRef]
22. Pincivero, D.M.; Gandaio, C.B.; Ito, Y. Gender-specific knee extensor torque, flexor torque, and muscle fatigue responses during maximal effort contractions. *Eur. J. Appl. Physiol.* **2003**, *89*, 134–141. [CrossRef] [PubMed]
23. Huston, L.J.; Wojtys, E.M. Neuromuscular performance characteristics in elite female athletes. *Am. J. Sports Med.* **1996**, *24*, 427–436. [CrossRef]
24. Stearns, K.M.; Keim, R.G.; Powers, C.M. Influence of relative hip and knee extensor muscle strength on landing biomechanics. *Med. Sci. Sports Exerc.* **2013**, *45*, 935–941. [CrossRef]
25. Claiborne, T.L.; Armstrong, C.W.; Gandhi, V.; Pincivero, D.M. Relationship between hip and knee strength and knee valgus during a single leg squat. *J. Appl. Biomech.* **2006**, *22*, 41–50. [CrossRef]
26. Cahalan, T.; Johnson, M.; Liu, S.; Chao, E. Quantitative measurements of hip strength in different age groups. *Clin. Orthop. Relat. Res. (1976–2007)* **1989**, *246*, 136–145. [CrossRef]
27. Hicks, A.L.; Kent-Braun, J.; Ditor, D.S. Sex differences in human skeletal muscle fatigue. *Exerc. Sport Sci. Rev.* **2001**, *29*, 109–112. [CrossRef]
28. Maughan, R.; Harmon, M.; Leiper, J.; Sale, D.; Delman, A. Endurance capacity of untrained males and females in isometric and dynamic muscular contractions. *Eur. J. Appl. Physiol. Occup. Physiol.* **1986**, *55*, 395–400. [CrossRef] [PubMed]
29. Cooke, D.M.; Haischer, M.H.; Carzoli, J.P.; Bazyler, C.D.; Johnson, T.K.; Varieur, R.; Zoeller, R.F.; Whitehurst, M.; Zourdos, M.C. Body mass and femur length are inversely related to repetitions performed in the back squat in well-trained lifters. *J. Strength Cond. Res.* **2019**, *33*, 890–895. [CrossRef] [PubMed]
30. Nimphius, S.; McBride, J.M.; Rice, P.E.; Goodman-Capps, C.L.; Capps, C.R. Comparison of quadriceps and hamstring muscle activity during an isometric squat between strength-matched men and women. *J. Sports Sci. Med.* **2019**, *18*, 101.
31. Hermens, H.J.; Freriks, B.; Disselhorst-Klug, C.; Rau, G. Development of recommendations for SEMG sensors and sensor placement procedures. *J. Electromyogr. Kinesiol.* **2000**, *10*, 361–374. [CrossRef]
32. Cohen, J. *Statistical Power Analysis for the Behavioral Sciences*; Lawrence Erlbaum Associates: Hillsdale, NJ, USA, 1988.

33. van den Tillaar, R.; Kristiansen, E.L.; Larsen, S. Is the Occurrence of the Sticking Region in Maximum Smith Machine Squats the Result of Diminishing Potentiation and Co-Contraction of the Prime Movers among Recreationally Resistance Trained Males? *Int. J. Environ. Res. Public Health* **2021**, *18*, 1366. [CrossRef] [PubMed]
34. van den Tillaar, R. Kinematics and muscle activation around the sticking region in free-weight barbell back squats/kinematika in misicna aktivacija okrog obmocja prevelikega odpora pri pocepih z bremenom zadaj med dvigovanjem utezi. *Kinesiol. Slov.* **2015**, *21*, 15.
35. Tesch, P.; Komi, P.; Jacobs, I.; Karlsson, J.; Viitasalo, J. Influence of lactate accumulation of EMG frequency spectrum during repeated concentric contractions. *Acta Physiol. Scand.* **1983**, *119*, 61–67. [CrossRef] [PubMed]
36. Hooper, D.R.; Szivak, T.K.; Comstock, B.A.; Dunn-Lewis, C.; Apicella, J.M.; Kelly, N.A.; Creighton, B.C.; Flanagan, S.D.; Looney, D.P.; Volek, J.S. Effects of fatigue from resistance training on barbell back squat biomechanics. *J. Strength Cond. Res.* **2014**, *28*, 1127–1134. [CrossRef] [PubMed]
37. Halperin, I.; Chapman, D.W.; Behm, D.G. Non-local muscle fatigue: Effects and possible mechanisms. *Eur. J. Appl. Physiol.* **2015**, *115*, 2031–2048. [CrossRef] [PubMed]
38. Bryanton, M.A.; Kennedy, M.D.; Carey, J.P.; Chiu, L.Z. Effect of squat depth and barbell load on relative muscular effort in squatting. *J. Strength Cond. Res.* **2012**, *26*, 2820–2828. [CrossRef] [PubMed]
39. Gorostiaga, E.M.; Navarro-Amezqueta, I.; Calbet, J.A.; Hellsten, Y.; Cusso, R.; Guerrero, M.; Granados, C.; Gonzalez-Izal, M.; Ibanez, J.; Izquierdo, M. Energy metabolism during repeated sets of leg press exercise leading to failure or not. *PLoS ONE* **2012**, *7*, e40621. [CrossRef]
40. Bloomer, R.J.; Falvo, M.J.; Fry, A.C.; Schilling, B.K.; Smith, W.A.; Moore, C.A. Oxidative stress response in trained men following repeated squats or sprints. *Med. Sci. Sports Exerc.* **2006**, *38*, 1436–1442. [CrossRef]
41. Baechle, T.R.; Earle, R.W. *Essentials of Strength Training and Conditioning*; Human kinetics: Champaign, IL, USA, 2008.

Disclaimer/Publisher's Note: The statements, opinions and data contained in all publications are solely those of the individual author(s) and contributor(s) and not of MDPI and/or the editor(s). MDPI and/or the editor(s) disclaim responsibility for any injury to people or property resulting from any ideas, methods, instructions or products referred to in the content.

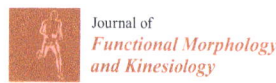

Article

The Acute Effect of Dynamic vs. Proprioceptive Neuromuscular Facilitation Stretching on Sprint and Jump Performance

Nor Fazila Abd Malek [1], Ali Md Nadzalan [1], Kevin Tan [2,3], Abdul Muiz Nor Azmi [2], Rajkumar Krishnan Vasanthi [4], Ratko Pavlović [5], Dana Badau [6,*] and Adela Badau [6]

1. Faculty of Sport Science and Coaching, Sultan Idris Education University, Tanjong Malim 35900, Perak, Malaysia; fazila.malek@fsskj.upsi.edu.my (N.F.A.M.); ali.nadzalan@fsskj.upsi.edu.my (A.M.N.)
2. Faculty of Psychology and Education, University Malaysia Sabah, Jalan UMS, Kota Kinabalu 88400, Sabah, Malaysia; k.tan@lboro.ac.uk (K.T.); abdulmuiz@ums.edu.my (A.M.N.A.)
3. School of Sport, Exercise and Health Sciences, Loughborough University, Epinal Way, Loughborough LE11 3TU, UK
4. Faculty of Health and Life Science, INTI International University, Nilai 71800, Negeri Sembilan, Malaysia; rajkumar.krishnan@newinti.edu.my
5. Faculty of Physical Education and Sport, University of East Sarajevo, Vuka Karadzica 30, 71126 East Sarajevo, Bosnia and Herzegovina; pavlovicratko@yahoo.com
6. Faculty of Physical Education and Mountain Sports, Transilvania University, 500068 Brasov, Romania; adela.badau@unitbv.ro
* Correspondence: dana.badau@unitbv.ro

Abstract: Participating in sports has been shown to promote overall wellness and, at the same time, reduce health risks. As more people are participating in sports, competitions have increased, and every aspect of the game has been focused by coaches and athletes in order to improve performance. One of these aspects is the warm-up session. The purpose of this study was to investigate the acute effect of a dynamic warm-up versus a proprioceptive neuromuscular facilitation (PNF) warm-up on the sprint and jump performance of recreationally active men. Thirty (n = 30) males were randomly assigned to undergo three sessions of different warm-up types, 72 h apart, involving either proprioceptive neuromuscular facilitation (PNF), dynamic stretching (DS), or no stretching session (control). The PNF and dynamic modes of stretching improved vertical jump performance, F (2.58) = 5.49, p = 0.046, to a certain extent (mean + 3.32% vs. control, p = 0.002 for dynamic and mean + 1.53% vs. control, p = 0.048 for PNF stretching). Dynamic stretching is best used to get a better vertical jump height. Sprint performance was also increased to a greater extent following the stretching session, F (2.58) = 5.60, p = 0.01. Sprint time was +1.05% faster vs. the control, with a value of p = 0.002 after dynamic stretching, while PNF stretching demonstrated a sprint time of +0.35% vs. the control, with a value of p = 0.049. Dynamic stretching showed a better sprint performance and also vertical jump height performance in this study. PNF and dynamic stretching prove to be equally efficacious in flexibility conditioning depending on the type of movement involved. This type of stretching should be utilized to help preserve or improve the performance output of physical activity, especially in sprinting and jumping events.

Keywords: stretching; warm-up; strength and conditioning; training protocol

Citation: Malek, N.F.A.; Nadzalan, A.M.; Tan, K.; Nor Azmi, A.M.; Krishnan Vasanthi, R.; Pavlović, R.; Badau, D.; Badau, A. The Acute Effect of Dynamic vs. Proprioceptive Neuromuscular Facilitation Stretching on Sprint and Jump Performance. *J. Funct. Morphol. Kinesiol.* **2024**, *9*, 42. https://doi.org/10.3390/jfmk9010042

Academic Editor: Diego Minciacchi

Received: 5 January 2024
Revised: 13 February 2024
Accepted: 24 February 2024
Published: 28 February 2024

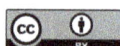

Copyright: © 2024 by the authors. Licensee MDPI, Basel, Switzerland. This article is an open access article distributed under the terms and conditions of the Creative Commons Attribution (CC BY) license (https://creativecommons.org/licenses/by/4.0/).

1. Introduction

Stretching prior to exercise is a norm among all athletes and the recreational population. It is a way for us to prepare our body for physical activity, training, or any sporting event by improving joint range of motion and muscle elasticity. Doing so can improve physical activity in terms of performance output and also reduce the chances of injury [1]. Consequently, it may also result in increased body core temperature in preparation for activities [1,2]. Coaches and athletes often include stretching exercises as a part of their training program or as a pre-event warm-up activity [3]. Stretching falls under the physical health components of flexibility. Flexibility, on the other hand, affects muscular performance [4]. It is recommended to do a stretching exercise for a healthy recreational population or athletes to prevent injury, for rehabilitation, and to increase athletic performance [5]. It was also suggested that the development of performance in the long term is related to an increase in stretching ability during activity and the tendency of a muscle to move in a flexible and less stiff way, which is an ideal condition for a resistance exercise to take place [6].

However, despite all the benefits, certain articles have speculated about the other proposed benefits stretching has to offer concerning the widespread acceptance and use of stretching [7–9]. Stretching, especially static or passive stretching, has been found in several studies to cause a considerable acute decline in various maximal muscle performances, such as force or power output [2,10–13], vertical jump performance [14,15], and sprinting performance [16]. These effects have ramifications for athletes who participate in power-based sports activities that demand strength and power generation, such as gymnastics, football, and sprinting, prompting some studies to advise avoiding static stretching before such events.

To overcome this issue, fitness enthusiasts, strength and conditioning coaches, and sports scientists have turned their attention to forming a combination form of stretching that could be utilized without a significant decrease in performance output. Various forms of active or dynamic warm-ups that incorporate movement while stretching have been designed and applied to prepare athletes during warm-up sessions [17]. Previous studies have shown that engaging in dynamic stretching exercises can lead to enhancements in physical activity performance, specifically in areas such as vertical jump performance and leg extension power [18,19]. Numerous studies also demonstrated an acute increase in power, sprint, or jump performance after dynamic stretches [20–24]. However, some studies contradict the idea that dynamic stretching is effective for performance development, such as by Nelson et al. [13], who found that dynamic stretching reduces the performance output of knee strength. This shows that a clear verdict on the effect of dynamic stretching has not been achieved.

Another type of stretching that is commonly used is proprioceptive neuromuscular facilitation (PNF) stretching. Static stimulation of the stretched muscle is used in PNF to produce optimal muscular relaxation [25]. Although studies on PNF are limited, there are interesting studies that have been obtained on the benefits of PNF stretching. PNF stretching is found to result in faster agility time because PNF has been shown to produce an increase in musculotendinous unit (MTU) stiffness [26]. An increase in muscular strength is also observed when PNF is done before sports practice with enough duration and consistency [27,28], and it also showed positive feedback on vertical jump performance [29]. Regardless, a study also indicated that PNF is shown to decrease performance before exercise with maximum effort [30–32] and it was also demonstrated to result in a negative effect when doing an isometric strength test [33].

Despite the acute effect of stretching on sports performance differing between types of stretching and movement, the PNF technique is considered to be one of the better methods to be utilized when compared with other stretching techniques, and studies not approving PNF are very few [34]. Furthermore, a significant portion of prior research has been focused on static stretching, with limited investigations conducted on the effects of two or more forms of stretching and their comparative outcomes.

This research endeavor is conducted with the aim of mitigating the persistent variability observed in various stretching protocols. This study also aims to add to the literature a comparison between techniques of stretching and their effects on physical activity performance. So, the purpose of this study is to see the immediate effect of PNF stretching and dynamic stretching on sprint and vertical jump performance among recreationally active individuals.

2. Materials and Methods

2.1. Participants

A total of thirty (n = 30) physically fit and active male individuals were recruited on a voluntary basis. The participants had an average age of 23.30 ± 3.33 years, a body height of 171.70 ± 2.84 cm, and a body mass of 76.43 ± 6.34 kg. Participants in this study involved male university students who had various sports backgrounds, whether recreational or competitive; they are also engaged in leisure-time physical activity at least three times per week. However, the requirement to be involved in this study does require participants to be experienced in jumping or sprinting [35,36]. In order to determine the required sample size for this study, a power analysis was conducted using G*Power software (version 3.1.9.4) for ANOVA repeated measures, within factors (small to medium effect size of 0.30, p-value of 0.05 and power of 0.80); the analysis revealed that a total sample size of n = 21 was adequate. Thus, n = 30 participants were recruited in this study, taking into account if any drop out occurred. They were randomly assigned to one of three experimental conditions, which included proprioceptive neuromuscular facilitation (PNF), dynamic stretching, and no stretching protocols. Prior to their involvement in this study, all participants were required to complete a Physical Activity Readiness Questionnaire (PAR-Q) and provide written informed permission. All individuals involved in the study were recreational sports players who engaged in physical activity three times per week. However, none of the participants had undergone any structured flexibility or strength training. The participants were devoid of any physical injuries during the assessment period and were given instructions to abstain from engaging in physically demanding activities for a duration of 24 h before the testing. The research study was carried out in adherence to the principles outlined in the Declaration of Helsinki, and the assessment methods were granted approval by the Ethics Committee for Human Testing at Sultan Idris Education University (Code: 2021-0442-01).

2.2. Study Design

Indicate methods and the purpose of their use: Participants were ready to be tested on 3 separate days, with at least 72 h between testing days to allow for a full recovery. Based on previous studies [37,38], duration of 48 to 72 h was recommended recovery time between sessions that involve plyometric and strength training exercise. Since this study does not involve heavy exercise, 72 h between testing days should be adequate. In the first session, the participant was familiarized with all the procedures. During the familiarization, the participants performed 3 sprint trials and 3 vertical jump trials to reduce the likelihood of a learning effect during the study [29,39]. On each data collection day, all the participants are required to complete a 10 min aerobic warm-up at 50 W using a stationary cycle ergometer [39]. Two (2) minutes of rest were given after the aerobic warm-up session. Each subject was then randomly assigned to perform 1 of 2 stretching protocols (i.e., dynamic or PNF) or a no-stretch control condition. The orders of the stretch protocol conditions were systematically varied for the 30 subjects. This modification was implemented to mitigate the impact of order effects, enabling every participant to complete both stretching procedures (Protocol A and Protocol B) as well as the control condition during the designated testing sessions. After the stretching session, the participant is required to undergo the vertical jump test and sprint test to measure their performance. The time period between the vertical jump test and sprint test was 5 min. Figure 1 shows flowchart for experiment protocol.

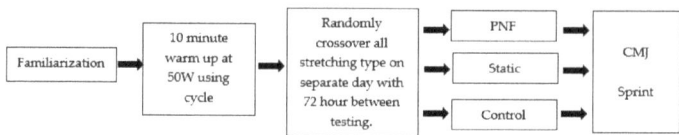

Figure 1. Flowchart of experiment protocol.

2.3. Experimental Protocols

2.3.1. PNF Stretching Protocols

The PNF stretching technique employed a "contract-relax-agonist-contraction" approach [40] necessitating the involvement of two individuals and requiring the subject to assume a supine position. The limb of choice was gradually and passively extended towards the maximum range of motion. The proprioceptive neuromuscular facilitation (PNF) stretch is commonly performed on the hamstring, gastrocnemius, gluteus, quadriceps, and hip flexor muscles. Subsequently, the participant endeavored to elicit maximal activation of the antagonist muscle groups associated with the favored limb, maintaining the leg in a fixed position for approximately 10 s. Following a brief 5 s period of rest, the participant is required to exert maximal activation of the agonist muscle groups. With the aid of the administrator, the limb is then maneuvered to achieve an enhanced range of motion (ROM) endpoint. The duration of this posture is 10 s [41,42]. This process is repeated another 2 times with 30 s of rest given between repetitions. PNF stretching involved in this study is shown in Table 1, consisting of (1) hamstring stretch, (2) quadricep stretch, (3) groin (butterfly) stretch, and (4) glute stretch. PNF implementation technique was based on studies from [43].

Table 1. PNF stretching protocol.

Muscle	Description
Hamstring stretch	Subject lies on their back with one leg extended and the other raised towards the ceiling. Assistant supports the raised leg and provides resistance by gently pushing the raised leg towards the subject's face as the subject pushes against the resistance.
Quadricep stretch	Subject in prone position with one leg bent at the knee, bringing the heel towards the buttocks. Assistant supports the raised foot and provides resistance by gently pushing the foot towards the buttocks as the subject pushes against the resistance.
Groin (butterfly) stretch	Subject sits on the floor with the soles of their feet together, knees bent out to the sides. Assistant provides resistance by gently pushing the knees towards the ground as the subject pushes against the resistance.
Glute stretch	Subject in supine position. Assistant assists by gently pushing the knee of the leg being stretched towards the opposite shoulder while the other person contracts the glute by pushing the knee away from the shoulder against the resistance.

2.3.2. Dynamic Stretching Protocol

The dynamic stretch encompasses the engagement and activation of muscles through the execution of rhythmic movements. The procedure involved the execution of a butt-kick exercise, wherein the participant repetitively and alternately brought the heel of each foot towards the buttocks while moving forward, with the objective of performing the exercise as swiftly as feasible. The procedure also involved the walking heel touch, where participants walk forward and touch their heel with both hands. The walking squat exercise involves the individual performing a squat at each stopping point while moving forward. The proposed exercise regimen includes walking lunges with a rotation, wherein the participant executes a substantial forward step while simultaneously performing a horizontal arm rotation. Additionally, the regimen incorporates a stretching exercise known as the hurdles leg raise, wherein participants ambulate with both hands extended anteriorly, palms facing downward, and proceed to elevate their extended leg towards the palm. The aforementioned technique was executed for a duration of 30 s on each occasion, with a total of 3 repetitions. Additionally, 20 s rest intervals between repetitions were given.

2.4. Measures

Vertical Jump Test. Participants stand with feet at shoulder width. Start in a standing position under the vertical jump equipment (Vertec, Sports Imports, Hilliard, OH, USA). Participants bend their knees and then jump vertically as high as possible, using both arms and legs to assist in projecting the body upwards. Participants try to reach the highest point possible on the Vertec equipment. The best of three attempts is recorded. The reliability of measurements obtained from the Vertec jumping equipment for vertical jump (VJ) height was assessed using intraclass correlation coefficients (ICCs). The ICC estimates and their corresponding 95% confidence intervals were calculated for three trials of VJ. The ICC estimates were as follows: ICC = 0.87, 95% CI = [0.43–0.87] for trial 1; ICC = 0.90, 95% CI = [0.85–0.95] for trial 2; and ICC = 0.92, 95% CI = [0.52–0.79] for trial 3. These results suggest good-to-excellent reliability [44] of the Vertec jumping equipment for measuring VJ height across multiple trials.

The 20 m Sprint Test. The experimental procedure entails the execution of a solitary maximal sprint covering a distance of 20 m, while employing a timing gate (Microgate, Bolzano, Italy) to accurately measure the duration of the sprint. The height of the timing gate was set at 1 m from ground due to the fact that the average height of adult male hip is at that height [45]. The participant assumes a standing split-stance start posture on the start line, with one foot positioned in front of the other. The position of the front foot is required to be situated posterior to the starting line. The initial position should be maintained for a duration of two seconds before commencing, and any swaying motions are prohibited. On the 'Go' signal, the participant must accelerate maximally to the finishing line. The reliability of sprint timing data obtained from timing gates was assessed using intraclass correlation coefficients (ICCs). Participants completed three sprint trials, and the timing data (in seconds) for each trial were recorded. The ICC estimates and standard errors of measurement (SEM) were calculated. Result of ICC = 0.92, SEM = 0.05 indicates excellent reliability [44] of the timing gates for measuring sprint times across the three trials.

2.5. Statistical Analysis

Data are reported as means and standard deviations. The assumption of normality was verified using the Shapiro–Wilk test. A repeated-measure analysis of variance (ANOVA) was used to compare the effects of different stretching types on sprint and vertical jump performance. A Bonferonni post-hoc test was applied to make a pairwise comparison between the data obtained when there was a significant effect detected. The statistical significance level for analyses was set at $p < 0.05$.

3. Results

Table 2 shows a test of the within-subject effect for vertical jumps. There is a significant effect in vertical jump performance among the three types of stretching protocol applied, F (2.58) = 5.49; $p = 0.046$, partial eta squared (η^2) = 0.05. Table 3 shows the pairwise comparison for vertical jumps between the three protocols.

In the vertical jump, performance was shown to be better after dynamic stretching compared to the PNF ($p = 0.046$) and control (no stretching) group ($p = 0.002$). PNF stretching was also shown to be significantly better compared to the control (no stretching) group ($p = 0.048$) (Table 4, Figure 2).

Table 2. Test of within-subject effect for vertical jump.

Source		Type III Sum of Square	df	Mean Square	F	Sig.	Observed Power
Test	Sphericity Assumed	25.400	2	12.700	5.49	0.046	0.253
Error (test)			58				

Table 3. Pairwise comparison for vertical jump (cm).

(I) Variable	(J) Variable	Mean Difference (I–J)	Std. Error	Sig.	95%CI Lower Bound	95%CI Upper Bound
Dynamic	PNF	0.700	0.990	0.046	−1.815	3.215
Dynamic	Control	1.300	1.009	0.002	−1.265	3.865
PNF	Control	0.600	0.338	0.048	−3.215	1.815

Table 4. Acute effects of different stretching conditions on vertical jump performance.

Group	Vertical Jump Test (cm)
Dynamic Stretching	40.40 ± 8.89 [bc]
PNF Stretching	39.70 ± 8.82 [c]
Control	39.10 ± 8.78 [ab]

PNF: [a] significant difference from dynamic stretching; [b] significant difference from PNF stretching; [c] significant difference from control; $p < 0.05$.

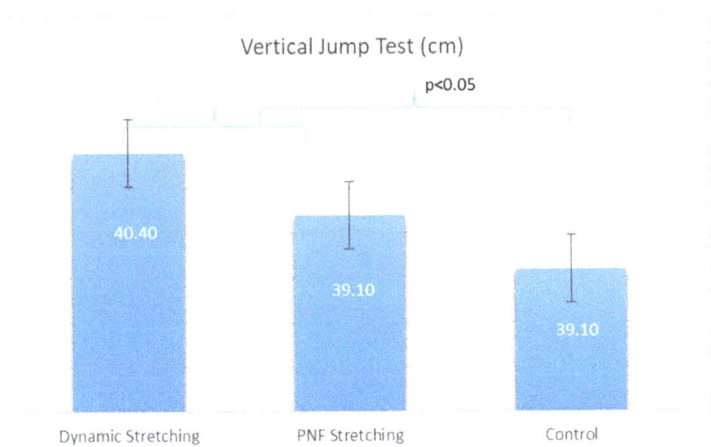

Figure 2. Acute effects of different stretching conditions on Vertical Jump Performance.

Table 5 shows the test of the within-subject effect for the 20 m sprint. There is a significant effect in sprint performance among the three types of stretching protocol applied, F (2.58) = 5.60; $p = 0.002$, partial eta squared (η^2) = 0.06. Table 6 shows the pairwise comparison for the 20 m sprint between the three protocols.

In the 20 m sprint, performance was shown to be significantly faster after dynamic stretching compared to PNF ($p = 0.002$) and no stretching ($p = 0.002$). On the other hand, PNF stretching was shown to be better compared to no stretching ($p = 0.049$). (Table 7, Figure 3).

Table 5. Test of within-subject effect for 20 m sprint (s).

Source		Type III Sum of Square	df	Mean Square	F	Sig.	Observed Power
Test	Sphericity Assumed	0.017	2	0.009	5.60	0.002	0.217
Error (test)			58				

Table 6. Pairwise comparison of 20 m sprint.

(I) Variable	(J) Variable	Mean Difference (I–J)	Std. Error	Sig.	95%CI Lower Bound	95%CI Upper Bound
Dynamic	PNF	−0.170	0.016	0.002	−0.057	0.023
Dynamic	Control	−0.034	0.025	0.002	−0.098	0.030
PNF	Control	−0.016	0.028	0.049	−0.088	0.056

Table 7. Acute effects of different stretching conditions on 20 m sprint performance.

Group	20 m Sprint Performance (s)
Dynamic Stretching	2.82 ± 0.22 [bc]
PNF Stretching	2.84 ± 0.23 [c]
Control	2.85 ± 0.23 [ab]

PNF: [a] significant difference from dynamic stretching; [b] significant difference from PNF stretching; [c] significant difference from control; $p < 0.05$.

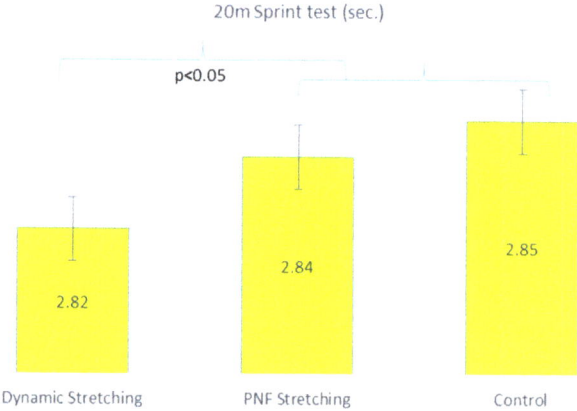

Figure 3. Acute effects of different stretching conditions on 20-m sprint performance.

4. Discussion

The adverse effect of static stretching has been reported by several studies; thus, the implementation of dynamic and other types of stretching should be considered. The objective of this study was to examine the immediate impact of dynamic stretching, PNF stretching, and a control condition on the sprint and jump performance of recreational male individuals. Specifically, the aim was to ascertain whether there are any notable disparities in performance output and performance comparison when different types of stretching are employed prior to exercise.

The main findings of the current study were that dynamic stretching and PNF stretching lead to significant increases in sprint time and also vertical jump height compared to no stretching. This is in support of previous findings that determined these two types of stretching help in increasing the performance output of an exercise [1,2] when compared with no stretching.

When comparing the dynamic and PNF stretch protocols in this study, it is discovered that the dynamic stretching protocols showed a better performance in sprinting time ($p = 0.002$) with a difference of 0.71% faster timing than the PNF stretching protocols group. In sprinting time, 0.02 s is a big difference. Vertical jump showed a 4.40% difference

(p = 0.046) in height, whereas the group with the dynamic warm-up protocols jumped higher than those in the PNF group. There is a difference of about 0.7 cm in height. Dynamic stretching gives an edge to the dynamic stretching group over the PNF stretching group. This result is backed by the data from numerous studies, which demonstrated an acute increase in power, sprint, or jump performance after dynamic stretches [20,24]. Dynamic stretching includes varieties of movements that are then combined with stretch movement. This type of movement, which incorporated more dynamic movement compared to PNF, can be considered as a warm-up movement by itself, thus bringing together the positive effect of a warm-up, which impacts core temperature and other temperature-related changes. Research has demonstrated that elevating muscle temperature leads to enhanced performance in activities requiring dynamic exertion over short durations [46].

PNF stretching by itself is developed to be a rehabilitation type of stretching and it is intended to be done on a person recovering from injury; thus, it requires less movement in its stretching protocol. It is somewhat similar to static stretching, but with assistance to increase flexibility. More movement protocols in dynamic stretching somewhat have a two-in-one function, promoting flexibility and elevating muscle temperature through active movement. An elevated muscle temperature usually occurs from the friction of intramuscular movement that occurs during exercise. When the muscle temperature is higher, it results in the increased transmission rate of an impulse, which is responsible for all our movement in exercise, and this will positively affect the force–velocity relationship, which is the core of performance output [46,47].

In contrast with the PNF stretching, the isometric contraction of the agonist muscle during PNF stretching serves as a key mechanism for enhancing flexibility and ROM, which may help to improve performance [48]. During proprioceptive neuromuscular facilitation (PNF) stretching, sustained isometric contraction of the stretched agonist muscle stimulates the neuromuscular spindle, leading to heightened muscle activation. This activation triggers impulses that directly influence the spinal motor neurons innervating the same muscle, intensifying the isometric contraction. Concurrently, inhibition of the antagonist muscle occurs, followed by a facilitation of the antagonist's concentric contraction. The "reversal of antagonists" method in PNF stretching entails an extended isometric contraction of the prelengthened agonist, which is believed to release fascia tension, enhancing the muscle's capacity to lengthen during subsequent antagonist concentric contractions. If the antagonist cannot further increase limb displacement, light pressure assists in augmenting the range of motion. Adjustment of both fascia and spindle to the new lengthened position occurs, with impulses inhibiting motor neurons to the agonist transmitted via branches. Additionally, tension elevation triggers impulses from the Golgi tendon organ (GTO), overriding neuromuscular spindle impulses, facilitating reflexive muscle relaxation (autogenic inhibition) and consequent muscle lengthening.

Even though the warm-up session is done before stretching, which resulted in a core temperature elevation, a study by Alemdaroğlu et al. [43] and Bradley et al. [29] showed that the sprint time and vertical jump height will return to normal levels after certain minutes of warming-up due to core temperature decrement. In the PNF condition, 20 m sprint performance returned to normal levels at 15 min post stretching, while 10 m performance took 20 min to recover. Bradley et al. [29] also showed a similar result, where the vertical jump performance returned to control values 15 min after stretching. Taking this into account, it can be said that the core temperature will gradually go down and this will affect performance during exercise. With this, dynamic stretching with more movement is deemed to be more useful in stretching while maintaining the core temperature at an optimum level for an exercise to produce a better performance output.

A better vertical jump height and faster sprint time when dynamic stretching is used could probably result from the effect of post-activation potentiation, which is produced from dynamic stretching [49–51]. The observed outcome is attributed to a temporary enhancement in muscular contractile ability subsequent to a deliberate voluntary contraction performed during the stretching process. In their study, Yamaguchi et al. [18] observed a reduction in the time required to reach peak torque and an augmentation in the rate of torque development subsequent to the implementation of dynamic stretching exercises. Based on the findings, it was determined that the occurrence of PAP is a possibility.

However, the literature also contains findings regarding compromised performance subsequent to engaging in dynamic stretching exercises [52–54]. However, it seems that the effect of the stretch is related and could be attributed to several factors, such as muscle group, stretching duration, stretching intensity or contraction type, and velocity. Further research on this needs to be done to add to the literature about all these determinants.

The strengths of the study were the following: comparative analysis of three groups of subjects, analysis of the impact of dynamic stretching vs. PNF on sprint and vertical jump performances; and the conception and implementation of two types of preparation protocols specific to the two types of stretching in the warm-up part. The limitations of the study were the following: the relatively small number of subjects included in the study, the non-inclusion of female subjects in the study, and the relatively short duration of the implementation of the two warm-up stretching protocols. In addition, neither core temperature nor joint range of motion was measured in this study, which is likely to be a mechanism of influencing factors on the improvement of jumping and sprinting performance.

5. Conclusions

Based on the aforementioned findings and the present outcomes, it can be concluded that dynamic stretches exhibit more efficacy compared to PNF stretches when employed in pre-activity warm-up routines to optimize sprint time and vertical jump height performance. There is a suggestion that including dynamic stretching into a pre-event warm-up routine may provide greater performance advantages compared to proprioceptive neuromuscular facilitation (PNF) stretching. Engaging in a brief session of dynamic stretching can lead to enhanced power output in activities such as vertical jumps and sprinting. This improvement in muscular power is notably more substantial compared to the effects of PNF stretching or the absence of stretching altogether. This knowledge may prove particularly valuable for players and coaches engaged in power-oriented sports, such as football and weightlifting.

Author Contributions: Conceptualization, N.F.A.M., A.M.N., K.T., A.M.N.A., R.K.V., R.P., D.B. and A.B.; methodology, N.F.A.M., A.M.N., K.T., A.M.N.A., R.K.V. and R.P.; formal analysis, N.F.A.M., A.M.N., K.T., A.M.N.A., R.K.V. and R.P.; investigation, N.F.A.M., A.M.N., K.T., A.M.N.A., R.K.V. and R.P.; data curation, N.F.A.M., A.M.N., K.T., A.M.N.A., R.K.V. and R.P.; writing—original draft preparation, N.F.A.M., A.M.N., K.T., A.M.N.A., R.K.V., R.P., D.B. and A.B.; writing—review and editing, N.F.A.M., A.M.N., K.T., A.M.N.A., R.K.V., R.P., D.B. and A.B. All authors have read and agreed to the published version of the manuscript.

Funding: This research received no external funding.

Institutional Review Board Statement: The research study was carried out in adherence to the principles outlined in the Declaration of Helsinki, and the assessment methods were granted approval by the Ethics Committee for Human Testing at Sultan Idris Education University (Code: 01.2021/2021-0442-01).

Informed Consent Statement: Informed consent was obtained from all subjects involved in the study.

Data Availability Statement: Data are contained within the article.

Acknowledgments: The authors would like to thank the Research Management and Innovation Center, Universiti Pendidikan Sultan Idris for the support provided on the publication of this manuscript.

Conflicts of Interest: The authors declare no conflicts of interest.

References

1. McGowan, C.J.; Pyne, D.B.; Thompson, K.G.; Rattray, B. Warm-Up Strategies for Sport and Exercise: Mechanisms and Applications. *Sports Med.* **2015**, *45*, 1523–1546. [CrossRef] [PubMed]
2. Behm, D.G.; Blazevich, A.J.; Kay, A.D.; McHugh, M. Acute effects of muscle stretching on physical performance, range of motion, and injury incidence in healthy active individuals: A systematic review. *Appl. Physiol. Nutr. Metab.* **2016**, *41*, 1–11. [CrossRef] [PubMed]
3. Gleim, G.W.; McHugh, M.P. Flexibility and its effects on sports injury and performance. *Sports Med.* **1997**, *24*, 289–299. [CrossRef] [PubMed]
4. Ferreira, G.N.; Teixeira-Salmela, L.F.; Guimarães, C.Q. Gains in flexibility related to measures of muscular performance: Impact of flexibility on muscular performance. *Clin. J. Sport Med.* **2007**, *17*, 276–281. [CrossRef] [PubMed]
5. Pescatello, L.S. *ACSM's Guidelines for Exercise Testing and Prescription*; Lippincott Williams & Wilkins: Philadelphia, PA, USA, 2014.
6. Young, W.B. The use of static stretching in warm-up for training and competition. *Int. J. Sports Physiol. Perform.* **2007**, *2*, 212–216. [CrossRef] [PubMed]
7. Shrier, I. Does stretching improve performance? A systematic and critical review of the literature. *Clin. J. Sport Med.* **2004**, *14*, 267–273. [CrossRef] [PubMed]
8. Weldon, S.M.; Hill, R.H. The efficacy of stretching for prevention of exercise-related injury: A systematic review of the literature. *Man. Ther.* **2003**, *8*, 141–150. [CrossRef]
9. Ingraham, S.J. The role of flexibility in injury prevention and athletic performance: Have we stretched the truth? *Minn. Med.* **2003**, *86*, 58–61.
10. Cramer, J.T.; Housh, T.J.; Johnson, G.O.; Miller, J.M.; Coburn, J.W.; Beck, T.W. Acute effects of static stretching on peak torque in women. *J. Strength Cond. Res.* **2004**, *18*, 236–241. [CrossRef]
11. Arntz, F.; Markov, A.; Behm, D.G.; Behrens, M.; Negra, Y.; Nakamura, M.; Moran, J.; Chaabene, H. Chronic Effects of Static Stretching Exercises on Muscle Strength and Power in Healthy Individuals Across the Lifespan: A Systematic Review with Multi-level Meta-analysis. *Sports Med.* **2023**, *53*, 723–745. [CrossRef]
12. Begovic, H.; Can, F.; Yağcıoğlu, S.; Ozturk, N. Passive stretching-induced changes detected during voluntary muscle contractions. *Physiother. Theory Pract.* **2020**, *36*, 731–740. [CrossRef] [PubMed]
13. Nelson, A.G.; Guillory, I.K.; Cornwell, C.; Kokkonen, J. Inhibition of maximal voluntary isokinetic torque production following stretching is velocity-specific. *J. Strength Cond. Res.* **2001**, *15*, 241–246. [PubMed]
14. Ryan, E.D.; Everett, K.L.; Smith, D.B.; Pollner, C.; Thompson, B.J.; Sobolewski, E.J.; Fiddler, R.E. Acute effects of different volumes of dynamic stretching on vertical jump performance, flexibility and muscular endurance. *Clin. Physiol. Funct. Imaging* **2014**, *34*, 485–492. [CrossRef] [PubMed]
15. Gesel, F.J.; Morenz, E.K.; Cleary, C.J.; LaRoche, D.P. Acute Effects of Static and Ballistic Stretching on Muscle-Tendon Unit Stiffness, Work Absorption, Strength, Power, and Vertical Jump Performance. *J. Strength Cond. Res.* **2022**, *36*, 2147–2155. [CrossRef] [PubMed]
16. Nelson, A.G.; Driscoll, N.M.; Landin, D.K.; Young, M.A.; Schexnayder, I.C. Acute effects of passive muscle stretching on sprint performance. *J. Sports Sci.* **2005**, *23*, 449–454. [CrossRef] [PubMed]
17. Hedrick, A. Dynamic flexibility training. *Strength Cond. J.* **2000**, *22*, 33. [CrossRef]
18. Yamaguchi, T.; Ishii, K. Effects of static stretching for 30 seconds and dynamic stretching on leg extension power. *J. Strength Cond. Res.* **2005**, *19*, 677–683. [CrossRef]
19. Turki, O.; Chaouachi, A.; Drinkwater, E.J.; Chtara, M.; Chamari, K.; Amri, M.; Behm, D.G. Ten minutes of dynamic stretching is sufficient to potentiate vertical jump performance characteristics. *J. Strength Cond. Res.* **2011**, *25*, 2453–2463. [CrossRef]
20. Li, F.Y.; Guo, C.G.; Li, H.S.; Xu, H.R.; Sun, P. A systematic review and net meta-analysis of the effects of different warm-up methods on the acute effects of lower limb explosive strength. *BMC Sports Sci. Med. Rehabil.* **2023**, *15*, 106. [CrossRef]
21. Opplert, J.; Babault, N. Acute Effects of Dynamic Stretching on Muscle Flexibility and Performance: An Analysis of the Current Literature. *Sports Med.* **2018**, *48*, 299–325. [CrossRef]
22. Takeuchi, K.; Nakamura, M.; Matsuo, S.; Akizuki, K.; Mizuno, T. Effects of Speed and Amplitude of Dynamic Stretching on the Flexibility and Strength of the Hamstrings. *J. Sports Sci. Med.* **2022**, *21*, 608–615. [CrossRef] [PubMed]
23. Pappas, P.T.; Paradisis, G.P.; Exell, T.A.; Smirniotou, A.S.; Tsolakis, C.K.; Arampatzis, A. Acute Effects of Stretching on Leg and Vertical Stiffness during Treadmill Running. *J. Strength Cond. Res.* **2017**, *31*, 3417–3424. [CrossRef] [PubMed]
24. Su, H.; Chang, N.J.; Wu, W.L.; Guo, L.Y.; Chu, I.H. Acute Effects of Foam Rolling, Static Stretching, and Dynamic Stretching During Warm-ups on Muscular Flexibility and Strength in Young Adults. *J. Sport Rehabil.* **2017**, *26*, 469–477. [CrossRef] [PubMed]
25. Rees, S.S.; Murphy, A.J.; Watsford, M.L.; McLachlan, K.A.; Coutts, A.J. Effects of proprioceptive neuromuscular facilitation stretching on stiffness and force-producing characteristics of the ankle in active women. *J. Strength Cond. Res.* **2007**, *21*, 572–577. [PubMed]
26. Jordan, J.B.; Korgaokar, A.D.; Farley, R.S.; Caputo, J.L. Acute effects of static and proprioceptive neuromuscular facilitation stretching on agility performance in elite youth soccer players. *Int. J. Exerc. Sci.* **2012**, *5*, 1–9.
27. Almeida, G.P.L.; Carneiro, K.K.A.; Morais, H.C.R.; Oliveira, J.B.B. Influence of stretching hamstring and quadriceps femoral muscles on knee peak torque and maximum power. *Fisioter. Pesqui.* **2009**, *16*, 346–351. [CrossRef]
28. de Oliveira, M.B.; Letieri, R.V.; de Holanda, F.J.; de Lima, I.H.V.; de Almeida Alves, T., Jr.; Furtado, G.E. Acute effect of flexibility exercises on vertical jump performance in young men: A pilot study/Efeito agudo de exercicios de flexibilidade no desempenho do salto vertical em homens: Um estudo piloto. *Motricidade* **2016**, *12*, 62–69.

29. Bradley, P.S.; Olsen, P.D.; Portas, M.D. The effect of static, ballistic, and proprioceptive neuromuscular facilitation stretching on vertical jump performance. *J. Strength Cond. Res.* **2007**, *21*, 223–226. [CrossRef]
30. Funk, D.C.; Swank, A.M.; Mikla, B.M.; Fagan, T.A.; Farr, B.K. Impact of prior exercise on hamstring flexibility: A comparison of proprioceptive neuromuscular facilitation and static stretching. *J. Strength Cond. Res.* **2003**, *17*, 489–492. [CrossRef]
31. Hindle, K.B.; Whitcomb, T.J.; Briggs, W.O.; Hong, J. Proprioceptive Neuromuscular Facilitation (PNF): Its Mechanisms and Effects on Range of Motion and Muscular Function. *J. Hum. Kinet.* **2012**, *31*, 105–113. [CrossRef]
32. Behm, D.G.; Alizadeh, S.; Daneshjoo, A.; Anvar, S.H.; Graham, A.; Zahiri, A.; Goudini, R.; Edwards, C.; Culleton, R.; Scharf, C.; et al. Acute Effects of Various Stretching Techniques on Range of Motion: A Systematic Review with Meta-Analysis. *Sports Med. Open* **2023**, *9*, 107. [CrossRef] [PubMed]
33. de Lima Costa, G.V.; da Silveira, A.L.B.; Di Masi, F.; Bentes, C.M.; de Sousa, M.D.S.C.; da Silva Novaes, J. Acute effect of different stretching methods on isometric muscle strength. *Acta Scientiarum. Health Sci.* **2014**, *36*, 51–57. [CrossRef]
34. Place, N.; Blum, Y.; Armand, S.; Maffiuletti, N.A.; Behm, D.G. Effects of a short proprioceptive neuromuscular facilitation stretching bout on quadriceps neuromuscular function, flexibility, and vertical jump performance. *J. Strength Cond. Res.* **2013**, *27*, 463–470. [CrossRef] [PubMed]
35. Lee, C.-L.; Hsu, W.-C.; Cheng, C.-F. Physiological adaptations to sprint interval training with matched exercise volume. *Med. Sci. Sports Exerc.* **2017**, *49*, 86–95. [CrossRef] [PubMed]
36. Nuzzo, J.L.; Anning, J.H.; Scharfenberg, J.M. The reliability of three devices used for measuring vertical jump height. *J. Strength Cond. Res.* **2011**, *25*, 2580–2590. [CrossRef] [PubMed]
37. Davies, G.; Riemann, B.L.; Manske, R. Current concepts of plyometric exercise. *Int. J. Sports Phys. Ther.* **2015**, *10*, 760. [PubMed]
38. Barahona-Fuentes, G.D.; Ojeda, Á.H.; Jerez-Mayorga, D. Effects of different methods of strength training on indicators of muscle fatigue during and after strength training: A systematic review. *Mot. Rev. Educ. Física* **2020**, *26*, e10200063. [CrossRef]
39. Hopkins, W.G.; Schabort, E.J.; Hawley, J.A. Reliability of power in physical performance tests. *Sports Med.* **2001**, *31*, 211–234. [CrossRef]
40. Chen, C.H.; Nosaka, K.; Chen, H.L.; Lin, M.J.; Tseng, K.W.; Chen, T.C. Effects of flexibility training on eccentric exercise-induced muscle damage. *Med. Sci. Sports Exerc.* **2011**, *43*, 491–500. [CrossRef]
41. Rowlands, A.V.; Marginson, V.F.; Lee, J. Chronic flexibility gains: Effect of isometric contraction duration during proprioceptive neuromuscular facilitation stretching techniques. *Res. Q. Exerc. Sport* **2003**, *74*, 47–51. [CrossRef]
42. Zaidi, S.; Ahamad, A.; Fatima, A.; Ahmad, I.; Malhotra, D.; Al Muslem, W.H.; Abdulaziz, S.; Nuhmani, S. Immediate and Long-Term Effectiveness of Proprioceptive Neuromuscular Facilitation and Static Stretching on Joint Range of Motion, Flexibility, and Electromyographic Activity of Knee Muscles in Older Adults. *J. Clin. Med.* **2023**, *12*, 2610. [CrossRef] [PubMed]
43. Alemdaroğlu, U.; Köklü, Y.; Koz, M. The acute effect of different stretching methods on sprint performance in taekwondo practitioners. *J. Sports Med. Phys. Fit.* **2016**, *57*, 1104–1110. [CrossRef] [PubMed]
44. Koo, T.K.; Li, M.Y. A guideline of selecting and reporting intraclass correlation coefficients for reliability research. *J. Chiropr. Med.* **2016**, *15*, 155–163. [CrossRef] [PubMed]
45. Reinhardt, L.; Schwesig, R.; Lauenroth, A.; Schulze, S.; Kurz, E. Enhanced sprint performance analysis in soccer: New insights from a GPS-based tracking system. *PLoS ONE* **2019**, *14*, e0217782. [CrossRef] [PubMed]
46. Bishop, D. Warm up I: Potential mechanisms and the effects of passive warm up on exercise performance. *Sports Med.* **2003**, *33*, 439–454. [CrossRef] [PubMed]
47. Badau, D.; Bacarea, A.; Ungur, R.N.; Badau, A.; Martoma, A.M. Biochemical and functional modifications in biathlon athletes at medium altitude training. *Rev. Romana Med. Lab.* **2016**, *24*, 327–335. [CrossRef]
48. Burke, D.G.; Holt, L.E.; Rasmussen, R.; MacKinnon, N.C.; Vossen, J.F.; Pelham, T.W. Effects of hot or cold water immersion and modified proprioceptive neuromuscular facilitation flexibility exercise on hamstring length. *J. Athl. Train.* **2001**, *36*, 16.
49. Hough, P.A.; Ross, E.Z.; Howatson, G. Effects of dynamic and static stretching on vertical jump performance and electromyographic activity. *J. Strength Cond. Res.* **2009**, *23*, 507–512. [CrossRef]
50. Matsuo, S.; Iwata, M.; Miyazaki, M.; Fukaya, T.; Yamanaka, E.; Nagata, K.; Tsuchida, W.; Asai, Y.; Suzuki, S. Acute and Prolonged Effects of 300 sec of Static, Dynamic, and Combined Stretching on Flexibility and Muscle Force. *J. Sports Sci. Med.* **2023**, *22*, 626–636. [CrossRef]
51. Mariscal, S.L.; Garcia, V.S.; Fernández-García, J.C.; de Villarreal, E.S. Acute effects of ballistic vs. passive static stretching involved in a prematch warm-up on vertical jump and linear sprint performance in soccer players. *J. Strength Cond. Res.* **2021**, *35*, 147–153. [CrossRef]
52. Paradisis, G.P.; Pappas, P.T.; Theodorou, A.S.; Zacharogiannis, E.G.; Skordilis, E.K.; Smirniotou, A.S. Effects of static and dynamic stretching on sprint and jump performance in boys and girls. *J. Strength Cond. Res.* **2014**, *28*, 154–160. [CrossRef]
53. Hernandez-Martinez, J.; Ramirez-Campillo, R.; Vera-Assaoka, T.; Castillo-Cerda, M.; Carter-Truillier, B.; Herrera-Valenzuela, T.; López-Fuenzalida, A.; Nobari, H.; Valdés-Badilla, P. Warm-up stretching exercises and physical performance of youth soccer players. *Front. Physiol.* **2023**, *14*, 1127669. [CrossRef]
54. Sá, M.A.; Neto, G.R.; Costa, P.B.; Gomes, T.M.; Bentes, C.M.; Brown, A.F.; Novaes, J.S. Acute effects of different stretching techniques on the number of repetitions in a single lower body resistance training session. *J. Hum. Kinet.* **2015**, *45*, 177–185. [CrossRef]

Disclaimer/Publisher's Note: The statements, opinions and data contained in all publications are solely those of the individual author(s) and contributor(s) and not of MDPI and/or the editor(s). MDPI and/or the editor(s) disclaim responsibility for any injury to people or property resulting from any ideas, methods, instructions or products referred to in the content.

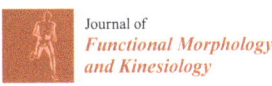

Journal of
Functional Morphology and Kinesiology

Article

Beyond Belief: Exploring the Alignment of Self-Efficacy, Self-Prediction, Self-Perception, and Actual Performance Measurement in a Squat Jump Performance—A Pilot Study

Alessandro Cudicio [1,*] and Valeria Agosti [2]

1. Department of Human and Social Sciences, University of Bergamo, 24129 Bergamo, Italy
2. Department of Humanities, Philosophy and Education, University of Salerno, 84084 Fisciano, Italy; vaagosti@unisa.it
* Correspondence: alessandro.cudicio@unibs.it; Tel.: +39-030-371-7457

Abstract: It is widely accepted that athletic performance emerges from a complex interaction between physical and cognitive features. Several studies highlighted self-efficacy (SE) in the cognitive domain of athletic performance, but no studies have correlated SE with sport-specific tasks. According to Bandura, this study explored SE and its relationship with self-prediction (SP), self-perception (PSJ), and actual performance in a squat jump (SJ). Thirty-nine healthy collegiate students were assessed using an SE questionnaire, an SP measurement tool, and a validated optical system for actual SJ performance. An SE score and an SE esteem index (SEE) were determined. The alignment between an individual's SP of their SJ performance and their SE beliefs was also examined. The data revealed a significant correlation between SE score and both SJ (r = 0.432; p = 0.006) and SP (r = 0.441; p = 0.005). Furthermore, disparities among the actual SJ, SP, and SEE were statistically non-significant, implying a congruence between self-belief and performance. With a deeper understanding of the interaction between SE, SP, and sport-specific tasks, sports professionals could develop targeted interventions to enhance athletes' overall athletic achievements and apply SE as a feature linking physical and cognitive athletic performance.

Keywords: athletic performance; self-efficacy; self-prediction; self-perception; squat jump

Citation: Cudicio, A.; Agosti, V. Beyond Belief: Exploring the Alignment of Self-Efficacy, Self-Prediction, Self-Perception, and Actual Performance Measurement in a Squat Jump Performance—A Pilot Study. *J. Funct. Morphol. Kinesiol.* **2024**, *9*, 16. https://doi.org/10.3390/jfmk9010016

Academic Editor: Giuseppe Musumeci

Received: 10 October 2023
Revised: 21 December 2023
Accepted: 28 December 2023
Published: 3 January 2024

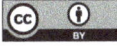

Copyright: © 2024 by the authors. Licensee MDPI, Basel, Switzerland. This article is an open access article distributed under the terms and conditions of the Creative Commons Attribution (CC BY) license (https://creativecommons.org/licenses/by/4.0/).

1. Introduction

Athletic performance is the result of a perfect balance among physical, cognitive, technical, and tactical elements that allow the athlete to achieve successful outcomes [1–3]. In athletic performance and in sport activities, cognitive functions and skills were identified as features useful to recognize information from the environment and link this to our background knowledge to better plan, organize, and execute the appropriate motor behavior [4,5]. An especially interesting and important cognitive feature in organizing athletic and sport performance is self-efficacy (SE), which refers to an individual's belief in their ability to effectively plan and carry out the necessary actions to achieve specific goals [6]. Indeed, SE is emerging as a psychological skill training tool to influence an athlete's performance [7] and sustain and ameliorate sport-specific performance over time [8,9]. Over the years, several studies have shown a positive correlation between SE and sport performance where, across various sporting and athletic endeavors, higher SE tends to be associated with enhanced performance outcomes [10–16]. On the other hand, Moritz et al. [10] outlined the limitations and perspectives of this relationship contrary to Bandura's idea of sport performance, referred to as an achievement that needs specific and objective (quantitative outcomes) descriptive criteria [6]. In this vein, for SE to be effective in athletic and sport performance, it should be considered as a qualitative skill that requires a quantitative outcome [6,10,17]. However, even if the quantitative component of the SE covers a significant importance in the realm of sport performance, it is also fundamental to not consider SE only as the actual performance (outcome) but rather as the judgment regarding what the individual can accomplish during the actual performance (goal). In this way, SE could be considered a cognitive feature useful to build subjective performance consistent with the environmental information and the sport-specific requirements [4,5,18]. To reduce discrepancies between goals and outcomes, Bandura outlined that it is crucial to introduce the athlete's own objective self-prediction (SP) of performance in the assessment measure [6]. Furthermore, to ensure valid and reliable outcomes, SE should be assessed in a task-specific manner; more specifically, the measures of SE and performance should be concordant [10]. To ensure this concordance, we chose the squat jump (SJ) as a useful task-specific performance for our study because it operates as a straightforward and effective test unaffected by physiological confounders [19].

SJ is a technique of the vertical jump beginning from a static, semi-squatting position useful in harnessing and releasing the elastic energy stored within the musculotendon complex, which sheds light on leg power capabilities [20]. SJ is a complex motor skill that requires complex motor coordination involving multiple joints but also requires perfect organization of motor behavior between the upper and lower body; no cognitive abilities are required. The height achieved in the SJ, both for inactive individuals and elite athletes, is indicative of explosive muscle strength and correlates with performance attributes like speed, agility, and power [21].

We assumed that shedding light on the intricate interplay between SE, SP, and actual SJ performance, also using a perceived SJ height (PSJ), could have potential implications for optimizing training and coaching cognitive strategies in sport science. To the best of our knowledge, no study has yet explored the nature of the relationship between SE and sport performance in a task-specific movement.

Designed as a pilot study, the aim of our research was to objectively assess the nature of the relationship between SE and sport performance in a task-specific movement and to identify the role of SE as a cognitive feature in sport performance.

2. Materials and Methods

2.1. Participants

A total of 39 healthy college students (27 M; 12 F), without any ongoing or history of neurological, orthopedic, and cardiac or systemic diseases that could interfere with physical performance, voluntarily participated during their curricular educational activities. All participants were assessed by anthropometric measurements with an electronic scale 872TM and a stadiometer 214TM (SECA, Hamburg, Germany) and physical activity level [22–25] (see Table 1). To ensure standardization within the group, only physically active individuals were included in the research. For this purpose, we utilized the IPAQ results to exclude individuals with a score below 700 MET/min/week [26]. Data were collected in adherence to all privacy policy procedures, and written informed consent was obtained from all participants in accordance with the Declaration of Helsinki [27].

Table 1. Demographic and descriptive data (yrs: years; m: male; f: female; kg: kilogram; cm: centimeters; BMI: body mass index; IPAQ: International Physical Activity Questionnaire; MET-min/wk: metabolic equivalent task minutes per week; SD: standard deviation).

Subjects Number	Sex (f/m)	Age (yrs) (Mean ±SD)	Weight (kg) (Mean ± SD)	Height (cm) (Mean ± SD)	BMI (Mean ± SD)	IPAQ (MET-min/wk) (Mean ± SD)
39	12/27	21.7 ± 1.8	70.2 ± 11.2	176 ± 9	22.6 ± 2.7	3797 ± 1979

The sample size for Pearson's correlation was determined using power analysis conducted in G-POWER (ver. 3.1.9.7, Düsseldorf, Germany) using an alpha of 0.05, a power of 0.90, and a medium effect size (rho = 0.5) for a two-tailed test. Based on the assumptions, the required minimum sample size was determined to be thirty-seven [28].

2.2. Experimental Procedure

Before starting, all participants were informed of the study's objectives and procedures. Subsequently, all participants underwent an SE, SP, SJ, and PSJ assessment conducted as follows (study timeline shown in Figure 1):

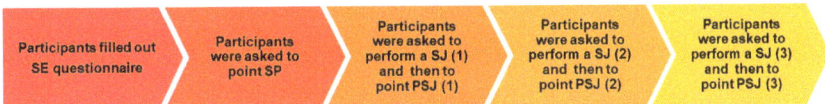

Figure 1. Study timeline. Self-efficacy (SE); self-prediction (SP); squat jump (SJ); perceived SJ (PSJ).

SE was assessed, according to Bandura [29], by an 8-item questionnaire using a five-level Likert scale (Q1–Q8), which was individually administered through Google Forms by means of their personal devices. The questionnaire was split into two sections. The first provided a graphic depiction of the correct technique for executing an SJ, consisting of a 6-item five-level Likert scale (Q1–Q6) graded from "not at all confident-1" to "extremely confident-5". This aimed to gauge the participants' confidence in performing an SJ at a specific height and confidence in their answers (height ranges were sex-specific). The second consisted of a 2-item five-level Likert scale (Q7), graded from "not good at all (below the 20th percentile)-1" to "extremely good (above the 80th percentile)-5", aimed to grade performance compared to their peers within the study group. The final item (Q8), a five-level Likert scale graded from "not at all confident-1" to "extremely confident-5", aimed to inquire about the participants' confidence in all their previous responses. To evaluate questionnaire results, two original SE scores were calculated, as explained in the subsequent statistical analysis section.

SP and PSJ were assessed by means of a custom-made vertical graduated rod, measured in centimeters (cm). SP, defined as the participants' subjective expectancy in jump height measure, was assessed only before the first jump, asking each participant to predict the maximum height they could achieve in an SJ by marking it on. PSJ, defined as the participant's self-perception in the height measure of the SJ performed, was assessed after each SJ trial, hence having experienced the execution, asking each participant to evaluate the perceived SJ height achieved in each performance. For both measurements, participants were asked to physically mark their predicted and perceived SJ height on the vertical graduated rod, illustrated in Figure 2, by simply pointing at it, transforming their SP and PSJ in a measurable (cm) outcome. To ensure both unbiased data collection and an uninfluenced response by external feedback, only the investigator had access to the gradations on the rod.

SJ performance was measured by means of a validated optical system (Optojump Microgate, Bolzano, Italy) [30]. After a warm-up that did not involve SJ, each participant completed three SJ trials, observing a rest period of 5 min between each trial to prevent fatigue from impacting muscle activation [31]. The protocol for executing the SJ was carried out following standardized procedures [32]. The height of each SJ trial and the average SJ height were used for the subsequent statistical analysis.

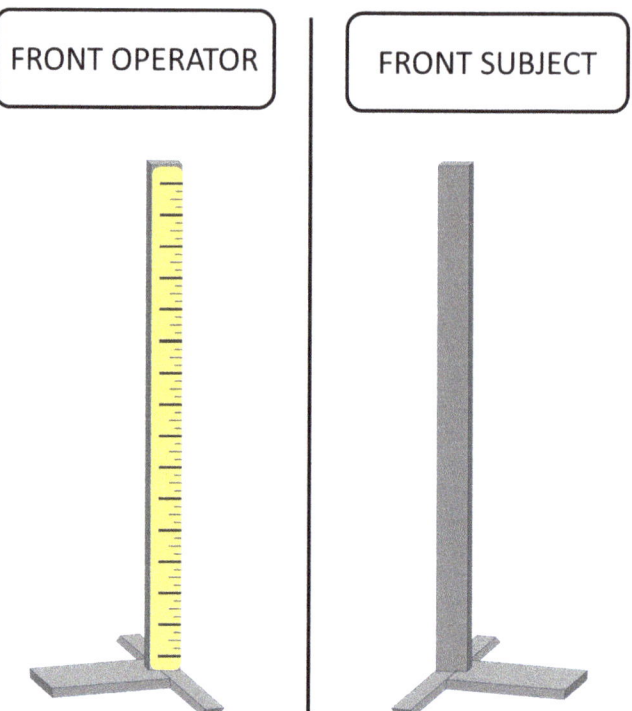

Figure 2. Graphical representation of the rod used to evaluate self-prediction and self-perception of the squat jump. On the left, the rod has been graduated to allow the operator to take the measurement; on the right, the smooth side of the rod shown to the subject during the evaluation.

2.3. Statistical Analysis

Descriptive and inferential statistical analyses were conducted using the Jamovi for Windows statistical package (ver. 2.3.23, Sydney, Australia). A type I error rate of 0.05 to establish statistical significance was applied.

The Shapiro–Wilk test was employed to assess the normality of the distributions of key variables. The test indicated that the distribution of weight and BMI does not significantly deviate from normality ($p = 0.288$ and $p = 0.090$, respectively). In contrast, height showed a slight but significant deviation from normality ($p = 0.046$). Age and IPAQ scores both exhibited significant departures from a normal distribution ($p < 0.001$ for both). Data are shown in Table 1. We applied parametric hypothesis tests even if the population is not normally distributed. Indeed, it was established that if the sample size is large enough ($n = 30$), the central limit theorem comes into effect and creates sampling distributions that are close to normal [33].

To evaluate the internal consistency of the SE questionnaire, Cronbach's α and McDonald's ω were assessed.

Before conducting repeated measures ANOVA and Pearson's statistical analysis, we calculate two SE values and two values showing the discrepancies between SP and SJ and between PSJ and SJ:

(1) The SE questionnaire score (SE score) was calculated to obtain a unique and comprehensive individual SE value. We calculated the value employing the following expression:

$$\text{SE score} = (((t - (Q1 + Q2 + Q3 + Q4 + Q5) + r - Q6 + r - Q7 + r - Q8 + |Q6 - Q8|) - y)/y) \times 100 \quad (1)$$

where (*t*) is a constant representing the maximum obtainable value; (*r*) is a constant corresponding to the maximum value of an answer; and Q1 to Q5 are questions related to an individual's confidence in performing a specific height jump; Q6 reflects the respondent's confidence in their answers from Q1 to Q5; Q7 assesses their self-evaluation compared to peers in the study group (self-reported percentile); Q8 pertains to their overall confidence in their previous responses; the absolute value of the difference between Q6 and Q8 represents the distance between the respondent's confidence in their answers from Q1 to Q5 and their overall confidence in their previous responses; (*y*) represents the highest achievable value. According to this equation, a higher value obtained in the SE score corresponds to subjects with higher SE.

(2) The SE esteem measure (SEE) was calculated to esteem the SJ height based on participants' confidence in performing an SJ at a specific height. We calculated the value employing the following expression:

$$SEE = (Q1 + Q2 + Q3 + Q4 + Q5) \times (c/r), \qquad (2)$$

where (*c*) is a constant denoting the maximum value within the range defined by the answer; (*r*) is a constant corresponding to the maximum value of an answer; and Q1 to Q5 are questions related to an individual's confidence in performing a specific height jump.

SEE allows the questionnaire data to be switched to measurable data in cm. A higher SEE corresponds to subjects with a higher SE jump-specific belief expressed in cm.

(3) The delta total error (DTE) was calculated to identify the error entity between SP and SJ or between PSJ and SJ. We calculated the value employing the following expression:

$$DTE = (SP\ or\ PSJ) - SJ, \qquad (3)$$

(4) The delta absolute error (DAE) was calculated to identify the absolute error entity between SP and SJ or between PSJ and SJ. We calculated the value employing the following expression:

$$DAE = |(SP\ or\ PSJ) - SJ|, \qquad (4)$$

The equations and delta values were used in the statistical analysis as follows.

A repeated measures ANOVA was performed to evaluate variations in SJ, SEE, and SP and variations in SP and PSJ errors among repetitions.

Pearson's *r* correlation was performed to investigate the associations between the SE score and both SP and actual SJ height, between SEE and SJ, between SEE and SP, and to compare the correlation between the self-reported percentile (Q7) and the SJ percentile.

3. Results

The 8-item SE questionnaire showed sufficient internal consistency and fit (Cronbach's $\alpha = 0.885$; McDonald's $\omega = 0.895$) for all the items.

The group results of the tests and questionnaires are reported in Table 2.

Table 2. Mean value and standard deviation for squat jump (SJ), self-efficacy score (SE score), self-efficacy esteem (SEE), self-prediction (SP), self-reported percentile (Q7), squat jump percentile (SJ percentile), and perceived squat jump (PSJ).

SJ (cm)	SE Score (%)	SEE (cm)	SP (cm)	Q7 (a.u.)	SJ Percentile (a.u.)	PSJ (cm)
36.5 ± 7.23	58.1 ± 10.55	37.5 ± 8.58	36.3 ± 9.7	3.1 ± 0.72	49.34 ± 29.8	36.28 ± 9.87

ANOVA repeated measure analysis showed no statistical differences ($p = 0.666$; $F(2.76) = 0.409$) in the measured values for SJ height, SP, and SEE, as illustrated in Figure 3.

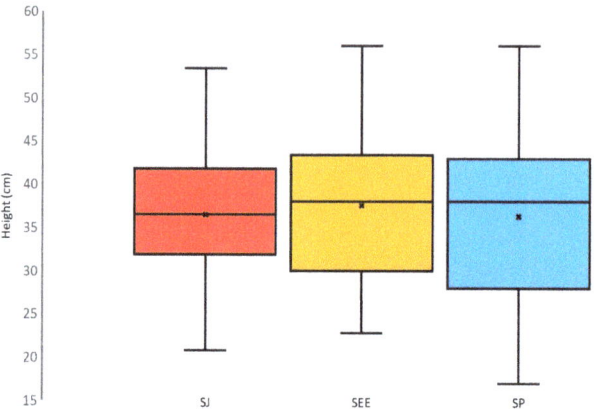

Figure 3. Boxplots of the distribution of SJ height measurements obtained during the SJ (in red), SSE (in yellow), and SP (in blue).

ANOVA repeated measure analysis showed no significant changes in DTE across different time points (p = 0.869; F (3.114) = 0.239), as depicted in Figure 4. The DTE measurements after each SJ exhibited a consistent trend, showing a decrease from the pre-assessment (PRE) to the first post-assessment (POST 1), further declining to the second post-assessment (POST 2), and ultimately stabilizing at the last post-assessment (POST 3). Moreover, when examining DAE values (p = 0.075; F (3.114) = 2.36), illustrated in Figure 5, a similar pattern emerged. DAE decreased from PRE to POST 1, followed by a further decline to POST 2, and eventually reaching the lowest point at POST 3. DTE and DAE means are reported in Table 3.

Table 3. Mean value and standard deviation for delta total error (DTE), delta absolute error (DAE), and pre-assessment (PRE) and after the first (POST 1), the second (POST 2), and the third (POST 3) squat jump.

DTE PRE (cm)	DTE POST 1 (cm)	DTE POST 2 (cm)	DTE POST 3 (cm)	DAE PRE (cm)	DAE POST 1 (cm)	DAE POST 2 (cm)	DAE POST 3 (cm)
−0.2 ± 9.89	−0.6 ± 8.28	−1.1 ± 7.47	−0.1 ± 6.12	7.6 ± 6.24	6.7 ± 4.76	5.9 ± 4.61	5.1 ± 3.40

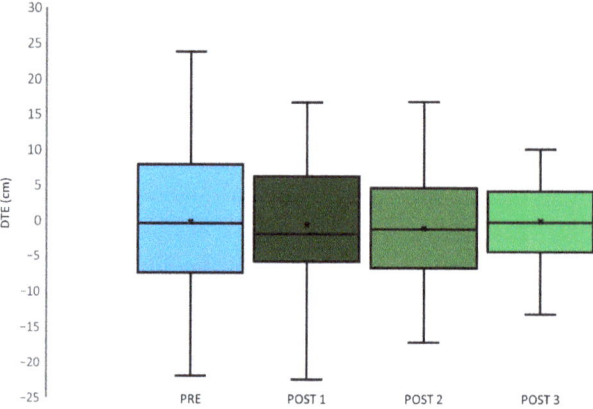

Figure 4. Boxplots depict distribution of DTE, PRE (light blue), POST 1 (dark green), POST 2 (green), and POST 3 (light green).

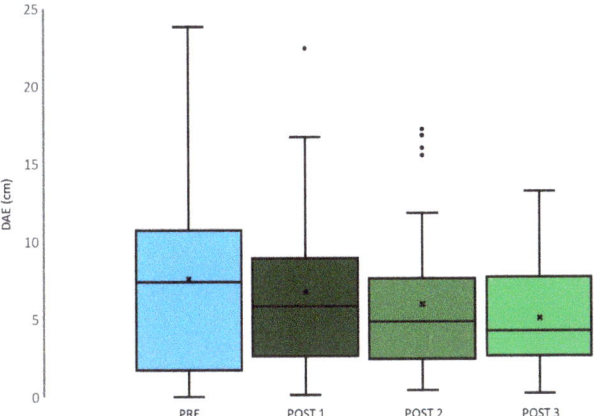

Figure 5. Boxplots depict distribution of DAE, PRE (light blue), POST 1 (dark green), POST 2 (green), and POST 3 (light green).

The coefficient of variation of DAE exhibited a gradual and consistent decrease across the four evaluations conducted (0.82, 0.71, 0.78, and 0.68).

Pearson's analysis showed a positive correlation between the self-reported percentile (Q7) and SJ percentile (r = 0.427; p = 0.007). The SE score exhibited significant correlations with both the SJ (r = 0.432; p = 0.006) (see Figure 6) and the SP (r = 0.441; p = 0.005) (see Figure 7). The SEE exhibited significant correlations with both the SJ (r = 0.440; p = 0.005) and the SP (r = 0.463; p = 0.002).

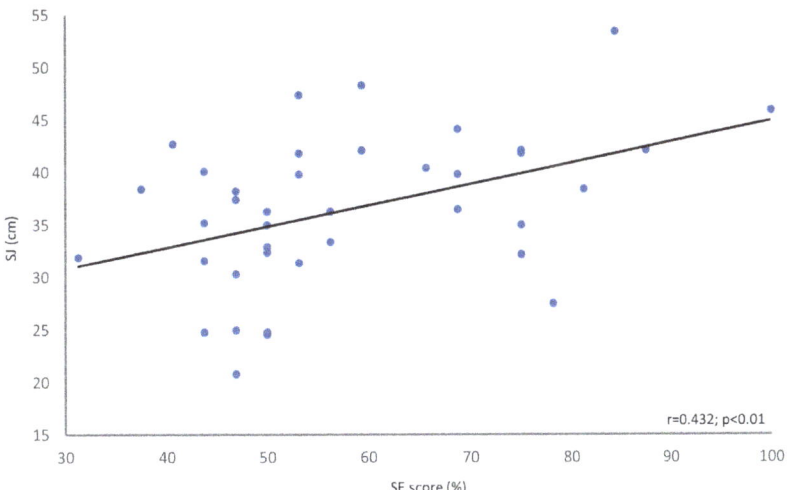

Figure 6. Linear correlation (solid black line) between the SE score (x-axis) and the SJ (y-axis). Each data point represents an individual subject.

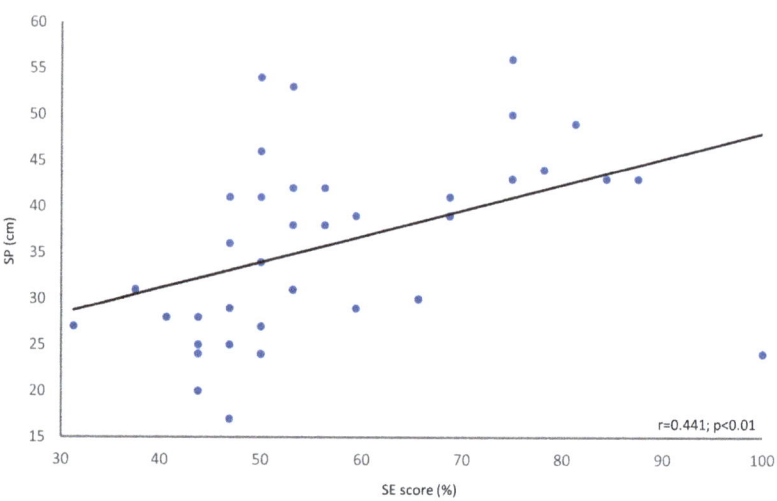

Figure 7. Linear correlation (solid black line) between the SE score (x-axis) and the SP (y-axis). Each data point represents an individual subject.

4. Discussion

As a pilot study, we presented preliminary findings in studying SE as a cognitive feature of sport performance. We started from Bandura's assumptions defining sport performance as "an objective outcome that must be specified by precise and objective descriptive indicators and measures that are generally quantitative and typically more based on results" and SE in sport performance as "a performer's belief that he or she can execute a behavior required to produce a certain outcome successfully" [6]. Due to the quantitative nature of sport performance, SE in sport fields must be contextualized in coherence and in its relationship with specific skills or tasks [10]. In this line, our study did not aim to investigate the trainability of SE or SJ but to objectively assess the nature of the relationship between SE and sport performance in a task-specific movement skill using original measures, scores, and procedures.

SJ is a fundamental athletic skill employed across a wide array of sports ranging from individual disciplines to team sports [34]. SJ has been widely shown to be an important tool in evaluating lower limb power, peripheral fatigue, elastic component compliance, and biomechanical domains to improve athletic performance. In our study, we used SJ measurements as an outcome to compare SE, SP, and PSJ.

SE is a cognitive feature widely investigated in sport and training contexts. However, previous studies highlighted the need for sports research employing the SE construct in relation to specific self-expectancy outcomes [35–38]. Previous studies also highlighted the need, in this area of the literature, for a univocal nomenclature required in assuming not only terminologies but also in defining original indices, measures, and procedures [39].

From these needs, as highlighted in previous studies, in our study, we explored SE using original scores and procedures in data collection. In detail, SP, PSJ, SE score, and SEE are values that we linked with actual performance in an SJ in order to better investigate the link between the motor task and the SE of the motor task. Furthermore, to obtain these values, we investigated the subjective perception of the motor task using two original methods of data collection: the first was organizing an 8-item five-level Likert scale SE questionnaire. We managed the questionnaire in two sections: one aimed to gauge the participants' confidence in performing an SJ at a specific height and confidence in their answers, the subsequent aimed to grade performance compared to their peers within the study group and also to inquire about the participants' confidence in all their previous responses; the second, using a custom-made vertical graduated rod transforming subjective SP and PSJ in a measurable (cm) outcome. This method, providing a tangible and standardized measure, we hypothesized that it might be useful to allow for a more in-depth understanding of participants' subjective experiences during the SJ performance and also ensure consistency in the participants' responses. This direct involvement of participants not only added a qualitative dimension to the data but also allowed for a more in-depth understanding of their subjective experiences during the jumping task. The use of a vertical graduated rod provided a tangible and standardized measure, ensuring consistency in the participants' responses. This detailed method not only captured the participants' objective performance but also delved into their perceptions, offering valuable insights into their self-assessment and confidence levels during the jumping trials.

An intriguing initial finding is that the SJ height, SP, and SEE results have shown an interesting interplay. As can be seen in Figure 3, these three parameters exhibited minimal differences. Contrary to expectations, these disparities were revealed to be not statistically significant, highlighting a compelling aspect of the study's findings ($p = 0.666$; $F(2,76) = 0.409$). This result suggested that participants' SJ performance was remarkably aligned with both their SEE and the SP. This congruence indicated a fascinating harmony between participants' beliefs in their abilities (as reflected in SEE) and the objective measurements of their performance. Such coherence between perception and reality not only underscores the participants' accurate self-assessment but also raises intriguing questions about the psychological factors influencing their confidence levels and performance outcomes. Moreover, this outcome supports the reliability of the method employed in this and in past [40] experimental setups. Then, it could serve as an encouraging revelation to include the evaluation of SE and SP during training, thereby enhancing athletes' self-awareness of their skills and, consequently, their overall performance.

Then, this study explored the alignment between individuals' DTA and DAE throughout multiple repetitions, objectively measured by an optical system, of an SJ execution. The results of the study did not uncover any significant disparities in DTE or DAE values over the various sampling times. However, an intriguing trend emerged as the coefficient of variation of DAE values decreased from the initial assessment to the final one. This decline in error suggests that with repeated attempts, individuals may enhance the accuracy of their SPJ assessments, indicating a potential alignment between SPJ and SE that develops over time. It is conceivable that the extended practice of SPJ over time could contribute to athletes improving their cognitive perception of their performance. Moreover, as outlined in previous studies [41,42], implementing a specialized training protocol like goal-plus-feedback has been proven effective in enhancing SE. This highlights the importance of urging trainers and professionals in sport and motor sciences to adopt tailored training practices from an educational point of view [43,44]. Emphasizing the significance of dedicated attention to improving SE can significantly enhance the overall training experience and outcomes. There are new needs in sport and skill learning directly linked with post-cognitive approaches [45]. The study of SE thus understood, which transcends the boundaries of a mechanistic view of the human organism and its movement organization and aligns with complex systems theory [46,47], allows us to view athletic and sport performance as an emergent property from the complex interaction between organism and a variable environment [48,49]. Therefore, the human body plays a central role in the realm of movement, and the individual is not merely a means of motion but rather the very essence of the movement itself. In this perspective, the person is not just a passive entity but an active protagonist, shaping and driving the entire process of physical activity. As highlighted by Balague and colleagues [50], "The emergence of self-organizing coordinated movement patterns occurring at all scales and in all types of situations in sport dilutes the extant boundaries between technique and tactics".

Furthermore, participants demonstrated the capability to gauge their performance level within the group. This observation remarked that participants' self-assessments were in line with their actual SJ performance, suggesting that they had a realistic understanding of their capabilities compared to peers. This aligns with the observations made by

Bandura [6] and Moritz [10], who emphasize the group's impact on SE assessment. This factor could have a significant role in shaping specific training regimens. Athletes looking to enhance their SE might find it more advantageous to engage in group training or regular competitive activities rather than pursuing solitary or isolated training methods.

The significant correlations observed between the SE score (as well as SEE) and both the SJ height and SP height indicate that SE plays a role in an individual's SJ performance. Although, in some cases, these interplays could be considered not extremely strong in terms of correlation strength, p-value < 0.01 and sample power stronger than 90% suggests that the found relationships are statistically significant and could be considered robust. This finding aligns with previous research that has demonstrated the influence of SE on various aspects of performance and achievement [10,11,16]. Athletes with higher SE tend to set more ambitious goals and exhibit greater determination to persist through rigorous training regimens. This confidence in their abilities translates into tangible improvements in athletic performance, as athletes approach competitions with a winning mindset and a belief in their capacity to excel [51–53]. The present study adds to this body of knowledge by highlighting the association between SE, SP, and SJ performance, providing further evidence of the transformative potential of SE in sport settings. The observed correlations between SE and SJ performance suggest that SE beliefs may serve as a predictor of an individual's jump height. To our opinion, this could play a crucial role in sport environments, especially in competitive and situational sports. This finding is consistent with Bandura's SE theory, which posits that individuals with stronger SE beliefs are more likely to engage in activities that lead to successful outcomes [10,11]. Therefore, assessing and enhancing SE beliefs could be a valuable strategy for coaches and sport professionals to optimize training programs and promote better performance outcomes.

The limitations of this study should be acknowledged. The study sample consisted of healthy young adults who were sport science students, which may limit the generalizability of the findings to other populations. Future research could include diverse samples with different age groups and athletic backgrounds to further explore the relationship between SE, SP, SPJ, and physical performance. Future studies could consider incorporating objective measures or observational assessments to complement self-report data. Additionally, the study focused on the SJ as the specific movement of interest. Including other jump techniques or different movements or skills could offer a more comprehensive and nuanced understanding of the subject matter.

However, to our knowledge, this is the first study exploring the intricate interplay between a specific movement, such as SJ, and individuals' SE, SP, and PSJ throughout multiple repetitions of SJ execution. Far from the aim to investigate the trainability of SE or SJ, our study aimed to respond to previous studies' requests to objectively assess the nature of the relationship between SE and sport performance in a task-specific movement skill using original measures, scores, and procedures.

5. Conclusions

As a pilot study, our research was conducted to test the practicality of methods and procedures for future application in larger-scale studies and to identify potential effects and associations that merit further exploration in a more extensive subsequent study [54]. SE was investigated as a cognitive feature useful to recognize information from the environment and link this to our background knowledge to better plan, organize, and execute the appropriate motor behavior.

In response to evolving requirements in sports and skill acquisition, it is essential to shift our focus to measuring and analyzing variables. Traditional methods often concentrate solely on either the individual or the external environment [55]. However, a more holistic approach is needed, one that considers the interaction between the athlete and their environment. Such a research approach aligns with the principles of post-cognitive theories [45]. These theories emphasize the importance of self-organization in addressing the challenges and problems encountered in performance tasks. Incorporating these concepts into sports training programs can lead to more effective learning designs that enhance the cognitive abilities of athletes.

Improving the knowledge of athletes' SE could hold the potential to greatly benefit training and coaching strategies, ultimately leading to improved performance outcomes. Additionally, the study's findings indicate that SP may benefit from repeated assessments and further training sessions, as evidenced by a decreasing coefficient of variation in error among the analyzed group. By gaining a deeper understanding of the relationship between SE, SP, PSJ, and physical performance, coaches and sport professionals could develop targeted interventions to enhance athletes' overall athletic achievements and also apply SE as a feature linking physical and cognitive athletic performance.

Author Contributions: Conceptualization, A.C.; methodology, A.C. and V.A.; formal analysis, A.C.; investigation, A.C.; data curation, A.C. and V.A.; writing—original draft preparation, A.C. and V.A.; writing—review and editing, A.C. and V.A.; supervision, V.A.; funding acquisition, V.A. All authors have read and agreed to the published version of the manuscript.

Funding: This research received no external funding.

Institutional Review Board Statement: Data were gathered during routine educational activities, aligning with the principles outlined in the Declaration of Helsinki. However, no sensitive data were collected. Given that this study focused on educational research and did not involve clinical data or treatment, ethical review and approval were waived.

Informed Consent Statement: Informed consent was obtained from all subjects involved in the study.

Data Availability Statement: The authors strongly encourage researchers with a vested interest to establish contact, as they are more than willing to share the data's content upon request.

Acknowledgments: We express our gratitude to J. Greig Inglis for his invaluable contribution to the English editing process.

Conflicts of Interest: The authors declare no conflicts of interest.

References

1. Madonna, G.; Agosti, V. Empathy and Sport Performance. *Ital. J. Health Educ. Sports Incl. Didact.* **2019**, *3*, 39–43. [CrossRef]
2. Almagro, B.J.; Sáenz-López, P.; Fierro-Suero, S.; Conde, C. Perceived Performance, Intrinsic Motivation and Adherence in Athletes. *Int. J. Environ. Res. Public Health* **2020**, *17*, 9441. [CrossRef] [PubMed]
3. Chow, J.Y.; Komar, J.; Seifert, L. The Role of Nonlinear Pedagogy in Supporting the Design of Modified Games in Junior Sports. *Front. Psychol.* **2021**, *12*, 744814. [CrossRef] [PubMed]
4. Kalén, A.; Bisagno, E.; Musculus, L.; Raab, M.; Pérez-Ferreirós, A.; Williams, A.M.; Araújo, D.; Lindwall, M.; Ivarsson, A. The Role of Domain-Specific and Domain-General Cognitive Functions and Skills in Sports Performance: A Meta-Analysis. *Psychol. Bull.* **2021**, *147*, 1290–1308. [CrossRef] [PubMed]
5. Trecroci, A.; Duca, M.; Cavaggioni, L.; Rossi, A.; Scurati, R.; Longo, S.; Merati, G.; Alberti, G.; Formenti, D. Relationship between Cognitive Functions and Sport-Specific Physical Performance in Youth Volleyball Players. *Brain Sci.* **2021**, *11*, 227. [CrossRef]
6. Bandura, A. *Self-Efficacy: The Exercise of Control*; Freeman, W.H., Ed.; Times Books; Henry Holt & Co.: New York, NY, USA, 1997.
7. Park, I.; Jeon, J. Psychological Skills Training for Athletes in Sports: Web of Science Bibliometric Analysis. *Healthcare* **2023**, *11*, 259. [CrossRef]
8. Toering, T.T.; Elferink-Gemser, M.T.; Jordet, G.; Visscher, C. Self-Regulation and Performance Level of Elite and Non-Elite Youth Soccer Players. *J. Sports Sci.* **2009**, *27*, 1509–1517. [CrossRef]
9. Zagórska, A.; Guszkowska, M. A Program to Support Self-Efficacy among Athletes. *Scand. J. Med. Sci. Sports* **2014**, *24*, e121-8. [CrossRef]
10. Moritz, S.E.; Feltz, D.L.; Fahrbach, K.R.; Mack, D.E. The Relation of Self-Efficacy Measures to Sport Performance: A Meta-Analytic Review. *Res. Q. Exerc. Sport* **2000**, *71*, 280–294. [CrossRef]
11. Rogowska, A.M.; Tataruch, R.; Niedźwiecki, K.; Wojciechowska-Maszkowska, B. The Mediating Role of Self-Efficacy in the Relationship between Approach Motivational System and Sports Success among Elite Speed Skating Athletes and Physical Education Students. *Int. J. Environ. Res. Public Health* **2022**, *19*, 2899. [CrossRef]
12. Valiante, G.; Morris, D.B. The Sources and Maintenance of Professional Golfers' Self-Efficacy Beliefs. *Sport Psychol.* **2013**, *27*, 130–142. [CrossRef]
13. Jenkins, S. Short Book Review: Self Efficacy in Sport: Research and Strategies for Working with Athletes, Teams and Coaches. *Int. J. Sports Sci. Coach.* **2008**, *3*, 293–295. [CrossRef]

14. Kitsantas, A.; Zimmerman, B.J. Comparing Self-Regulatory Processes Among Novice, Non-Expert, and Expert Volleyball Players: A Microanalytic Study. *J. Appl. Sport Psychol.* **2002**, *14*, 91–105. [CrossRef]
15. Treasure, D.C.; Monson, J.; Lox, C.L. Relationship between Self-Efficacy, Wrestling Performance, and Affect Prior to Competition. *Sport Psychol.* **1996**, *10*, 73–83. [CrossRef]
16. Theodorakis, Y. Effects of Self-Efficacy, Satisfaction, and Personal Goals on Swimming Performance. *Sport Psychol.* **1995**, *9*, 245–253. [CrossRef]
17. Feltz, D.L.; Short, S.E.; Sullivan, P.J. *Self-Efficacy in Sport*; Human Kinetics: Champaign, IL, USA, 2008; ISBN 0736059997.
18. McAuley, E. The Role of Efficacy Cognitions in the Prediction of Exercise Behavior in Middle-Aged Adults. *J. Behav. Med.* **1992**, *15*, 65–88. [CrossRef] [PubMed]
19. Caseiro-Filho, L.C.; Girasol, C.E.; Rinaldi, M.L.; Lemos, T.W.; Guirro, R.R.J. Analysis of the Accuracy and Reliability of Vertical Jump Evaluation Using a Low-Cost Acquisition System. *BMC Sports Sci. Med. Rehabil.* **2023**, *15*, 107. [CrossRef]
20. Van Hooren, B.; Zolotarjova, J. The Difference Between Countermovement and Squat Jump Performances: A Review of Underlying Mechanisms with Practical Applications. *J. Strength Cond. Res.* **2017**, *31*, 2011–2020. [CrossRef]
21. Nishiumi, D.; Nishioka, T.; Saito, H.; Kurokawa, T.; Hirose, N. Associations of Eccentric Force Variables during Jumping and Eccentric Lower-Limb Strength with Vertical Jump Performance: A Systematic Review. *PLoS ONE* **2023**, *18*, e0289631. [CrossRef]
22. Bassett, D.R. International Physical Activity Questionnaire: 12-Country Reliability and Validity. *Med. Sci. Sports Exerc.* **2003**, *35*, 1396. [CrossRef]
23. Lee, P.H.; Macfarlane, D.J.; Lam, T.; Stewart, S.M. Validity of the International Physical Activity Questionnaire Short Form (IPAQ-SF): A Systematic Review. *Int. J. Behav. Nutr. Phys. Act.* **2011**, *8*, 115. [CrossRef] [PubMed]
24. Minetto, M.A.; Motta, G.; Gorji, N.E.; Lucini, D.; Biolo, G.; Pigozzi, F.; Portincasa, P.; Maffiuletti, N.A. Reproducibility and Validity of the Italian Version of the International Physical Activity Questionnaire in Obese and Diabetic Patients. *J. Endocrinol. Investig.* **2018**, *41*, 343–349. [CrossRef] [PubMed]
25. Hallal, P.C.; Victora, C.G. Reliability and Validity of the International Physical Activity Questionnaire (IPAQ). *Med. Sci. Sports Exerc.* **2004**, *36*, 556. [CrossRef] [PubMed]
26. Craig, C.L.; Marshall, A.L.; Sjöström, M.; Bauman, A.E.; Booth, M.L.; Ainsworth, B.E.; Pratt, M.; Ekelund, U.; Yngve, A.; Sallis, J.F.; et al. International Physical Activity Questionnaire: 12-Country Reliability and Validity. *Med. Sci. Sports Exerc.* **2003**, *35*, 1381–1395. [CrossRef] [PubMed]
27. World Medical Association. World Medical Association Declaration of Helsinki: Ethical Principles for Medical Research Involving Human Subjects. *JAMA* **2013**, *310*, 2191–2194. [CrossRef] [PubMed]
28. Faul, F.; Erdfelder, E.; Buchner, A.; Lang, A.-G. Statistical Power Analyses Using G*Power 3.1: Tests for Correlation and Regression Analyses. *Behav. Res. Methods* **2009**, *41*, 1149–1160. [CrossRef] [PubMed]
29. Bandura, A. *Self-Efficacy Beliefs of Adolescents (Guide for Constructing Self-Efficacy Scales)*; Information Age Publishing: Charlotte, NC, USA, 2005; pp. 307–337.
30. Glatthorn, J.F.; Gouge, S.; Nussbaumer, S.; Stauffacher, S.; Impellizzeri, F.M.; Maffiuletti, N.A. Validity and Reliability of Optojump Photoelectric Cells for Estimating Vertical Jump Height. *J. Strength Cond. Res.* **2011**, *25*, 556–560. [CrossRef]
31. Marcolin, G.; Cogliati, M.; Cudicio, A.; Negro, F.; Tonin, R.; Orizio, C.; Paoli, A. Neuromuscular Fatigue Affects Calf Muscle Activation Strategies, but Not Dynamic Postural Balance Control in Healthy Young Adults. *Front. Physiol.* **2022**, *13*, 799565. [CrossRef]
32. Petrigna, L.; Karsten, B.; Marcolin, G.; Paoli, A.; D'Antona, G.; Palma, A.; Bianco, A. A Review of Countermovement and Squat Jump Testing Methods in the Context of Public Health Examination in Adolescence: Reliability and Feasibility of Current Testing Procedures. *Front. Physiol.* **2019**, *10*, 1384. [CrossRef]
33. Gregory, W.C.; Dale, I.F. *Nonparametric Statistics for Non-Statisticians: A Step-by-Step Approach*; John Wiley & Sons, Inc.: New Jersey, NJ, USA, 2009.
34. Chalitsios, C.; Nikodelis, T.; Panoutsakopoulos, V.; Chassanidis, C.; Kollias, I. Classification of Soccer and Basketball Players' Jumping Performance Characteristics: A Logistic Regression Approach. *Sports* **2019**, *7*, 163. [CrossRef]
35. Cataldo, R.; John, J.; Chandran, L.; Pati, S.; Shroyer, A.L.W. Impact of Physical Activity Intervention Programs on Self-Efficacy in Youths: A Systematic Review. *ISRN Obes.* **2013**, *2013*, 586497. [CrossRef] [PubMed]
36. Gao, Z.; Xiang, P.; Lee, A.M.; Harrison, L. Self-Efficacy and Outcome Expectancy in Beginning Weight Training Class: Their Relations to Students' Behavioral Intention and Actual Behavior. *Res. Q. Exerc. Sport* **2008**, *79*, 92–100. [CrossRef] [PubMed]
37. Gao, Z.; Lee, A.M.; Harrison, L. Understanding Students' Motivation in Sport and Physical Education: From the Expectancy-Value Model and Self-Efficacy Theory Perspectives. *Quest* **2008**, *60*, 236–254. [CrossRef]
38. Wurtele, S.K. Self-Efficacy and Athletic Performance: A Review. *J. Soc. Clin. Psychol.* **1986**, *4*, 290–301. [CrossRef]
39. Lochbaum, M.; Sherburn, M.; Sisneros, C.; Cooper, S.; Lane, A.M.; Terry, P.C. Revisiting the Self-Confidence and Sport Performance Relationship: A Systematic Review with Meta-Analysis. *Int. J. Environ. Res. Public. Health* **2022**, *19*, 6381. [CrossRef]
40. Cudicio, A.; Agosti, V. The Link between Physical Performance and Self-Efficacy: How Much Can I Jump? *Ital. J. Health Educ. Sports Incl. Didact.* **2023**, *7*, 830. [CrossRef]
41. Schunk, D.H. Self-Efficacy, Motivation, and Performance. *J. Appl. Sport Psychol.* **1995**, *7*, 112–137. [CrossRef]
42. Tanaka, K.; Watanabe, K. Overestimation and Underestimation in Learning and Transfer. In Proceedings of the 2011 International Conference on Biometrics and Kansei Engineering, Takamatsu, Japan, 19–22 September 2011; pp. 81–86.

43. Woods, C.T.; McKeown, I.; Rothwell, M.; Araújo, D.; Robertson, S.; Davids, K. Sport Practitioners as Sport Ecology Designers: How Ecological Dynamics Has Progressively Changed Perceptions of Skill "Acquisition" in the Sporting Habitat. *Front Psychol.* **2020**, *11*, 654. [CrossRef]
44. Sibilio, M. Simplex Didactics: A Non-Linear Trajectory for Research in Education. *Rev. Synth* **2015**, *136*, 477–493. [CrossRef]
45. Avilés, C.; Navia, J.A.; Ruiz-Pérez, L.-M.; Zapatero-Ayuso, J.A. How Enaction and Ecological Approaches Can Contribute to Sports and Skill Learning. *Front. Psychol* **2020**, *11*, 3691. [CrossRef]
46. Davids, K.; Hristovski, R.; Araújo, D.; Balague Serre, N.; Button, C.; Passos, P. *Complex Systems in Sport*; Routledge: London, UK, 2013; ISBN 9781136482151.
47. Morin, E. Le Défi de La Complexité. *Chimères* **1988**, *5*, 1–18. [CrossRef]
48. Agosti, V.; Autuori, M. Fencing Functional Training System (Ffts): A New Pedagogical-Educational Training Project. *Sport Sci.* **2020**, *13*, 118–122.
49. Balagué, N.; Torrents, C.; Hristovski, R.; Kelso, J.A.S. Sport Science Integration: An Evolutionary Synthesis. *Eur. J. Sport Sci.* **2017**, *17*, 51–62. [CrossRef] [PubMed]
50. Balague, N.; Torrents, C.; Hristovski, R.; Davids, K.; Araújo, D. Overview of Complex Systems in Sport. *J. Syst. Sci. Complex* **2013**, *26*, 4–13. [CrossRef]
51. Burns, L.; Weissensteiner, J.R.; Cohen, M. Lifestyles and Mindsets of Olympic, Paralympic and World Champions: Is an Integrated Approach the Key to Elite Performance? *Br. J. Sports Med.* **2019**, *53*, 818–824. [CrossRef]
52. Gee, C.J. How Does Sport Psychology Actually Improve Athletic Performance? A Framework to Facilitate Athletes' and Coaches' Understanding. *Behav. Modif.* **2010**, *34*, 386–402. [CrossRef]
53. Sklett, V.H.; Lorås, H.W.; Sigmundsson, H. Self-Efficacy, Flow, Affect, Worry and Performance in Elite World Cup Ski Jumping. *Front. Psychol.* **2018**, *9*, 1215. [CrossRef]
54. Thabane, L.; Ma, J.; Chu, R.; Cheng, J.; Ismaila, A.; Rios, L.P.; Robson, R.; Thabane, M.; Giangregorio, L.; Goldsmith, C.H. A Tutorial on Pilot Studies: The What, Why and How. *BMC Med. Res. Methodol.* **2010**, *10*, 1. [CrossRef]
55. Araújo, D.; Davids, K.; Renshaw, I. Cognition, Emotion and Action in Sport. In *Handbook of Sport Psychology*; Wiley: Hoboken, NJ, USA, 2020; pp. 535–555.

Disclaimer/Publisher's Note: The statements, opinions and data contained in all publications are solely those of the individual author(s) and contributor(s) and not of MDPI and/or the editor(s). MDPI and/or the editor(s) disclaim responsibility for any injury to people or property resulting from any ideas, methods, instructions or products referred to in the content.

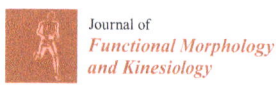

Article

Analysis of the Performance and Sailing Variables of the Optimist Class in a Variety of Wind Conditions

Israel Caraballo [1,2,*], Luka Pezelj [3] and Juan José Ramos-Álvarez [4]

[1] GALENO Research Group, Department of Physical Education, Faculty of Education Sciences, University of Cádiz, 11519 Puerto Real, Spain
[2] Instituto de Investigación e Innovación Biomédica de Cádiz (INiBICA), 11009 Cádiz, Spain
[3] Faculty of Maritime Studies, University of Split, 21000 Split, Croatia; lpezelj@pfst.hr
[4] Escuela de Medicina Deportiva, Departamento de Radiología, Rehabilitación y Fisioterapia, Universidad Complutense de Madrid, 28040 Madrid, Spain; jjramosa@med.ucm.es
* Correspondence: israel.caraballo@uca.es

Abstract: The aim of this study was to analyse the variables that determine the performance of the Optimist class during a regatta in different wind conditions. A total of 203 elite sailors of the Optimist class (121 boys and 82 girls) participated in the study. According to their ranking in the regatta, the sample was divided into four performance groups. In a regatta with 11 races, the velocity made good (VMG), the distance and the manoeuvres were evaluated by means of GNSS equipment in three different courses. The boys performed a greater number of upwind and running manoeuvres than the girls. The very-low-level sailors obtained a lower VMG in all the courses analysed compared with the rest of the groups of sailors of higher levels. Upwind manoeuvres, broad reach and running VMG were significant variables for establishing differences in performance level when the wind speed was in a range of 5 to ≤8 knots. When the wind speed was in the >8 to ≤12 knot range, upwind distance was the key variable in determining performance differences. VMG, upwind and broad reach distance and broad reach manoeuvres were the most important variables when the wind speed was in the >12 to 15 knots range. The boys performed more manoeuvres than the girls in the upwind and running courses.

Keywords: GPS; sailors; sport performance; tactics; elite; GNSS

Citation: Caraballo, I.; Pezelj, L.; Ramos-Álvarez, J.J. Analysis of the Performance and Sailing Variables of the Optimist Class in a Variety of Wind Conditions. *J. Funct. Morphol. Kinesiol.* **2024**, *9*, 18. https://doi.org/10.3390/jfmk9010018

Academic Editor: Carl Foster

Received: 16 November 2023
Revised: 20 December 2023
Accepted: 31 December 2023
Published: 3 January 2024

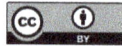

Copyright: © 2024 by the authors. Licensee MDPI, Basel, Switzerland. This article is an open access article distributed under the terms and conditions of the Creative Commons Attribution (CC BY) license (https://creativecommons.org/licenses/by/4.0/).

1. Introduction

Among the different dinghy sailing classes, the Optimist class is part of the monohull category and is crewed by a single sailor. This class is governed by the class rules and uses a boat with a weight of 35 kg, a length of 2.36 m, a beam of 1.12 m and a main sail area of 3.32 m^2. In the Optimist class, boys and girls up to the age of 15 years compete together [1]. This class has been proposed by the International Sailing Federation and has its own organisation at the international level: The International Optimist Dinghy Association. In the course racing discipline, the sailors must complete a race in the shortest time possible, sailing upwind, on a broad reach and running in a course marked by buoys.

Dinghy sailing is a multifaceted sport where performance is determined by numerous factors, such as morphology, psychological and physical fitness, and technical and tactical skills [2,3]. Moreover, performance is also influenced by the characteristics of the boat and the weather conditions [4,5]. The factors that determine performance in a regatta are technique (speed) and tactics (distance and manoeuvres) [6,7]. The most important variable in a regatta is the speed of the boat and the velocity made good (VMG) on the windward and leeward courses [8]. Other studies have shown that elite sailors complete the course using a shorter distance [9,10]. Where manoeuvres are concerned, studies have shown that the most successful sailors perform fewer upwind manoeuvres [11,12].

Regarding performance, several studies have analysed the relationship between performance and technical and tactical skills in the windsurfing [6,11], Laser class [8,13], 2.4mR class [7] and Formula Kite class [14,15]. However, to our knowledge, not all aspects of technical and tactical performance have been thoroughly examined in the Optimist class. Therefore, the aim of our study was to identify the variables that determine sport performance in Optimist class sailors under different wind conditions.

2. Materials and Methods

2.1. Participants

The study sample consisted of 203 international elite sailors (82 girls) of the Optimist class, with an age range of 9 to 15 years, who competed in an international regatta. The data were collected from World-Sailing, and they were obtained from a publicly accessible website [16]. Thus, ethical approval and written/informed consent from all participants were not necessary. To perform the analysis based on wind speed, the total sample of 203 sailors was divided into four performance groups according to the ranking of the sailors in the regatta: high-level sailors (P_{25}), medium-level sailors (P_{50}), low-level sailors (P_{75}) and very-low-level sailors (P_{99}). The percentile values in the ranking (25th, 50th and 75th) were used to divide the sample into P_{25} ($n = 51$; 18 girls), P_{50} ($n = 51$; 22 girls), P_{75} ($n = 51$; 16 girls) and P_{99} ($n = 50$; 26 girls).

2.2. Regatta

The analysed regatta was the Travemünder Woche 2017. This regatta was an international competition and it was a qualifying competition for the World Cup, although only the results obtained in the ranking of this regatta were used. The average values of the velocity made good (knots), distance (km) and manoeuvres (number of manoeuvres) variables during the upwind, broad reach and running courses were obtained through a SAP-Sailing application [17]. This application uses a global navigation satellite system device (GNSS) placed on the sailor's boat. From this device, data are transmitted and processed in real time by the application, obtaining information about those variables. The average values of variables during each course were obtained from the regatta and the races. Furthermore, wind speed was analysed in all races of the regatta. The ranking in the regatta and a single race was used to determine the performance of the sailors, which allowed classifying the athletes in the different performance groups. A total of 11 races were analysed. The race course consisted of four legs: two upwind, one broad reach and one running (Figure 1). The wind speed in the regatta ranged between 2.8 and 16.4 knots. Wind speed was categorised in each race according to the Royal Yachting Association [18]: 5 to ≤8 knots (light wind), >8 to ≤12 knots (medium wind) and >12 to 15 knots (strong wind). Wind speed was measured continuously and the maximum and minimum values were used to calculate the average for each race.

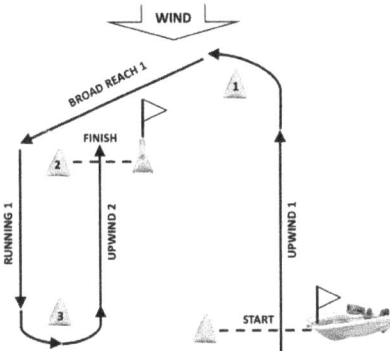

Figure 1. Regatta race course.

2.3. Statistical Analysis

The data are presented as mean and standard deviations (SD). The level of significance was set at $p < 0.05$. SPSS v20.0 software (SPSS Lead Technologies Inc., Chicago, IL, USA) was used for the statistical analyses. The data were subjected to a descriptive analysis and inferences. The normality of all variables was verified using the Kolmogorov–Smirnov test and the Levene´s test was used to evaluate the homogeneity of variance. ANOVA was used to determine the possible differences, based on sex (males and females) and performance level (P_{25}, P_{50}, P_{75} and P_{99}). Under the assumption of equal variances, a Bonferroni post hoc test was used when statistically significant differences were detected and a Games–Howell post hoc was applied to establish differences for variables with unequal variances. The effect size was calculated using partial eta-squared (η_p^2), considering <0.25, 0.26–0.63, and >0.63 as small, medium, and large effect size, respectively [19,20]. The ranges in wind speed in each of the races were analysed to study the effect of the interaction between the performance level and wind speed on performance.

3. Results

Table 1 shows the descriptive statistics of the variables for the total sample and by sex in the regatta. It was observed that the boys performed a larger number of manoeuvres in the upwind and running courses compared to the girls. No statistically significant differences were observed in the variables age, upwind VMG, upwind distance, broad reach VMG, broad reach distance, broad reach manoeuvres, running VMG, running distance, or ranking.

Table 1. Mean ± SD of the variables analysed in all sailors and in girls and boys.

Variable	Total Sample (n = 203)	Girls (n = 82)	Boys (n = 121)	ANOVA p-Value	E_R^2
Age (years)	13.1 ± 1.2	13.2 ± 1	13 ± 1.3	0.229	0.00
Upwind VMG (knots)	1.6 ± 0.3	1.6 ± 0.2	1.6 ± 0.3	0.334	0.04
Upwind distance (km)	1.2 ± 0.1	1.2 ± 0.1	1.3 ± 0.1	0.942	0.00
Upwind manoeuvres (number)	9.3 ± 2.1	8.7 ± 2.1	9.5 ± 1.9 *	0.005	0.03
Broad reach VMG (knots)	3.5 ± 0.4	3.5 ± 0.4	3.5 ± 0.4	0.194	0.01
Broad reach distance (km)	0.9 ± 0.1	0.9 ± 0.1	0.9 ± 0.1	0.690	0.00
Broad reach manoeuvres (number)	0.4 ± 0.3	0.4 ± 0.4	0.4 ± 0.3	0.962	0.00
Running VMG (knots)	3.4 ± 0.4	3.4 ± 0.4	3.4 ± 0.3	0.157	0.01
Running distance (km)	0.8 ± 0.1	0.7 ± 0.1	0.8 ± 0.1	0.103	0.01
Running manoeuvres (number)	3.5 ± 1	3.3 ± 1.1	3.6 ± 0.1 *	0.022	0.02
Ranking	102 ± 58.7	107.8 ± 60.2	98.1 ± 57.6	0.247	0.00

Note: VMG: Velocity Made Good; E_R^2 = effect size. *: Statistically significant difference between boys and girls ($p < 0.05$).

Figure 2 shows the analysis for each of the groups of sailors according to their level of performance in the regatta. It was observed that, in the upwind (1.7 ± 0.2 vs. 1.5 ± 0.2 knots; $p < 0.01$), broad reach (3.7 ± 0.4 vs. 3.2 ± 0.4 knots; $p < 0.01$) and running (3.6 ± 0.3 vs. 3.2 ± 0.4 knots; $p < 0.01$) courses, the high-level sailors obtained greater VMG compared to the very-low-level sailors. Medium-level sailors had a greater VMG compared to the very-low-level sailors in the upwind (1.6 ± 0.1 vs. 1.5 ± 0.2 knots; $p < 0.05$), broad reach (3.6 ± 0.3 vs. 3.2 ± 0.4 knots; $p < 0.01$) and running (3.5 ± 0.3 vs. 3.2 ± 0.4 knots; $p < 0.01$). Similarly, the VMG was higher in the low-level sailors compared to the very-low-level group in the upwind (1.6 ± 0.2 vs. 1.5 ± 0.2 knots; $p < 0.01$) and broad reach (3.54 ± 0.4 vs. 3.2 ± 0.4 knots; $p < 0.05$). With regard to the broad reach distance in the regatta, the very-low-level sailors travelled a shorter distance compared to the high-level sailors (0.9 ± 0.1 vs. 0.8 ± 0.1 km; $p < 0.05$). No statistically significant differences were observed in the other variables.

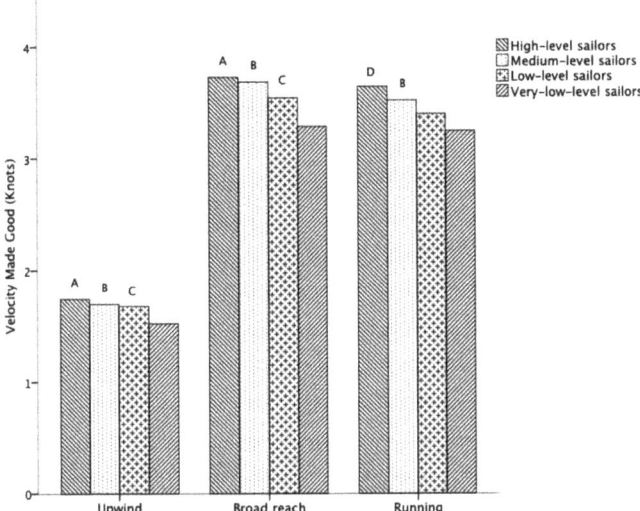

Figure 2. Comparison between the groups of sailors with different performance levels in upwind, broad reach and running courses for velocity made good. Note: **A**: statistically significant difference between high-level and very-low-level sailors; **B**: statistically significant difference between medium-level and very-low-level sailors; **C**: statistically significant difference between low-level and very-low-level sailors; **D**: statistically significant difference between high-level and low-level and very-low-level sailors; statistical significance level: $p < 0.05$.

When the races were assessed, the results showed that the high-level sailors had a greater VMG in the broad reach (3.3 ± 0.9 vs. 2.9 ± 1.3 knots; $p < 0.01$) and running (3.1 ± 0.8 vs. 2.7 ± 1.2 knots; $p < 0.01$) courses compared to the very-low-level sailors in a light wind (Table 2). Regarding strong wind conditions, the high-level sailors presented a higher value of upwind VMG compared to the medium-level (1.9 ± 0.3 vs. 1.8 ± 0.3 knots; $p < 0.05$), low-level (1.9 ± 0.3 vs. 1.7 ± 0.4 knots; $p < 0.01$) and very-low-level (1.9 ± 0.3 vs. 1.6 ± 0.4 knots; $p < 0.01$) sailors. In all the wind conditions analysed, higher VMG values were achieved. When analysing the distances travelled in the different wind speed conditions, it was observed that the high-level sailors travelled a shorter upwind distance than the very-low-level (1.3 ± 0.3 vs. 1.4 ± 0.3 km; $p < 0.05$) sailors in a medium wind. In strong wind conditions, the results showed that the upwind distance was shorter in the high-level sailors (1.3 ± 0.2 vs. 1.4 ± 0.3 km; $p < 0.05$) compared to the very-low-level sailors. However, the high-level sailors travelled a longer broad reach distance in strong wind conditions compared to the low-level (1.1 ± 0.2 vs. 1 ± 0.2 km; $p < 0.01$) and very-low-level sailors (1.1 ± 0.2 vs. 1 ± 0.2 km; $p < 0.01$). With respect to the number of manoeuvres, compared to the very-low-level sailors, the high-level sailors presented a larger number of upwind manoeuvres in a light wind (14.3 ± 7.6 vs. 12.2 ± 9.1 number; $p < 0.05$). Nevertheless, when the number of manoeuvres was analysed in strong wind conditions, it was observed that the high-level sailors had a greater value of broad reach manoeuvres compared to the medium-level (0.6 ± 0.8 vs. 0.3 ± 0.7 manoeuvres; $p < 0.01$) and low-level (0.6 ± 0.8 vs. 0.3 ± 0.8 manoeuvres; $p < 0.01$) sailors.

Table 2. Mean ± SD of the variables analysed in the percentile groups according to wind speed in races.

Wind Speed	Variable	P_{25} (n = 51)	P_{50} (n = 51)	P_{75} (n = 51)	P_{99} (n = 50)	ANOVA p-Value	E_R^2
5 to ≤8 (knots)	Upwind VMG (knots)	1.6 ± 0.5	1.6 ± 0.4	1.6 ± 2.5	1.3 ± 0.6	0.083	0.01
	Upwind distance (km)	1 ± 0.3	1 ± 0.3	1.1 ± 0.4	1.1 ± 0.4	0.190	0.00
	Upwind manoeuvres (number)	14.3 ± 7.6 [E]	14 ± 7.4	12.8 ± 7.9	12.2 ± 9.1	0.021	0.01
	Broad reach VMG (knots)	3.3 ± 0.9 [E]	3.2 ± 0.8 [G]	3.2 ± 1.1	2.9 ± 1.3	0.001	0.02
	Broad reach distance (km)	0.8 ± 0.2	0.8 ± 0.2 [F]	0.8 ± 0.3	0.7 ± 0.3	0.011	0.01
	Broad reach manoeuvres (number)	0.4 ± 0.9	0.5 ± 1.9	0.5 ± 1.5	0.5 ± 2	0.697	0.00
	Running VMG (knots)	3.1 ± 0.8 [E]	3 ± 0.8 [G]	2.9 ± 1	2.7 ± 1.2	0.000	0.02
	Running distance (km)	0.6 ± 0.3	0.6 ± 0.3	0.5 ± 0.3	0.5 ± 0.3	0.069	0.01
	Running manoeuvres (number)	2.7 ± 2.8	2.7 ± 3	2.5 ± 3.1	2.6 ± 3.1	0.857	0.00
>8 to ≤12 (knots)	Upwind VMG (knots)	1.6 ± 0.4	1.6 ± 0.3	1.6 ± 0.3	1.5 ± 0.4	0.297	0.00
	Upwind distance (km)	1.3 ± 0.3 [E]	1.4 ± 0.3	1.4 ± 0.2	1.4 ± 0.3	0.027	0.01
	Upwind manoeuvres (number)	21 ± 8.1	22 ± 8.1	21.2 ± 8.9	21.2 ± 9	0.620	0.00
	Broad reach VMG (knots)	3.8 ± 0.9	3.8 ± 0.9	3.8 ± 0.8	3.7 ± 1	0.470	0.00
	Broad reach distance (km)	0.8 ± 0.2	0.8 ± 0.1	0.8 ± 0.1	0.8 ± 0.2	0.764	0.00
	Broad reach manoeuvres (number)	0.2 ± 0.5	0.1 ± 0.4	0.2 ± 0.7	0.3 ± 1.7	0.270	0.00
	Running VMG (knots)	3.4 ± 0.9	3.4 ± 0.8	3.5 ± 0.7	3.3 ± 0.9	0.588	0.00
	Running distance (km)	0.8 ± 0.2	0.8 ± 0.2	0.9 ± 0.1	0.8 ± 0.2	0.561	0.00
	Running manoeuvres (number)	4.4 ± 3.3	4.1 ± 2.7 [F]	5.1 ± 3.1	4.7 ± 3.1	0.029	0.01
>12 to 15 (knots)	Upwind VMG (knots)	1.9 ± 0.3 [A]	1.8 ± 0.3 [G]	1.7 ± 0.4	1.6 ± 0.4	0.000	0.02
	Upwind distance (km)	1.3 ± 0.2 [E]	1.4 ± 0.2	1.4 ± 0.3	1.4 ± 0.3	0.021	0.01
	Upwind manoeuvres (number)	20.8 ± 7.7	20.7 ± 8.1	21.2 ± 7.9	22.3 ± 8	0.178	0.00
	Broad reach VMG (knots)	4 ± 0.7 [C]	3.9 ± 0.8 [H]	3.6 ± 1.1 [I]	3.3 ± 1.2	0.000	0.07
	Broad reach distance (km)	1.1 ± 0.2 [C]	1 ± 0.2	1 ± 0.2	1 ± 0.2	0.00	0.02
	Broad reach manoeuvres (number)	0.6 ± 0.8 [B]	0.3 ± 0.7	0.3 ± 0.8	0.5 ± 1.1	0.01	0.01
	Running VMG (knots)	4 ± 0.7 [C]	3.9 ± 0.8 [H]	3.9 ± 0.9	3.6 ± 1.2	0.00	0.06
	Running distance (km)	0.9 ± 0.1	0.9 ± 0.2	0.9 ± 0.2	0.9 ± 0.2	0.170	0.00
	Running manoeuvres (number)	3.3 ± 2.2	3.7 ± 2.4	3.6 ± 2.7	3.5 ± 2.5	0.369	0.00

Note: VMG: Velocity Made Good; [A]: statistically significant difference between P_{25} vs. P_{50}, P_{75} and P_{99}; [B]: statistically significant difference between P_{25} vs. P_{50} and P_{75}; [C] statistically significant difference between P_{25} vs. P_{75} and P_{99}; [E]: statistically significant difference between P_{25} and P_{99}; [F]: statistically significant difference between P_{50} and P_{75}; [G]: statistically significant difference between P_{50} and P_{99}; [H]: statistically significant difference between P_{50} vs. P_{75} and P_{99}; [I]: statistically significant difference between P_{75} and P_{99}; P_{25}: high-level sailors; P_{50}: medium-level sailors; P_{75}: low-level sailors; P_{99}: very-low-level sailors; E_R^2 = effect size; statistical significance level: $p < 0.05$.

4. Discussion

The aim of this study was to identify the variables that determine a sailor's performance in different wind conditions.

The results of our study showed that the boys performed a larger number of upwind manoeuvres and running manoeuvres in comparison to the girls. VMG is the variable that differentiates sailors according to their level of performance on the three courses analysed. In terms of wind speed, statistical differences in upwind manoeuvres, broad reach VMG and running VMG were reported between the high-level and low-level sailors in light wind conditions (5 to ≤8 knots). In medium wind conditions (>8 to ≤12 knots), it was observed that the high-level sailors covered a shorter upwind distance than the very-low-level sailors. When the wind was strong (>12 to15 knots), the results showed that the high-level sailors achieved a higher VMG on all courses, travelled a shorter distance upwind, covered a shorter distance in broad reach, and performed fewer broad reach manoeuvres.

Regarding sex, statistically significant differences were only found in the number of manoeuvres in upwind and running, with the boys performing more manoeuvres than the girls. Although it has been observed that the larger the number of manoeuvres that were performed, the greater was the effort required by the sailor [12], with this action reducing the velocity of the boat [21], the larger the number of manoeuvres that were performed, the better was the orientation of the boat to reach the buoy [13,22]. This could explain the larger number of manoeuvres in the upwind and running courses performed by the boys compared to the girls. In this regatta, both boys and girls sailed the same course; thus, they were exposed to the same wind speed and wave conditions. Therefore, these results could be relevant to coaches when planning the training of sailors based on sex. To the best of our knowledge, this is the first study to compare the technical and tactical variables of elite Optimist sailors by sex during a regatta.

The data obtained from our sailors in the regatta showed that the high-level sailors achieved the highest VMG in each of the courses (upwind, broad reach and running) compared to the very-low-level sailors. Similarly, the higher-level groups of sailors sailed faster (VMG) in the upwind, broad reach and running courses compared to the lower-level sailors. VMG as a performance factor in the courses of upwind, broad reach and running, in terms of average VMG, has also been confirmed in other classes, such as Formula Kite, Windsurfing and Laser [8–10,14]. This could suggest that the most successful group of sailors have a better technical level, which would allow them to reach higher speeds in each of the courses [23]. Therefore, and based on our results, we would assert that, in our Optimist class sailors, the higher the level of the sailor is, the greater is the VMG achieved in the upwind, broad reach and running courses. The results of our study could be very interesting for coaches and sailors, since they indicate that the VMG of the elite sailor is not affected by a specific course. Thus, improving the VMG in each of the courses might be the target of the training sessions.

Analysing the wind speed in each of the races, it was found that the variables that determine performance in dinghy sailing would be different depending on the wind speed in the regatta. In light winds (5 to ≤8 knots), our results suggest that upwind manoeuvres, broad reach VMG and running VMG may be the variables that determine sailor performance. The high-level and medium-level sailors had a higher VMG than the very-low-level sailors. This may also mean that the most successful sailors handle the boat more efficiently [24]. With regard to the number of manoeuvres, in the Laser class, it has been observed that the number of manoeuvres performed by the sailor in upwind increases in light wind conditions [22]. In these wind conditions, the sailor must make a larger number of tacks to find the most favourable wind zones that will allow him/her to advance until he/she reaches the windward buoy. Moreover, it has been shown that the angle between the wind and the bow must be approximately 40° in order to reduce the distance travelled by the board against the wind [24]. In medium wind conditions (>8 to ≤12 knots), it was observed that the most successful sailors sailed a shorter distance upwind compared to the less successful sailors. Our results are in line with those of sailors in the windsurfing class [9,10]. Our data showed no statistically significant differences in VMG or manoeuvres. We can thereby confirm that, in these wind conditions, it is the upwind distance which determines performance in the Optimist class. The most successful sailors would use better tactics to complete the course in a shorter distance [8,25]. Therefore, our results suggest that training for the Optimist class could be focused on improving upwind distance when the wind speed is between >8 and ≤12 knots. When the wind speed was between >12 and 15 knots, our results showed that the most successful sailors had a higher VMG in all courses, although it should be noted that the high-level sailors had a higher upwind speed compared to the other three groups. Previous studies have also shown that VMG is considered an important variable in regattas, with more successful sailors having a higher VMG in both upwind and running legs [26]. Thus, our findings suggest that VMG in the upwind course could be a variable that determines the performance of the sailor in the Optimist class in strong wind speeds. As with >8 to ≤12 knot winds, the high-level sailors covered a shorter distance upwind, although they covered a longer distance in broad reach compared to the low-level sailors. In a similar way to the windsurfing class, it can be assumed that the longer distance travelled by the top sailors is compensated for by their higher speed, which allows them to reach their destination in a shorter time [11]. In broad reach, to achieve a better planning of the boat and thus a higher speed, the sailor can change the orientation of the boat in relation to the wind, although this increased angle may also increase the distance travelled. Regarding manoeuvres, it was observed that the high-level sailors performed a greater number of manoeuvres in broad reach compared to the rest of the sailors. In Laser class sailors, it has been observed that the number of downwind manoeuvres increased with the increase in wind speed [13]. Our results could be explained by the fact that, in strong winds, the technical action of hiking puts pressure on the abdominal and quadriceps muscles, restricting blood flow and increasing muscle fatigue. When the sailor performs manoeuvres, he/she changes position, reducing the pressure on the muscles and increasing blood flow [27,28]. This reduces muscle fatigue by increasing oxygen consumption in the abdominal and quadriceps muscles. Therefore, and considering that the manoeuvres reduce the speed of the boat and can also lead to greater fatigue in the sailor [11,22], the latter must train to increase efficiency in the manoeuvres and thus reduce the loss of speed of the boat in strong wind conditions [24]. Our results are consistent with those obtained by Chun et al. [6], and we can therefore confirm that the technical and tactical variables played an important role when starting in strong wind conditions.

5. Strengths and Limitations

Our study is not exempt from limitations. Firstly, the anthropometric characteristics of the sailors were not collected. It is possible that the performance of the sailor may be influenced by the variables in weight and height. Unfortunately, it was not possible to include such data in this study, although it would have been interesting to analyse these variables, which could provide additional information to better explain results. Secondly, it would be interesting to assess some of the relevant aspects involved in the physical performance and physiological demands of Optimist course racing. In addition, future studies could focus on analysing these variables in different wind conditions and specifically analyse each of the races that make up the regatta.

To our knowledge, this is the first study to evaluate VMG, distance and manoeuvres in a real regatta situation as a function of the performance of the sailors, specifically in Optimist class sailors, and it is also the first study to analyse the three types of courses developed during a regatta (upwind, broad reach and running).

6. Conclusions

In the Optimist class, sailor performance is determined by upwind, broad reach and running VMG in all types of wind speed conditions. Performance in the Optimist class is determined by the distance travelled upwind in winds between 8 and 12 knots.

Author Contributions: Conceptualisation, I.C. and L.P.; methodology, I.C. and J.J.R.-Á.; software, I.C.; validation, I.C., L.P. and J.J.R.-Á.; formal analysis, I.C. and L.P.; investigation, I.C.; resources, L.P.; data curation, I.C. and J.J.R.-Á.; writing—original draft preparation, I.C. and L.P.; writing—review and editing, I.C., L.P. and J.J.R.-Á.; visualisation, I.C.; supervision, I.C. and L.P; project administration, I.C.; funding acquisition, L.P. All authors have read and agreed to the published version of the manuscript.

Funding: This research received no external funding.

Institutional Review Board Statement: Ethical review and approval were waived for this study, since all the data used in this study are publicly accessible in World-Sailing® and SAP-Sailing®.

Informed Consent Statement: Patient consent was waived, since all the data used in this study are publicly accessible in World-Sailing® and SAP-Sailing®.

Data Availability Statement: Publicly available datasets were analysed in this study. These data can be found in https://www.sapsailing.com/gwt/Home.html#EventsPlace: (accessed on 12 February 2021).

Acknowledgments: The authors would like to thank L. Pezelj from the University of Split for their cooperation and keen interest in the study design.

Conflicts of Interest: The authors declare no conflicts of interest.

References

1. Callewaert, M.; Boone, J.; Celie, B.; De Clercq, D.; Bourgois, J.G. Cardiorespiratory and muscular responses to simulated upwind sailing exercise in Optimist sailors. *Pediatr. Exerc. Sci.* **2014**, *26*, 56–63. [CrossRef] [PubMed]
2. Tan, B.; Aziz, A.R.; Spurway, N.C.; Toh, C.; Mackie, H.; Xie, W.; Wong, J.; Fuss, F.K.; Teh, K.C. Indicators of maximal hiking performance in Laser sailors. *Eur. J. Appl. Physiol.* **2006**, *98*, 169–176. [CrossRef] [PubMed]
3. Bojsen-Moller, J.; Larsson, B.; Magnusson, P.; Aagaard, P. Yatch type and crew-specific differences in anthropometric, aerobic capacity, and muscle strength parameters among international Olympic class sailors. *J. Sports Sci.* **2007**, *25*, 1117–1128. [CrossRef] [PubMed]
4. Pluijms, J.; Cañal-Bruland, C.; Kats, S.; Savelsbergh, G. Translating key methodological issues into technological advancements when running in-situ experiments in sports: An example from sailing. *Int. J. Sports Sci. Coach.* **2013**, *8*, 90–103. [CrossRef]
5. Bernardi, M.; Quattrini, F.M.; Rodio, A.; Fontana, G.; Madaffari, A.; Brugnoli, M.; Marchetti, M. Phsyiological characteristics of America´s Cup sailors. *J. Sports Sci.* **2007**, *25*, 1141–1152. [CrossRef] [PubMed]
6. Chun, S.; Park, J.; Kim, T.; Kim, Y. Performance analysis based on GPS data of Olympic class windsurfing. *Int. J. Perform. Anal. Sport* **2022**, *22*, 332–342. [CrossRef]
7. Caraballo, I.; Cruz Leon, C.; Pérez-Bey, A.; Gutiérrez-Manzanedo, J.V. Performance analysis of paralympic 2.4 mR class sailing. *J. Sports Sci.* **2021**, *39*, 109–115. [CrossRef]
8. Caraballo, I.; Conde-Caveda, J.; Pezelj, L.; Milavić, B.; Castro-Piñero, J. GNSS applications to assess performance in Olympic sailors: Laser Class. *Appl. Sci.* **2021**, *11*, 264. [CrossRef]
9. Hagiwara, M.; Ishii, Y. Analysis of racing factors in windsurfing under light wind. *Med. Sci. Sports Exerc.* **2016**, *48*, 1040. [CrossRef]
10. Anastasiou, A.; Jones, T.; Mullan, P.; Ross, E.; Howatson, G. Descriptive analysis of Olympic class windsurfing competition during the 2017–2018 regatta season. *Int. J. Perform. Anal. Sport* **2019**, *19*, 517–529. [CrossRef]
11. Caraballo, I.; Domínguez, R.; Felipe, J.L.; Sánchez-Oliver, J. Key performance indicators of Olympic windsurfers during a World Cup: RS:X class®. *J. Sports Sci.* **2022**, *40*, 2645–2653. [CrossRef] [PubMed]
12. Bay, J.; Bojsen-Moller, J.; Nordsborg, N.B. Reliable and sensitive physical testing of elite trapeze sailors. *Scan. J. Med. Sci. Sports* **2018**, *28*, 919–927. [CrossRef] [PubMed]
13. Pan, D.; Sun, K. Analysis of sailing variables and performance of laser sailors with different rankings under the condition of certain wind speed. *Heliyon* **2022**, *8*, e11682. [CrossRef] [PubMed]
14. Caraballo, I.; González-Montesinos, J.L.; Casado-Rodríguez, F.; Gutiérrez-Manzanedo, J.V. Performance analysis in Olympic sailors of the Formula Kite Class using GPS. *Sensor* **2021**, *21*, 574. [CrossRef] [PubMed]
15. Caimmi, G.; Semprini, G. Heart rate and GPS data analysis of kiteboard course racing during the Italian Championship. *Sport Sci. Health* **2017**, *13*, 79–85. [CrossRef]
16. Travemünder Woche 2017 Final Overall Results. Available online: https://www.manage2sail.com/nl/Home/DownloadReport/event/94c64512-e3ae-43a2-99b8-9fd7912d7c4d/report/033c5ec4-4562-4ec1-aabe-c1170e241250 (accessed on 21 March 2022).
17. SAP Sailing. Optimist (International German Youth Championship). Available online: https://tw2017.sapsailing.com/gwt/Home.html#/regatta/overview/:eventId=7784129f-7832-49f1-a5f0-b8d66aa5560c&regattaId=TW2017 (accessed on 21 March 2022).
18. Olympic Classes Speed Charts. Available online: https://www.rya.org.uk/racing/race-officials/resource-centre/forms-data-diagrams-graphics/Pages/data-reference.aspx (accessed on 21 March 2022).
19. Tomczak, M.; Tomczak, E. The need to report effect size estimates revisited. An overview of some recommended measures of effect size. *Trend Sport Sci.* **2014**, *1*, 19–25.
20. Ferguson, C.J. An effect size primer: A guide for clinicians and researchers. *Prof. Psychol. Res. Pract.* **2009**, *40*, 532–538. [CrossRef]
21. Bojsen-Møller, J.; Larsson, B.; Aagaard, P. Physical requirements in Olympic sailing. *Eur. J. Sport. Sci.* **2015**, *15*, 220–227. [CrossRef]
22. Winchcombe, C.; Goods, P.; Binnie, M.; Doyle, M.; Peeling, P. Workload demands of Laser class sailing regattas. *Int. J. Perform. Anal. Sport* **2021**, *21*, 663–678. [CrossRef]
23. Gourlay, T.; Martellotta, J. Aero-hydrodynamics of an RS: X Olympic racing sailboard. *CMST Cent. Mar. Sci. Technol. Res. Rep.* **2011**, *1*, 1–17. Available online: https://www.perthhydro.com/pdf/Gourlay2011Aero-hydroRsx.pdf (accessed on 12 February 2021).
24. Castagna, O.; Brisswalter, J.; Lacour, J.R.; Vogiatzis, I. Physiological demands of different sailing techniques of the new Olympic windsurfing class. *Eur. J. Appl. Physiol.* **2008**, *104*, 1061–1067. [CrossRef] [PubMed]
25. Walls, J.; Bertrand, L.; Gale, T.; Saunders, N. Assessment of upwind dinghy sailing performance using a virtual reality dinghy sailing simulator. *J. Sci. Med. Sport* **1998**, *1*, 61–72. [CrossRef] [PubMed]
26. Day, A.H. Performance prediction for sailing dinghies. *Ocean. Eng.* **2017**, *136*, 67–79. [CrossRef]
27. Spurway, N.C. Hiking physiology and the "quasi-isometric" concept. *J. Sports Sci.* **2007**, *25*, 1081–1093. [CrossRef]
28. Vogiatzis, I.; Tzineris, D.; Athanasopoulos, D.; Georgiadou, O.; Geladas, N. Quadriceps oxygenation during isometric exercise in sailing. *Int. J. Sports Med.* **2008**, *29*, 11–15. [CrossRef]

Disclaimer/Publisher's Note: The statements, opinions and data contained in all publications are solely those of the individual author(s) and contributor(s) and not of MDPI and/or the editor(s). MDPI and/or the editor(s) disclaim responsibility for any injury to people or property resulting from any ideas, methods, instructions or products referred to in the content.

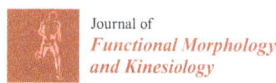

Article

The Influence of Unstable Load and Traditional Free-Weight Back Squat Exercise on Subsequent Countermovement Jump Performance

Renata Jirovska [1], Anthony D. Kay [2], Themistoklis Tsatalas [3], Alex J. Van Enis [1], Christos Kokkotis [4], Giannis Giakas [3,*] and Minas A. Mina [1,*]

[1] Department of Sport, Outdoor and Exercise Science, School of Human Sciences & Human Sciences Research Centre, University of Derby, Kedleston Road, Derby DE22 1GB, UK; renca274@gmail.com (R.J.); a.vanenis@derby.ac.uk (A.J.V.E.)
[2] Sport, Exercise & Life Sciences, University of Northampton, Northampton NN1 5PH, UK; tony.kay@northampton.ac.uk
[3] Department of Physical Education and Sport Science, University of Thessaly, Karyes, 42100 Trikala, Greece; ttsatalas@uth.gr
[4] Department of Physical Education and Sport Science, Democritus University of Thrace, 69100 Komotini, Greece; ckokkoti@affil.duth.gr
* Correspondence: ggiakas@uth.gr (G.G.); m.mina@derby.ac.uk (M.A.M.)

Abstract: The purpose of the present study was to examine the effects of a back squat exercise with unstable load (UN) and traditional free-weight resistance (FWR) on subsequent countermovement jump (CMJ) performance. After familiarisation, thirteen physically active males with experience in resistance training visited the laboratory on two occasions during either experimental (UN) or control (FWR) conditions separated by at least 72 h. In both sessions, participants completed a task-specific warm-up routine followed by three maximum CMJs (pre-intervention; baseline) and a set of three repetitions of either UN or FWR back squat exercise at 85% 1-RM. During the UN condition, the unstable load was suspended from the bar with elastic bands and accounted for 15% of the total load. Post-intervention, three maximum CMJs were performed at 30 s, 4 min, 8 min and 12 min after the last repetition of the intervention. The highest CMJ for each participant was identified for each timepoint. No significant increases ($p > 0.05$) in jump height, peak concentric power, or peak rate of force development (RFD) were found after the FWR or UN conditions at any timepoint. The lack of improvements following both FWR and UN conditions may be a consequence of the low percentage of unstable load and the inclusion of a comprehensive task-specific warm-up. Further research is required to explore higher UN load percentages (>15%) and the chronic effects following the implementation of a resistance training programme.

Keywords: conditioning contractions; explosive strength; elastic bands; vertical jump; warm-up; post-activation performance enhancement (PAPE)

1. Introduction

Warm-up protocols can precondition the neuromuscular system by manipulating different loading strategies to reduce the risk of injury and enhance performance in subsequent high-intensity activities [1–3]. Performing maximal or sub-maximal contractions can acutely increase force production and athletic performance as well as enhance mechanical power above previous voluntary performance, which is usually referred to as post-activation potentiation (PAP) although not synonymous with "classic" PAP (i.e., electrically elicited twitch contraction [4]). The term PAP and its associated mechanisms (including increased muscle temperature [5], myofilament calcium sensitivity [6], and neural drive [7]) have been misinterpreted in the literature and often used to describe an enhancement in voluntary muscle function instead of increases in electrically induced twitch force. However, acute

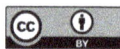

enhancement in performance has been more recently reported as post-activation performance enhancement (PAPE) [8] following high-intensity voluntary muscular contractions and, importantly, can be incorporated in the design of warm-up strategies [9].

Whilst classical PAP is apparent for <3 min following the conditioning contraction [10], peak voluntary contraction (PAPE) occurs 6–10 min following the conditioning contraction [11]. Therefore, acute enhancements in voluntary performance are unlikely to be associated with classical PAP but rather the PAPE phenomenon. The mechanisms underpinning the PAPE phenomenon include (a) rapid increases in muscle temperature in response to a brief intense conditioning activity, which is associated with a greater rate of force development (RFD) and contraction velocity [12]; (b) a high-intensity stimulus (i.e., heavy-load exercise) increases H-reflex potentiation, the excitability of alpha motor neurons and the recruitment of higher-order motor units [13] to increase the efficiency of the neuromuscular system [14]; (c) increases in muscle blood flow and muscle fibre water content may also consequently increase Ca^{2+} sensitivity and thus enhance muscle force output and contraction velocity [15]; however, increases in motivation and acute improvements in motor control strategies cannot be discounted [9].

Warm-up is the process of physical preparation before sporting participation [16] and is considered to enhance subsequent performance [17]. Different limited warm-up strategies have been explored to acutely augment athletic performance ranging from no warm-up at all [4] to stretching, cycling, running, and sub-maximal repetitions of the task [3,18]. Jo et al. [3] found that recovery duration (5–20 min) failed to influence performance after a heavy-load back squat exercise with limited warm-up consisting of cycling for 10 min followed by a Wingate Test. Duthie et al. [18] implemented a standardised warm-up including cycling followed by static stretching and found a significant difference in power performance in jump squats using contrast training methods in athletes with higher strength levels compared to complex training methods. However, Hamada et al. [4] used no warm-up and found a greater potentiation response in Type I muscle fibres following a twitch maximum voluntary contraction. A "comprehensive task-specific" warm-up (including progressively intense task-specific conditioning contractions) has not been commonly used prior to a specific activity being tested [2]. Consequently, as warm-up strategies have been implemented to potentiate muscular force production to enhance subsequent performance following a conditioning activity, it is unclear whether any acute enhancements in performance are due to the warm-up or the conditioning activity itself [19].

The modalities necessary to elicit a PAPE effect remain relatively unexplored: particularly, varying repetitions and sets (volume), exercise intensity and rest periods [20]. Dynamic [21] and isometric voluntary contractions (MVCs) [22] have been used as conditioning contractions to elicit a PAPE response. The volume of conditioning contractions plays a key role in the onset and magnitude of PAPE for strength and conditioning practitioners on improving subsequent jump performance [23]. Rixon et al. [24] compared isometric vs. dynamic conditioning contractions and found an increase in CMJ height and peak power 3 min following three isometric MVC back squats; although 3 min after the 3RM dynamic back squats, there was no increase in CMJ height, and an increase in peak power was observed. However, the two conditioning activities were not identical in terms of volume to allow a direct comparison. Gourgoulis et al. [25] observed a significantly increased vertical jump performance following half squats with sub-maximal loads. In contrast, Hanson et al. [26] observed no significant increase in vertical jump performance following light (40%) and heavy (80%) load. Lower conditioning volumes may induce less fatigue and an earlier PAPE effect, although higher volumes may cause excessive fatigue and may delay the onset of PAPE or negate its presence [27,28]. The varied methodologies across studies, intensities and duration, as well as the equivocal findings in the literature, highlight the difficulty of comparing findings to determine an effective protocol to elicit PAPE.

Generating instability during a back squat exercise by suspending part of the total load from the barbell using elastic bands allows a higher activation of the stabilising muscles, as the lifter is likely to put greater effort into stabilising and controlling the bar [29]. The unstable load can negatively affect the range and speed of motion when compared to stable conditions to reduce force and power output [30]. However, Lawrence and Carlson [31] investigated the changes in force output and muscle activation during a back squat exercise at 60% of their 1-RM using unstable (i.e., elastic bands) and stable (i.e., free-weight) load and found a significant increase in muscle activity of the stabilising muscles (rectus abdominis, external obliques, and soleus). Therefore, the unstable load during the squat exercise incorporated as part of a warm-up can allow a greater activation of the stabilising muscles that may possibly contribute to subsequent performance enhancement.

The back squat exercise is commonly used to improve jump performance with Mina et al. [2] reporting that variable resistance (i.e., elastic bands attached equidistant to the sides of the bar and anchored to the floor) during a back squat exercise improved subsequent countermovement jump (CMJ) performance at 30 s, 4 min, 8 min, and 12 min compared to free-weight resistance alone. The increased muscle activation of vastus lateralis observed by Mina et al. [2] may have contributed to the increase in jump height, given the variation in muscle force requirements imposed by the use of variable resistance influenced the muscle recruitment patterns [2,9]. Therefore, the manipulation of different loading strategies during warm-up exercises may alter muscle recruitment amplitude, allowing increases in performance compared to traditional free-weight resistance alone [31,32].

It is of great importance for strength and conditioning practitioners to examine different variable resistance techniques as part of a warm-up routine to potentiate acute performance, enhance mechanical stimulus and muscle activity. However, no study to date has investigated the potential of suspending part of the total load from the barbell using elastic bands (i.e., unstable but constant load) in performance enhancement programmes. Therefore, the purpose of this study was to compare the influence of two back squat conditions; free-weight resistance (FWR) and unstable load (UN) suspended from the bar using elastic bands, following a comprehensive task-specific warm-up on subsequent CMJ performance. Given the improvements in performance previously reported after warm-up and conditioning contractions [1,2,31,32], it was hypothesised that (a) FWR and UN load would significantly improve subsequent CMJ performance (jump height, peak concentric power and RFD), and (b) the UN condition would provide significantly greater improvements than FWR condition.

2. Materials and Methods

2.1. Participants

Thirteen physically active men with more than two years' resistance training experience (mean ± SD: age = 23.6 ± 1.6 years, height = 179.0 ± 9.2 cm, mass = 86.5 ± 10.0 kg) volunteered to take part in the current study. Inclusion criteria for participation were actively engaged with resistance training with experience in squat exercise and optimal training volume of 3–5 times per week but with no experience of using unstable load as part of their training program. The participants had to report no recent illness or lower limb injuries and refrained from engaging in strenuous activities and using stimulants for at least 48 h before the initial commencement of testing until completion of all testing sessions. Prior to the commencement of testing, all participants provided a written informed consent and completed a pre-medical questionnaire. Across all sessions, participants were instructed to wear the same footwear and were prohibited from using any supportive equipment. The study received ethical approval from the ethics committee at the University of Derby, United Kingdom, with approval reference ETH2122-0282.

To ensure an adequate population to reach statistical power (set at 0.8) was recruited, effect sizes were calculated for jump height (ES = 1.5), peak power (ES = 1.5) and RFD (ES = 1.3) using similar previous studies [2,33,34] with the measure with the smallest ES (i.e., RFD [ES = 1.3]) used to calculate sample size. The total sample size was estimated through a priori power analysis, using the G power V 3.1.9.7 software (Heinrich-Heine-Universität, Düsseldorf, Germany). The following input parameters were applied using a repeated-measure design: effect size f $\approx$ 1.34, α = 0.05, power = 0.80. The analysis revealed that the initial sample size required for statistical power was 10; therefore, considering the possibility of participant withdrawal and data loss, 15 participants were recruited with 13 participants completing the study.

2.2. Protocol Overview

To examine the acute effects of two different back squat conditions, control (FWR) or experimental (UN), a randomised crossover design was used on three separate occasions. Participants visited the laboratory for the familiarisation session and then either the FWR and UN conditions with a minimum separation of 72 h between each visit. Prior to all sessions, a comprehensive task-specific warm up was performed. During the familiarisation session, anthropometric data were collected, participants were familiarised with the testing protocols, and their one-repetition maximum (1-RM) back squat was assessed (please see below). In the experimental conditions, a prescribed warm-up routine was performed followed by three pre-intervention CMJs and then a set of three repetitions of back squat at 85% 1-RM (FWR and UN) followed by three post-intervention CMJs at 30 s, 4 min, 8 min, and 12 min.

2.3. Familiarisation Session and One Repetition Maximum (1-RM) Back Squat Assessment

During the familiarisation session, the participant's 1-RM was assessed following a previously validated protocol designed by Sheppard and Tripplet [35]. Participants warmed up 5 min on a cycle ergometer (Monark 874E, Varberg, Sweden) at 65 rpm with a 1 kg load followed by 2 min rest and then performed two sets of 10 repetitions of unloaded back squat with a 20 kg Olympic bar with 2 min rest between sets. Participants then performed 8 to 10 repetitions at 50% of their previously determined 1-RM, and after a further 2 min rest, the load was increased by 10–20% for one set of 3 to 5 repetitions. Following a further 2 min rest, participants increased the load by 10–20% and performed one set of 2 to 3 repetitions. After 2–4 min rest, the load was increased by 10% and loads ~5% were added for each consecutive set of one repetition until failure to complete a lift. Their last successful lift was recorded as their 1-RM (144.23 $\pm$ 6.17 kg).

2.4. Comprehensive Warm-Up and Countermovement Jump Trials

In the FWR and UN conditions, a comprehensive task-specific warm-up was adopted from Mina et al. [2]. Participants performed a 5-min warm-up on a cycle ergometer at 60 rpm with a 1 kg load followed by 5 continuous body weight squats at 2:2 s tempo (eccentric/concentric). Following a 30 s rest period, participants performed another 5 continuous body weight squats at a 1:1 s tempo (eccentric/concentric). After a 20 s rest, 5 continuous CMJs at 70% of their perceived maximum were performed, and after a further 30 s rest, maximal CMJs were performed every 30 s until three consecutive jumps were performed within 3% of jump height. All participants completed 4–7 jumps in all trials. The CMJ was initiated from an upright position (keeping the hands on the hips at all times) and squatted downwards with the knees and hips flexed and jumped as high as possible, trying to reach maximal height [36]. To establish baseline (i.e., after warm-up) performance, data were collected 2 min later from three maximal pre-intervention CMJs. The procedures described above were followed by one of the conditioning contractions (described later), and a series of three maximum CMJ trials was performed at 30 s, 4 min, 8 min, and 12 min after the intervention with active recovery (i.e., walking) between each timepoint (see Table 1).

Table 1. Timeline of the study design.

Task	Intensity/Effort	Time [min]
5-min cycling	60 rpm	0–5.0
5 BW squats	2:2 s tempo	5.0–5.5
5 BW squats	1:1 s tempo	6.0–6.5
5 CMJs	70% perceived maximum	7.0–7.5
Single CMJs every 30 s	Maximum (100%)	8.0–8.5
CMJs (pre-intervention test)	Maximum (100%)	10.5–11.5
FWR or UN squats	85% 1-RM	12.5–13.0
CMJs (post-intervention test)	Maximum (100%)	13.5, 17.5, 21.5, 25.5

BW = body weight; CMJ = countermovement jump; FWR = free-weight resistance; UN = unstable load; 1-RM—one repetition maximum.

2.5. Intervention

In the FWR and UN conditions, participants performed one set of 3 repetitions of the back squat with the load set at 85% 1-RM. In the FWR condition, traditional load was added to the Olympic bar (20 kg) using weight plates set at 85% 1-RM ((0.85 × 1-RM load) − 20 kg) to determine the load on the bar. In the UN condition, the unstable load was set at 15% (0.15 × 0.85 × 1-RM load) and the remaining 85% load ((0.85 × 0.85 × 1-RM load) − 20 kg) was added using the traditional loading pattern (i.e., Olympic bar and weight plates). For example, where 1-RM is 100 kg load, in the FWR condition, this would equate to 85% 1-RM (85 kg) subtracting 20 kg (bar weight), leaving 65 kg on the bar. In the UN condition, the unstable load (15%) will require 13 kg of unstable load and the remaining 85% will be 72 kg, subtracting the 20 kg bar leaving 52 kg weight on the bar. The unstable load was suspended from the bar with the elastic bands placed next to the lifting collar with small diameter Eleiko plates hanging from the bar so that the load during the back squat exercise was not in contact with the floor. A super mini Pullum elastic band with ranging resistance of 10–50 lb resistance, 19 mm wide, 1041 mm long and with approximate distance from the bar at 60 cm on either side of the bar was used in this study (see Figure 1). Total loads in both experimental conditions were equal for each individual.

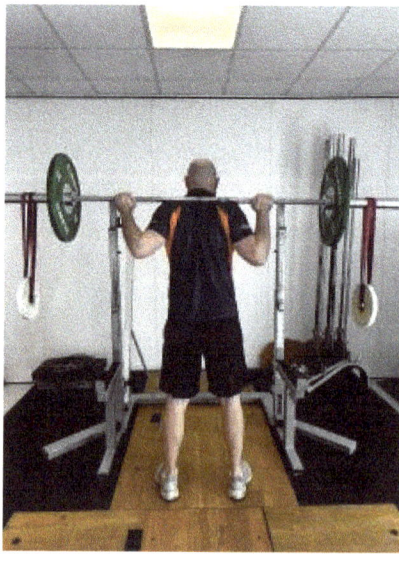

Figure 1. Unstable load from elastic bands hanging from the barbell during the back squat exercise.

2.6. Force Platform Analyses

The kinetic data analyses were similar to Mina et al. [2]. During all CMJ trials, body mass was initially calculated with the participants standing stationary on the platform (Bertec, FP4060-10-2000, Bertec Corporation, Columbus, OH, USA) with ground reaction forces collected at a sampling frequency of 1000 Hz. Data processing initially included the participant's weighting phase (i.e., body weight) [37], which was identified prior to the execution of each CMJ trial when the participants were stationary. The body weight was calculated by averaging the vertical ground reaction forces (GRFs) from each platform over a 2 s period and was divided by 9.81 to obtain each participant's body mass. The net vertical force was calculated by subtracting the average body weight value from the vertical GRF value at each timepoint. Initiation of the jump (i.e., the beginning of the eccentric phase) was determined using the point when net vertical GRF decreased by two standard deviations (SD) below the mean baseline force (i.e., participant's weight at rest) [2]. Vertical GRF was integrated during the eccentric and concentric phases of the jump using the trapezoid method. Impulse, which is equivalent to the change in momentum of the body, was then directly quantified by integrating the applied force over time using the following equation [38]:

$$J = \int F dt = \Delta p, \quad (1)$$

where J = impulse, F = force, t = time and Δp = change in momentum.

Take-off velocity was then determined from impulse data by dividing by body mass, with jump height calculated from take-off velocity using standard equations for motion [39]. Since the force, mass, and initial velocity conditions were known, instantaneous velocity could be calculated. The instantaneous power was calculated as force × velocity, and the peak values were determined for the propulsive phase of the CMJ [2,38]:

$$V_{(0)} = 0, \quad (2)$$

$$F_{(i)}t = m(v_{(i+1)} - v_{(i)}), \quad (3)$$

$$\Delta v = (F_{(i)}t)/m, \quad (4)$$

$$P_{(i)} = F_{(i)} \times V_{(i)}, \quad (5)$$

where F = force, t = 1/sampling frequency, m = mass of body, load, v = velocity, i = index value of the time series, and P = power.

The normalised (to body weight) peak RFD was calculated (eccentric and concentric phase) using a moving 20 ms time window from the first rise in force during the eccentric phase (2). The highest CMJ for each participant was identified at each of the five timepoints and the corresponding kinetic data were used for statistical analyses.

2.7. Statistical Analysis

The data obtained from the study were analysed using the SPSS statistical software (version 27.0; IBM, Armonk, NY, USA). All data are reported as mean ± standard error (SE) with eta squared (η_p^2) and Cohen's d used to calculate effect sizes (ES) for the analysis of variance (ANOVA) and post hoc t-tests, respectively. Boundary intervals for η_p^2 effect sizes were <0.10 (negligible), 0.10–0.24 (small), 0.25–0.40 (medium), and ≥0.40 (large) for Cohen's d boundary intervals were <0.2 (negligible), 0.2–0.49 (small), 0.5–0.79 (medium), and ≥0.8 (large) [40]. The Shapiro–Wilk test was used to assess normal distribution; no significant difference ($p > 0.05$) was observed in any variable indicating a normal distribution across all data sets. Mauchley's tests were used to assess homogeneity of variance and where sphericity was violated, Greenhouse–Geisser (Epsilon ≤ 0.75) or Huynh–Feldt (Epsilon > 0.75) correction factors were used [40]. To determine differences in

(a) jump height, (b) peak concentric power, and (c) RFD 20 ms, separate two-way repeated measures ANOVAs (time × condition) were performed. Where significant differences were detected, post hoc analyses with Bonferroni and Sidak corrections proved too conservative (i.e., masked the location of the difference); thus Tukey's, LSD correction was used to determine the location of the differences. Statistical significance was set at $p < 0.05$ for all tests.

3. Results

3.1. Reliability

Within-session reliability for all measures was determined during pre-intervention (baseline) CMJ measures. No significant differences ($p > 0.05$) were detected in any data set with interclass correlation coefficients (ICCs) calculated for jump height (0.93), peak concentric power (0.89) and peak RFD (0.76) indicating good-to-excellent reliability with low coefficients of variance (CV) calculated for jump height (4.2%), peak concentric power (2.0%) and peak RFD (4.7%).

3.2. Jump Height

The two-way repeated measures ANOVA revealed no significant interaction effect ($F_{2.06, 24.74} = 0.368$, $p = 0.702$, $\eta_p^2 = 0.030$) for jump height, while a significant main effect of time ($F_{2.22, 26.63} = 3.493$, $p = 0.041$, $\eta_p^2 = 0.225$) but not of condition ($F_{1, 12} = 1.873$, $p = 0.196$, $\eta_p^2 = 0.135$) was detected. Post hoc pairwise comparisons revealed that Bonferroni and Sidak corrections were too conservative, as no significant difference at any timepoint was detected.

Tukey's LSD revealed no significant difference at any timepoint (30 s, 4 min, 8 min, or 12 min) compared to pre-intervention (data collapsed across conditions: mean range = −1.7 to 3.2% ($d = −0.35$ to 0.36); FWR condition: mean range = −1.0 to 4.1% ($d = −0.26$ to 0.46); UN condition: mean range = −1.2 to 2.3% ($d = 0.00$ to 0.79)) (see Figure 2). However, pairwise comparisons revealed jump height was significantly higher at 30 s than at 8 min (data collapsed across conditions = 2.0 ± 1.2% ($d = 0.35$); FWR condition = 3.0 ± 2.0% ($d = 0.48$); UN condition = 1.0 ± 1.4% ($d = 0.20$)) and 12 min (data collapsed across conditions = 3.2 ± 1.2% ($d = 0.58$); FWR condition = 4.4 ± 2.0% ($d = 0.68$); UN condition = 2.1 ± 1.3% ($d = 0.47$)).

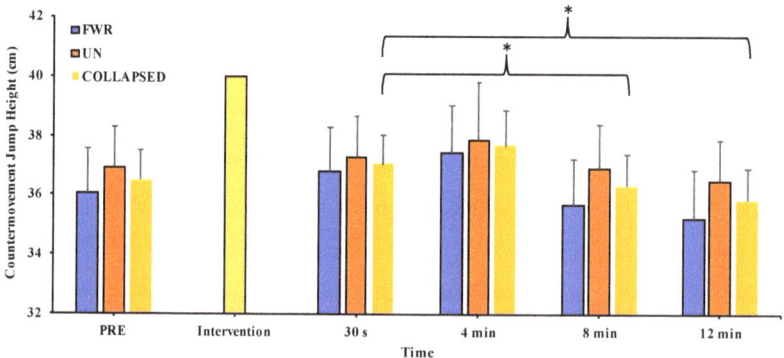

Figure 2. Measures of countermovement jump performance pre-intervention (PRE) and across all timepoints following the free weight resistance (FWR) and unstable (UN) conditioning interventions (collapsed data also shown). Values are presented as mean ± SE; * $p < 0.05$.

3.3. Peak Power

No significant interaction effect ($F_{4, 48} = 0.510$, $p = 0.729$, $\eta_p^2 = 0.041$) was revealed for peak power, while a significant main effect of time ($F_{4, 48} = 3.126$, $p = 0.023$, $\eta_p^2 = 0.207$) but not of condition ($F_{1, 12} = 3.400$, $p = 0.090$, $\eta_p^2 = 0.221$) was detected. Post hoc pairwise comparisons revealed that Bonferroni and Sidak corrections were too conservative, as no significant difference at any timepoint was detected. Tukey's LSD revealed no significant difference at any timepoint (30 s, 4 min, 8 min, or 12 min) compared to pre-intervention (data collapsed across conditions: mean range = −2.1 to 2.4% (d = −0.39 to 0.32); FWR condition: mean range = −0.3 to 3.6% (d = 0.06 to 0.36); UN condition: mean range = −4.0 to 1.3% (d = 0.12 to 0.74)) (see Figure 3). However, pairwise comparisons revealed peak power was significantly greater at 4 min (data collapsed across conditions = 4.2 ± 1.4% (d = 0.80); FWR condition = 3.3 ± 1.4% (d = 0.64); UN condition = 5.1 ± 1.4% (d = 0.94)) and 8 min (data collapsed across conditions = 2.3 ± 0.9% (d = 0.52); FWR condition = 0.9 ± 0.8% (d = 0.35); UN condition = 3.7 ± 1.6% (d = 0.67)) than at 12 min.

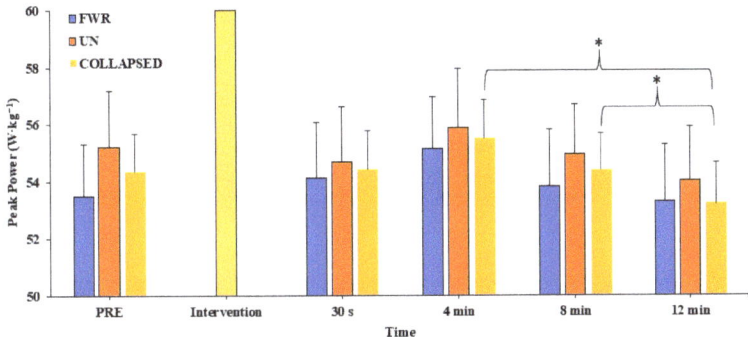

Figure 3. Measure of peak power pre-intervention (PRE) and across all timepoints following the free weight resistance (FWR) and unstable (UN) conditioning interventions (collapsed data also shown). Values are presented as mean ± SE; * $p < 0.05$.

3.4. Peak RFD

No significant interaction effect ($F_{4, 48}$ = 1.447, p = 0.233, η_p^2 = 0.108) or main effects of time ($F_{4, 48}$ = 0.294, p = 0.881, η_p^2 = 0.024) or condition ($F_{1, 4}$ = 0.252, p = 0.625, η_p^2 = 0.021) were detected for peak RFD (see Figure 4).

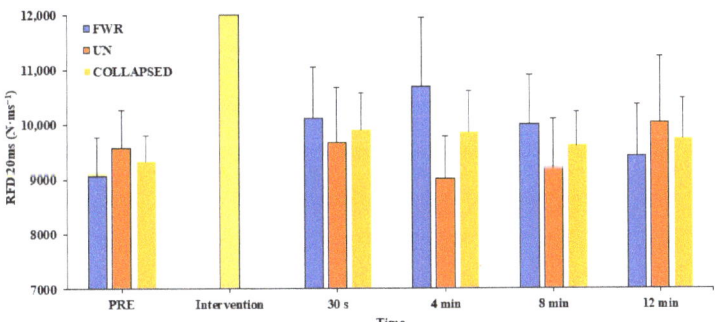

Figure 4. Measure of peak rate of force development (RFD) pre-intervention (PRE) and across all timepoints in the free weight resistance (FWR) and unstable (UN) conditioning interventions (collapsed data also shown). Values are presented as mean ± SE.

4. Discussion

The current study investigated the magnitude and time-course of changes in countermovement jump (CMJ) performance after free-weight resistance (FWR) and unstable load (UN) back squat exercise performed following a comprehensive task-specific warm-up routine. In the FWR and UN conditions, no significant interaction or differences between conditions were detected at any timepoint. Using collapsed data (main effects analyses), compared to baseline, no significant changes were found in CMJ height, peak concentric power, or peak RFD at any timepoint (30 s, 4 min, 8 min, and 12 min), which is indicative of no potentiating effects of either intervention on CMJ performance. Thus, the hypotheses were rejected as neither the stable load during FWR or the unstable load during UN back squat exercise interventions enhanced CMJ performance. However, jump height at 12 min and 8 min was significantly lower compared to 30 s with peak power at 12 min also significantly lower compared to 4 min and 8 min. These reductions at 8 min and 12 min cannot be explained by fatigue, as no reduction was apparent at any earlier timepoint compared with baseline, and thus they are likely attributable to the participants losing motivation at 8 min and 12 min to perform numerous maximal CMJs at several timepoints. Regardless, the hypotheses were rejected, as neither the stable load during FWR or the unstable load during UN back squat exercise interventions enhanced CMJ performance. The lack of improvement compared to baseline in any measure following the FWR and UN condition after a comprehensive task-specific warm-up suggests that no additional benefit (i.e., PAP/PAPE effect) was derived from the inclusion of intense loading, which is consistent with previous research where an absence of change in CMJ performance was found when dynamic warm-up exercise (10 m lunge walks × 2, 10 body-squats × 2) was performed following high-intensity free weight contractions [41]. However, inconsistencies in PAPE responses [25,36,41] may depend on fatigue potentiation or perseveration potentiation interactions on subsequent performance.

Since this was the first PAPE study examining the impact of implementing unstable loads during the back squat exercise on jump performance, certain methodological approaches in this study could possibly explain the lack of significant changes following the UN condition. In the present study, the percentage of unstable loading was 15% of the 85% total load during the UN condition, which may be too low to sufficiently amplify potentiation and improve subsequent CMJ performance. Lawrence and Carlson [31] compared stable squats (traditional free-weights) and unstable squats (load suspended from the bar) with a load set at 60% of 1-RM and found an increased muscle activation of the torso (i.e., stabilising muscles), and during the pilot, >60% of 1-RM of five repetitions was perceived challenging for subjects to complete. Similarly, Ostrowski et al. [42] investigated stable and unstable bench press at two different intensities (60% and 80%) with greater muscle activation at 80% load in the concentric phase. This suggests that unstable loading techniques may vary across different exercises. However, previous research has extensively investigated variable resistance (i.e., chains and elastic bands) ranging 10–30% of the overall load [43,44]. Ebben and Jensen (2002) investigated elastic band and chain-loaded resistance set at 10% and found no significant effect on EMG or lifting kinetics [43]. Further, Stevenson et al. (2010) examined elastic band resistance set at 15% or 30% and failed to find a significant increase in power compared to FWR alone [44]. In contrast, which in combination with free-weights, they found no significant differences, although variable resistance set at higher percentages (35% load) has shown potentiating effects on squat performance [1,2,45,46]. In the present study, the amount of unstable load used was set at 15% of the total 85% given the challenging tolerance of using unstable loads alone at higher percentages [31,42], and the low proportion of unstable load failed to amplify potentiation.

Although the use of unstable load may require a greater muscle activation by the stabilising muscles, it can be more challenging for those who lack regular free-weight resistance training. In the present study, we used experienced weight-trained individuals, which could have allowed more control over the unstable load; hence, they may not have been unstable enough to elicit a potentiation response [47–49]. Therefore, the combination of unstable load with free-weight resistance can foster stability and reduce the degree of difficulty compared to unstable loads alone. Possible factors for this lack of difference could be the level of instability, intensity, elasticity of the bands suspending the load, movement tempo and the proportion of stable/unstable load. While power analysis was conducted, further study needs to be conducted with a larger sample size to confirm these data. Another limitation is that the participants had no previous experience with unstable load; thus, future investigations should allow a longer familiarisation period with unstable load. In addition, research is required to examine the electromyographic (EMG) activity of the stabilising muscles during stable and unstable load of the back squat exercise and how these may yield acute improvements in subsequent performance. In addition, considerations ought to include the type of conditioning contractions, including bench press, deadlift, etc. as well as participant characteristics (i.e., experienced versus novice lifters) to confirm the effectiveness of unstable load as a performance enhancement technique.

5. Conclusions

The use of FWR and UN load during the back squat exercise following a comprehensive task-specific warm-up failed to alter CMJ height and force/power production. These findings are suggestive that the proportion of unstable load used in the present study in combination with free-weights was insufficient to augment subsequent CMJ performance. Given the individuals that took part in the present study had over 2 years' experience in weight training may have allowed a greater control over the unstable load; thus, the amount of unstable load may have been low to elicit a potentiation response. Further research is required to clearly understand how a higher proportion of unstable load in combination with free-weights during the back squat exercise can sufficiently challenge the musculature, the level of difficulty emanating from the unstable load, and the ability to maintain balance during the execution of the exercise to possibly increase subsequent performance.

Author Contributions: Conceptualization, R.J., M.A.M. and A.D.K.; methodology, R.J., M.A.M., A.D.K. and T.T.; software, C.K. and A.J.V.E.; validation, M.A.M., A.D.K. and T.T.; formal analysis, R.J., A.J.V.E. and A.D.K.; investigation, R.J.; data curation, R.J and A.J.V.E.; writing—original draft preparation, R.J. and M.A.M.; writing—review and editing, M.A.M., A.D.K. and T.T.; visualization, G.G. and M.A.M.; supervision, M.A.M. and A.D.K.; project administration, G.G. and C.K. All authors have read and agreed to the published version of the manuscript.

Funding: This research received no external funding.

Institutional Review Board Statement: The study was conducted in accordance with the Declaration of Helsinki and approved by the Institutional Review Board (or Ethics Committee) of The University of Derby (protocol code ETH2122-0282 and date of approval 7 November 2021).

Informed Consent Statement: Informed consent was obtained from all participants involved in the study. Written informed consent has been obtained from the participants to publish this paper.

Data Availability Statement: Data are available upon request.

Acknowledgments: Antonia D. Mina assisted with proofreading, suggesting revisions and formatting the manuscript.

Conflicts of Interest: The authors declare no conflict of interest.

References

1. Mina, M.A.; Blazevich, A.J.; Giakas, G.; Seitz, L.B.; Kay, A.D. Chain-Loaded Variable Resistance Warm-up Improves Free-Weight Maximal Back Squat Performance. *Eur. J. Sport Sci.* **2016**, *16*, 932–939. [CrossRef] [PubMed]
2. Mina, M.A.; Blazevich, A.J.; Tsatalas, T.; Giakas, G.; Seitz, L.B.; Kay, A.D. Variable, but Not Free-weight, Resistance Back Squat Exercise Potentiates Jump Performance Following a Comprehensive Task-specific Warm-up. *Scand. J. Med. Sci. Sports* **2019**, *29*, 380–392. [CrossRef] [PubMed]
3. Jo, E.; Judelson, D.A.; Brown, L.E.; Coburn, J.W.; Dabbs, N.C. Influence of Recovery Duration after a Potentiating Stimulus on Muscular Power in Recreationally Trained Individuals. *J. Strength Cond. Res.* **2010**, *24*, 343–347. [CrossRef] [PubMed]
4. Hamada, T.; Sale, D.G.; MacDougall, J.D.; Tarnopolsky, M.A. Postactivation Potentiation, Fiber Type, and Twitch Contraction Time in Human Knee Extensor Muscles. *J. Appl. Physiol.* **2000**, *88*, 2131–2137. [CrossRef] [PubMed]
5. Racinais, S.; Oksa, J. Temperature and Neuromuscular Function. *Scand. J. Med. Sci. Sports* **2010**, *20*, 1–18. [CrossRef] [PubMed]
6. Moore, R.L.; Stull, J.T. Myosin Light Chain Phosphorylation in Fast and Slow Skeletal Muscles in Situ. *Am. J. Physiol. Cell Physiol.* **1984**, *247*, C462–C471. [CrossRef] [PubMed]
7. Trimble, M.H.; Harp, S.S. Postexercise Potentiation of the H-Reflex Humans. *Med. Sci. Sports Exerc.* **1998**, *30*, 933–941.

8. Cuenca-Fernández, F.; Smith, I.C.; Jordan, M.J.; MacIntosh, B.R.; López-Contreras, G.; Arellano, R.; Herzog, W. Nonlocalized Postactivation Performance Enhancement (PAPE) Effects in Trained Athletes: A Pilot Study. *Appl. Physiol. Nutr. Metab.* **2017**, *42*, 1122–1125. [CrossRef]
9. Blazevich, A.J.; Babault, N. Post-Activation Potentiation versus Post-Activation Performance Enhancement in Humans: Historical Perspective, Underlying Mechanisms, and Current Issues. *Front. Physiol.* **2019**, *10*, 1359. [CrossRef]
10. Vandervoort, A.; Quinlan, J.; McComas, A. Twitch Potentiation after Voluntary Contraction. *Exp. Neurol.* **1983**, *81*, 141–152. [CrossRef]
11. Wilson, J.M.; Duncan, N.M.; Marin, P.J.; Brown, L.E.; Loenneke, J.P.; Wilson, S.M.; Jo, E.; Lowery, R.P.; Ugrinowitsch, C. Meta-Analysis of Postactivation Potentiation and Power: Effects of Conditioning Activity, Volume, Gender, Rest Periods, and Training Status. *J. Strength Cond. Res.* **2013**, *27*, 854–859. [CrossRef] [PubMed]
12. Stein, R.; Gordon, T.; Shriver, J. Temperature Dependence of Mammalian Muscle Contractions and ATPase Activities. *Biophys. J.* **1982**, *40*, 97–107. [CrossRef] [PubMed]
13. Folland, J.P.; Wakamatsu, T.; Fimland, M.S. The Influence of Maximal Isometric Activity on Twitch and H-Reflex Potentiation, and Quadriceps Femoris Performance. *Eur. J. Appl. Physiol.* **2008**, *104*, 739–748. [CrossRef] [PubMed]
14. Hodgson, M.; Docherty, D.; Robbins, D. Post-Activation Potentiation: Underlying Physiology and Implications for Motor Performance. *J. Sports Med.* **2005**, *35*, 585–595. [CrossRef] [PubMed]
15. Edman, K.; Andersson, K.-E. The Variation in Active Tension with Sarcomere Length in Vertebrate Skeletal Muscle and Its Relation to Fibre Width. *Experientia* **1968**, *24*, 134–136. [CrossRef] [PubMed]
16. Jeffreys, I. Warm up Revisited–the 'Ramp'Method of Optimising Performance Preparation. *UKSCA J.* **2006**, *6*, 15–19.
17. Bishop, D. Warm up II: Performance Changes Following Active Warm up and How to Structure the Warm Up. *J. Sports Med.* **2003**, *33*, 483–498. [CrossRef] [PubMed]
18. Duthie, G.M.; Young, W.B.; Aitken, D.A. The Acute Effects of Heavy Loads on Jump Squat Performance: An Evaluation of the Complex and Contrast Methods of Power Development. *J. Strength Cond. Res.* **2002**, *16*, 530–538. [CrossRef]
19. MacIntosh, B.R.; Robillard, M.-E.; Tomaras, E.K. Should Postactivation Potentiation Be the Goal of Your Warm-Up? *Appl. Physiol. Nutr. Metab.* **2012**, *37*, 546–550. [CrossRef]
20. Tillin, N.A.; Bishop, D. Factors Modulating Post-Activation Potentiation and Its Effect on Performance of Subsequent Explosive Activities. *J. Sports Med.* **2009**, *39*, 147–166. [CrossRef]
21. Masamoto, N.; Larson, R.; Gates, T.; Faigenbaum, A. Acute Effects of Plyometric Exercise on Maximum Squat Performance in Male Athletes. *J. Strength Cond. Res.* **2003**, *17*, 68–71. [PubMed]
22. French, D.N.; Kraemer, W.J.; Cooke, C.B. Changes in Dynamic Exercise Performance Following a Sequence of Preconditioning Isometric Muscle Actions. *J. Strength Cond. Res.* **2003**, *17*, 678–685. [PubMed]
23. de Keijzer, K.L.; McErlain-Naylor, S.A.; Dello Iacono, A.; Beato, M. Effect of Volume on Eccentric Overload-Induced Postactivation Potentiation of Jumps. *Int. J. Sports Physiol. Perform.* **2020**, *15*, 976–981. [CrossRef] [PubMed]
24. Rixon, K.P.; Lamont, H.S.; Bemben, M.G. Influence of Type of Muscle Contraction, Gender, and Lifting Experience on Postactivation Potentiation Performance. *J. Strength Cond. Res.* **2007**, *21*, 500–505. [CrossRef] [PubMed]
25. Gourgoulis, V.; Aggeloussis, N.; Kasimatis, P.; Mavromatis, G.; Garas, A. Effect of a Submaximal Half-Squats Warm-up Program on Vertical Jumping Ability. *J. Strength Cond. Res.* **2003**, *17*, 342–344. [PubMed]
26. Hanson, E.D.; Leigh, S.; Mynark, R.G. Acute Effects of Heavy-and Light-Load Squat Exercise on the Kinetic Measures of Vertical Jumping. *J. Strength Cond. Res.* **2007**, *21*, 1012–1017. [CrossRef]
27. Wallace, B.J.; Shapiro, R.; Wallace, K.L.; Abel, M.G.; Symons, T.B. Muscular and Neural Contributions to Postactivation Potentiation. *J. Strength Cond. Res.* **2019**, *33*, 615–625. [CrossRef]
28. Seitz, L.B.; Haff, G.G. Factors Modulating Post-Activation Potentiation of Jump, Sprint, Throw, and Upper-Body Ballistic Performances: A Systematic Review with Meta-Analysis. *J. Sports Med.* **2016**, *46*, 231–240. [CrossRef]
29. Kohler, J.M.; Flanagan, S.P.; Whiting, W.C. Muscle Activation Patterns While Lifting Stable and Unstable Loads on Stable and Unstable Surfaces. *J. Strength Cond. Res.* **2010**, *24*, 313–321. [CrossRef]
30. Anderson, K.G.; Behm, D.G. Maintenance of EMG Activity and Loss of Force Output with Instability. *J. Strength Cond. Res.* **2004**, *18*, 637–640.
31. Lawrence, M.A.; Carlson, L.A. Effects of an Unstable Load on Force and Muscle Activation during a Parallel Back Squat. *J. Strength Cond. Res.* **2015**, *29*, 2949–2953. [CrossRef] [PubMed]
32. Israetel, M.A.; McBride, J.M.; Nuzzo, J.L.; Skinner, J.W.; Dayne, A.M. Kinetic and Kinematic Differences Between Squats Performed with and without Elastic Bands. *J. Strength Cond. Res.* **2010**, *24*, 190–194. [CrossRef] [PubMed]
33. Argus, C.K.; Gill, N.D.; Keogh, J.W.; Blazevich, A.J.; Hopkins, W.G. Kinetic and Training Comparisons Between Assisted, Resisted, and Free Countermovement Jumps. *J. Strength Cond. Res.* **2011**, *25*, 2219–2227. [CrossRef] [PubMed]
34. Gołaś, A.; Maszczyk, A.; Zajac, A.; Mikołajec, K.; Stastny, P. Optimizing Post Activation Potentiation for Explosive Activities in Competitive Sports. *J. Hum. Kinet.* **2016**, *52*, 95. [CrossRef]
35. Sheppard, J.M.; Triplett, N.T. Program Design for Resistance Training. In *Essentials of Strength Training and Conditioning*, 4th ed.; Haff, G.G., Triplett, N.T., Eds.; Human Kinetics: Champaign, IL, USA, 2016; pp. 439–470.
36. Young, W.B.; Jenner, A.; Griffiths, K. Acute Enhancement of Power Performance from Heavy Load Squats. *J. Strength Cond. Res.* **1998**, *12*, 82–84.

37. McMahon, J.J.; Suchomel, T.J.; Lake, J.P.; Comfort, P. Understanding the Key Phases of the Countermovement Jump Force-Time Curve. *Strength Cond. J.* **2018**, *40*, 96–106. [CrossRef]
38. Linthorne, N.P. Analysis of Standing Vertical Jumps Using a Force Platform. *Am. J. Phys.* **2001**, *69*, 1198–1204. [CrossRef]
39. Kibele, A. Possibilities and Limitations in the Biomechanical Analysis of Countermovement Jumps: A Methodological Study. *J. Appl. Biomech.* **1998**, *14*, 105–117. [CrossRef]
40. Field, A. *Discovering Statistics Using IBM SPSS Statistics*, 5th ed.; SAGE Publications Ltd.: Thousand Oaks, CA, USA, 2018; pp. 64–72.
41. Witmer, C.A.; Davis, S.E.; Moir, G.L. The Acute Effects Of Back Squats On Mechanical Variables During Countermovement Vertical Jump Performance In Women: 1493: Board# 149 June 2 9: 30 AM–11: 00 AM. *Med. Sci. Sports Exerc.* **2010**, *42*, 294.
42. Ostrowski, S.J.; Carlson, L.A.; Lawrence, M.A. Effect of an Unstable Load on Primary and Stabilizing Muscles during the Bench Press. *J. Strength Cond. Res.* **2017**, *31*, 430–434. [CrossRef]
43. Ebben, W.E.; Jensen, R.L. Electromyographic and Kinetic Analysis of Traditional, Chain, and Elastic Band Squats. *J. Strength Cond. Res.* **2002**, *16*, 547–550. [PubMed]
44. Stevenson, M.W.; Warpeha, J.M.; Dietz, C.C.; Giveans, R.M.; Erdman, A.G. Acute Effects of Elastic Bands during the Free-Weight Barbell Back Squat Exercise on Velocity, Power, and Force Production. *J. Strength Cond. Res.* **2010**, *24*, 2944–2954. [CrossRef] [PubMed]
45. Mina, M.A.; Blazevich, A.J.; Giakas, G.; Kay, A.D. Influence of Variable Resistance Loading on Subsequent Free Weight Maximal Back Squat Performance. *J. Strength Cond. Res.* **2014**, *28*, 2988–2995. [CrossRef] [PubMed]
46. Wallace, B.J.; Winchester, J.B.; McGuigan, M.R. Effects of Elastic Bands on Force and Power Characteristics during the Back Squat Exercise. *J. Strength Cond. Res.* **2006**, *20*, 268–272.
47. Dunnick, D.D.; Brown, L.E.; Coburn, J.W.; Lynn, S.K.; Barillas, S.R. Bench Press Upper-Body Muscle Activation between Stable and Unstable Loads. *J. Strength Cond. Res.* **2015**, *29*, 3279–3283. [CrossRef]
48. Masel, S.; Maciejczyk, M. Effects of Post-Activation Performance Enhancement on Jump Performance in Elite Volleyball Players. *Appl. Sci.* **2022**, *12*, 9054. [CrossRef]
49. Sañudo, B.; de Hoyo, M.; Haff, G.G.; Muñoz-López, A. Influence of Strength Level on the Acute Post-Activation Performance Enhancement Following Flywheel and Free Weight Resistance Training. *Sensors* **2020**, *20*, 7156. [CrossRef]

Disclaimer/Publisher's Note: The statements, opinions and data contained in all publications are solely those of the individual author(s) and contributor(s) and not of MDPI and/or the editor(s). MDPI and/or the editor(s) disclaim responsibility for any injury to people or property resulting from any ideas, methods, instructions or products referred to in the content.

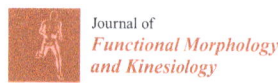

Article

Reactive Strength Index, Rate of Torque Development, and Performance in Well-Trained Weightlifters: A Pilot Study

Giorgos Anastasiou [1], Marios Hadjicharalambous [1], Gerasimos Terzis [2] and Nikolaos Zaras [1,*]

[1] Human Performance Laboratory, Department of Life Sciences, School of Life and Health Sciences, University of Nicosia, Nicosia 2417, Cyprus; hadjicharalambous.m@unic.ac.cy (M.H.)
[2] Sports Performance Laboratory, School of Physical Education and Sport Science, National and Kapodistrian University of Athens, 157 72 Athens, Greece; gterzis@phed.uoa.gr
* Correspondence: zaras.n@unic.ac.cy

Abstract: The purpose of this study was to investigate the correlation between the reactive strength index (RSI) using the drop jump (DJ) and the isometric rate of torque development (RTD) with weightlifting performance in national-level weightlifters. Seven male weightlifters (age: 28.3 ± 5.7 years, body mass: 80.5 ± 6.7 kg, body height: 1.73 ± 0.07 m) participated in this study. Measurements were performed 2 weeks prior to the national championship and included the countermovement jump (CMJ), the squat jump (SJ), the DJ from three different drop heights (20, 30, and 40 cm), and the isometric peak torque (IPT) and RTD. Performance in CMJ and SJ was significantly correlated with weightlifting performance (r ranging from 0.756 to 0.892). Significant correlations were found between weightlifting performance with DJ contact time (r ranging from −0.759 to −0.899) and RSI (r ranging from 0.790 to 0.922). Moreover, the best RSI was significantly correlated with the snatch (r = 0.921, p = 0.003) and total performance (r = 0.832, p = 0.020). Small to very large correlations were found between IPT and RTD with weightlifting performance (r ranging from 0.254 to 0.796). These results suggest that RSI and contact time variables from DJ may predict weightlifting performance in well-trained weightlifters. Additionally, IPT and RTD may provide useful insights into the neuromuscular fitness condition of the weightlifter.

Keywords: snatch; clean and jerk; contact time; power

Citation: Anastasiou, G.; Hadjicharalambous, M.; Terzis, G.; Zaras, N. Reactive Strength Index, Rate of Torque Development, and Performance in Well-Trained Weightlifters: A Pilot Study. *J. Funct. Morphol. Kinesiol.* **2023**, *8*, 161. https://doi.org/10.3390/jfmk8040161

Academic Editor: Giuseppe Musumeci

Received: 24 September 2023
Revised: 29 October 2023
Accepted: 7 November 2023
Published: 20 November 2023

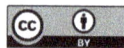

Copyright: © 2023 by the authors. Licensee MDPI, Basel, Switzerland. This article is an open access article distributed under the terms and conditions of the Creative Commons Attribution (CC BY) license (https://creativecommons.org/licenses/by/4.0/).

1. Introduction

Olympic weightlifting is a power-demanding sport consisting of two lifts: the snatch and the clean and jerk. During the snatch, the athlete is required to lift the barbell from the ground and overhead in one consecutive movement [1]. In addition, the clean and jerk consists of two different movements: the clean, which requires the athlete to lift the barbell from the ground to the shoulders, and the jerk, which requires the athlete to bring the barbell from the shoulders to overhead [2]. Both the snatch and clean and jerk lifts are highly technical multi-joint movements where the entire neuromuscular system of the weightlifter must be simultaneously activated for a successful lifting attempt [3].

In Olympic weightlifting training, athletes routinely utilize heavy loads (≥80% of 1 repetition maximum (RM)), with an intentionally fast movement of lifting velocity [4], to attempt to enhance performance during main competitions. This strategy is not only applied in the snatch and the clean and jerk but also in other weightlifting derivatives (back squat, front squat, pulls, etc.). This type of training may lead to a significant increase in power (i.e., vertical jumps) and in the rate of force development (RFD) [5–7]. Several studies, for example, have shown that vertical jumps such as the countermovement jump (CMJ), the deep squat CMJ, and the squat jump (SJ) may significantly predict performance in the snatch and clean and jerk. Indeed, a significant correlation was observed between weightlifting performance and CMJ variables [6–11], whereas deep CMJ and SJ may also be valid predictors of weightlifting performance [8,12,13]. Furthermore, a recent meta-analysis revealed that CMJ and SJ power production had a significant correlation magnitude to weightlifting performance, reaching nearly perfect values (r = 0.92) [14]. Although the link between CMJ and SJ with weightlifting performance has been extensively researched, the correlation between drop jump (DJ) capability and weightlifting performance remains largely unexplored. The DJ is considered a fast stretch–shortening cycle movement that produces a rapid eccentric phase and a faster transition to the concentric phase [15], which is similar to the weightlifting movements. A crucial variable derived from the DJ analysis is the reactive strength index (RSI), which can be calculated as the quotient of DJ height and ground contact time [16,17]. A previous study on male NCAA Division I basketball players showed that the RSI was correlated with the vertical stiffness of the lower musculoskeletal system during various DJ heights [17]. Although data are scarce for weightlifters, it could be hypothesized that the DJ may be a useful test to predict weightlifting performance, even though such a premise needs further investigation.

Performance in weightlifting requires a high RFD in short time frames ranging from 0 to 250 milliseconds [18–20]. The RFD is a parameter that shows how quickly an athlete can apply his/her maximum force, and it is calculated by the force–time curve [7,21,22]. Significant correlations have been found between weightlifting performance with RFD measured through mid-thigh pull [9,13,21] and isometric leg press [7,10,11]. In addition, a recent meta-analysis showed that the RFD calculated from mid-thigh pulls may have a significant correlation magnitude to weightlifting performance, reaching large values (r ranging from 0.51 to 0.60) [14]. Although these tests are multi-joint and sports-specific, several laboratories are equipped with isokinetic machines that can measure angular velocities in single-joint movements with high accuracy [23]. Additionally, it is a common strategy to evaluate athletes' preparedness before competitions through isokinetic measurements. However, data are scarce regarding the correlation between single-joint movements, like the isometric knee extension and weightlifting performance. A study of sixty-seven adolescent weightlifters showed significant correlations between weightlifting performance and isokinetic knee extension force at 60, 90, and 180 deg/sec (r = 0.597, 0.693, and 0.725, respectively) [23], but no correlation was presented between the rate of torque development (RTD) and weightlifting performance. Consequently, whether a correlation exists between the knee extension isometric peak torque (IPT) and the RTD with weightlifting performance remains unexplored.

The aim of the present study was to investigate the correlation (a) between RSI and weightlifting performance and (b) between knee extension IPT and RTD with weightlifting performance. It was hypothesized that the RSI and knee extension IPT and RTD might be valid predictors of weightlifting performance.

2. Materials and Methods

2.1. Participants

Seven male weightlifters (N = 7, age: 28.3 ± 5.7 years, body mass: 80.5 ± 6.7 kg, body height: 1.72 ± 0.07 m, personal best in snatch: 105.6 ± 14.2 kg, personal best in clean and jerk: 131.5 ± 19.6 kg) with 4.6 ± 2.2 years of competitive experience participated in the study. Three of the athletes were members of the national weightlifting team and holders of the national records in their individual bodyweight categories. All athletes participated in national and international weightlifting competitions. Inclusion criteria were as follows: (a) absence of any cardiovascular, orthopedic, and neuromuscular issues; (b) systematic weightlifting training and regular participation in competitions; (c) absence of any illegal drug use. Athletes were fully informed of the risks and benefits of the study prior to entry, and they signed an institutionally approved informed consent. All procedures were in accordance with the 1975 Declaration of Helsinki as revised in 2000 and were approved by the national ethics committee of Cyprus (project number EEBK/EΠ/2020/55).

2.2. Design

This study focused on the investigation of correlations between the DJ, the knee extension IPT, and RTD with weightlifting performance. Seven well-trained male weightlifters visited the laboratory on two different occasions within a week. During the first visit, anthropometric characteristics and a familiarization session of the vertical jumps and the knee extension isometric test were performed. During the second visit, measurements of the CMJ, the SJ, the DJ, and the knee extension isometric test were performed. On a different day, all athletes performed the 1-RM test in the snatch and clean and jerk in their training facilities. A correlation analysis was performed to investigate the relationships between variables.

2.3. Olympic Weightlifting Performance

Performance in weightlifting (snatch and clean and jerk) was measured at the training facilities of the athletes during the afternoon hours at a standard temperature of ~24 °C [24]. Athletes performed the 1-RM test in the snatch and clean and jerk according to the international regulations of the International Weightlifting Federation. Specifically, the 1-RM test started with the snatch. After a self-selected warm-up with static and dynamic stretching exercises, athletes performed 3–4 sets of 5–6 repetitions with an empty barbell. Then, the athletes performed 2 sets of 5 repetitions with 50% of the predicted 1-RM and 1 set of 2–3 repetitions at 65%, 75%, and 85% of the predicted 1-RM. Then, single repetitions were performed at 90% and 95% of the predicted 1-RM. Three maximum attempts were given to athletes after 95% of their individual predicted 1RM for achieving their maximum effort. Fifteen minutes after the snatch, the 1-RM test in the clean and jerk was performed, similarly to 1-RM snatch test, as described above. During the 1-RM attempts, a certified weightlifting coach was present to provide feedback to the athletes. The best performance in the snatch and in the clean and jerk was used for the statistical analysis. Total performance was expressed as the sum of the snatch and the clean and jerk in kilograms.

2.4. Countermovement Jumps

Laboratory measurements began with the CMJs. Briefly, after 5 min warm-up on a stationary bicycle and following several dynamic stretching exercises, athletes performed 3 sub-maximal intensity CMJs. Following 3 min of rest, the athletes performed 4 maximal CMJs (Optojump Modular System, Warwickshire, UK) with 2 min rest between each attempt. More specifically, the athletes remained in a standing position with arms akimbo; from this position, the athletes performed an individual self-selected semi-squat and jumped as high as possible. Data were recorded and analyzed to calculate the maximum vertical jump height, the power output [Power = (51.9·CMJ height in cm) + (48.9·Body Mass in kg) − 2007], and the power per body mass [25]. The highest jump height was used in the statistical analysis. The intra-class correlation coefficients (ICC) for the CMJ height, the power production, and the power per body mass were 0.989 [95% Confident intervals (CI): Lower = 0.957, Upper = 0.997], 0.980 (95% CI: Lower = 0.985, Upper = 0.990), and 0.981 (95% CI: Lower = 0.978, Upper = 0.991), respectively.

2.5. Squat Jumps

Following the CMJs, athletes performed the SJs. Similarly to the CMJs test, athletes performed 3 SJs attempts with sub-maximal intensity followed by 4 SJs attempts with maximal intensity. More specifically, the athletes remained in a standing position with arms akimbo; then, the athletes performed an individual self-selected semi-squat and remained motionless until the researcher gave them the instruction to jump. No countermovement was allowed. The highest jump height was used in the statistical analysis. Data were recorded and analyzed (Optojump Next, Warwickshire, UK) for calculating the maximum vertical jump height, the power output [Power = (60.7·SJ height in cm) + (45.3·Body Mass in kg) − 2055], and the power per body mass [25]. The ICC for the SJ height, the power production, and the power per body mass were 0.979 (95% CI: Lower = 0.962, Upper = 0.998), 0.985 (95% CI: Lower = 0.989, Upper = 0.991), and 0.989 (95% CI: Lower = 0.968, Upper = 0.995), respectively.

2.6. Drop Jumps

Ten minutes after the SJ test, the athletes performed the DJ test. Three different drop heights were used: 20, 30, and 40 cm. All athletes were familiar with the technique of the DJ since they had performed it before, in previous similar measurements, in the same laboratory. For warming-up purposes, two DJ attempts with sub-maximal intensity were allowed from 20 cm drop height for all athletes, and after 3 min, the athletes performed 3 DJ attempts with maximal intensity with arms akimbo from all drop heights with a randomized order (Optojump Modular System, Warwickshire, UK). Two minutes of rest were allowed between each attempt. Athletes stepped on the box with arms akimbo and projected their limb of choice in front of them and outside the box. Then, they were instructed to let their body fall down with both their feet touching the ground simultaneously. Researchers also instructed the athletes to minimize the ground contact time as much as possible (floor is lava) and then to jump as high as possible. Data were recorded and analyzed to calculate the time flight, the contact time, the jump height, the RSI, and the reactive strength ratio (RSR) [26]. The DJ with the best RSI was used for the statistical analysis [27]. The ICCs for the time flight, the contact time, the jump height, the RSI, and the RSR were 0.987 (95% CI: Lower = 0.934, Upper = 0.998), 0.961 (95% CI: Lower = 0.795, Upper = 0.993), 0.987 (95% CI: Lower = 0.934, Upper = 0.998), 0.995 (95% CI: Lower = 0.971, Upper = 0.999), and 0.996 (95% CI: Lower = 0.980, Upper = 0.999), respectively.

2.7. Isokinetic Knee Extension Peak Torque and Rate of Torque Development

Fifteen minutes after the DJs, athletes performed the isometric knee extension measurement on an isokinetic dynamometer (HUMAC NORM isokinetic extremity system, Massachusetts, USA) for the evaluation of the quadriceps maximum IPT and RTD. The athletes were seated on the isokinetic dynamometer chair, and straps were used to ensure the stable position of the shoulders, the hips, and the non-tested leg. The tested leg was determined during the familiarization session [28]. Additionally, both hips were at 110° flexion while the knee angle was set at 60° flexion (0° = full extension) [29,30]. Three submaximal effort trials were performed with progressively increasing force, and then 3 maximal effort trials were performed. Athletes were instructed to apply their maximum force as fast as possible and to sustain it for 3 s. Real-time visual feedback of the torque applied was provided for each effort via a computer monitor placed just in front of the athlete, while athletes received verbal encouragement to apply their maximum force. Data from the isometric measurement were recorded and analyzed from the isometric torque–time curve. Maximum IPT was calculated as the greater torque generated from the torque–time curve, while RTD was calculated as the mean tangential slope of the torque–time curve in specific windows of 0–20, 0–40, 0–60, 0–80, 0–100, 0–120, 0–150, 0–200, and 0–250 milliseconds. The ICC for the IPT was 0.990 (95% CI: Lower = 0.964, Upper = 0.998), and for the RTD, it was 0.893 (95% CI: Lower = 0.649, Upper = 0.972).

2.8. Statistical Analysis

All data are presented as means ± SD. Performance in the snatch, the clean and jerk, and the total were collected as absolute values and transformed according to the Sinclair formula, which is a polynomial equation for weightlifters and is used as a method of obviating body mass differences in weightlifting total [13,31]. Pearson's r product-moment correlation coefficient was used to explore the relationships between the weightlifting performance (Sinclair values) with the CMJ, the SQJ, the DJ, the IPT, and the RTD. In addition, Hopkins scales were used to investigate the magnitude of effect for the correlations: trivial < 0.10; small < 0.10–0.29; moderate ≤ 0.30–0.49; large ≤ 0.50–0.69; very large ≤ 0.70–0.89; and nearly perfect ≥ 0.9 [32]. A three-way analysis of variance for repeated measures was used to examine differences between the DJ heights (20, 30 40 cm) with a Bonferroni correction.

Due to the small sample size, the Hedges g effect size was calculated. Reliability for all measurements was performed using a two-way random effect ICC with 95% CI. Significance was accepted at $p \leq 0.05$.

3. Results

All weightlifters completed all performance tests without experiencing any injury. Table 1 presents the results from the snatch, the clean and jerk, and the total expressed both with absolute and Sinclair values, as well as the variables calculated from the CMJ, the SJ, the IPT, and the RTD.

Table 1. Weightlifting performance expressed both in absolute (kg) and Sinclair values: countermovement jump, squat jump, lower body isometric peak torque, and rate of torque development results.

Snatch (kg)	100.1 ± 11.2
Clean and Jerk (kg)	124.0 ± 16.0
Total (kg)	224.1 ± 26.1
Snatch (Sinclair)	122.3 ± 12.0
Clean and Jerk (Sinclair)	151.6 ± 18.0
Total (Sinclair)	274.0 ± 28.6
CMJ height (cm)	48.6 ± 9.9
CMJ power (W)	4448.2 ± 659.1
CMJ power/body mass (W/kg)	55.2 ± 6.2
SJ height (cm)	44.3 ± 10.0
SJ power (W)	4278.7 ± 744.0
SJ power per body mass (W/kg)	53.1 ± 7.3
IPT (N·m^{-1})	331.4 ± 51.7
RTD40 (N·m^{-1}·s^{-1})	1873.1 ± 444.6
RTD60 (N·m^{-1}·s^{-1})	1946.6 ± 439.8
RTD80 (N·m^{-1}·s^{-1})	1978.3 ± 397.3
RTD100 (N·m^{-1}·s^{-1})	1848.4 ± 331.8
RTD120 (N·m^{-1}·s^{-1})	1770.6 ± 342.0
RTD150 (N·m^{-1}·s^{-1})	1651.2 ± 314.4
RTD200 (N·m^{-1}·s^{-1})	1403.6 ± 255.6
RTD250 (N·m^{-1}·s^{-1})	1173.3 ± 215.6

SJ = squat jump, CMJ = countermovement jump, IPT = isometric peak torque, RTD = rate of torque development.

Results from the DJ are presented in Figure 1. Specifically, the flight time was significantly longer for the 40 cm condition compared with 20 cm ($p = 0.013$, $g = 0.888$), but not when compared with the 30 cm drop height ($p = 0.065$, $g = 0.436$). No significant difference was found for contact time between conditions ($p = 0.058$). Jump height was significantly greater for the 40 cm compared with the 20 cm condition ($p = 0.015$, $g = 0.848$), but not when compared with the 30 cm drop height ($p = 0.072$, $g = 0.428$). No significant difference was found for the RSI ($p = 0.128$) and the RSR ($p = 0.102$) between all conditions. Almost all athletes achieved their best RSI and RSR from the 40 cm drop height, except for one who achieved his best RSI and RSR from the 20 cm drop height. Consequently, the optimum average drop height for the best RSI for all athletes was 37.1 ± 7.6 cm.

All variables from the CMJ and the SJ were significantly positively correlated with weightlifting performance (Table 2). In addition, the contact time, the RSI, and the RSR from the DJs were largely correlated with weightlifting performance (Table 3). Trivial to small correlations were found between the flight time and the jump height from the DJs with weightlifting performance (r ranging from −0.037 to 0.258). In addition, significant positive correlations were found between the snatch and the total with the best individual RSI (Figure 2), while the correlation between the clean and jerk with the RSI was almost significant (r = 0.736, $p = 0.059$, very large). Similarly, significant positive correlations were found between the RSR with the snatch (r = 0.923, $p = 0.003$, nearly perfect), with the total (r = 0.844, $p = 0.017$, very large), and almost with the clean and jerk (r = 0.731, $p = 0.062$, very large).

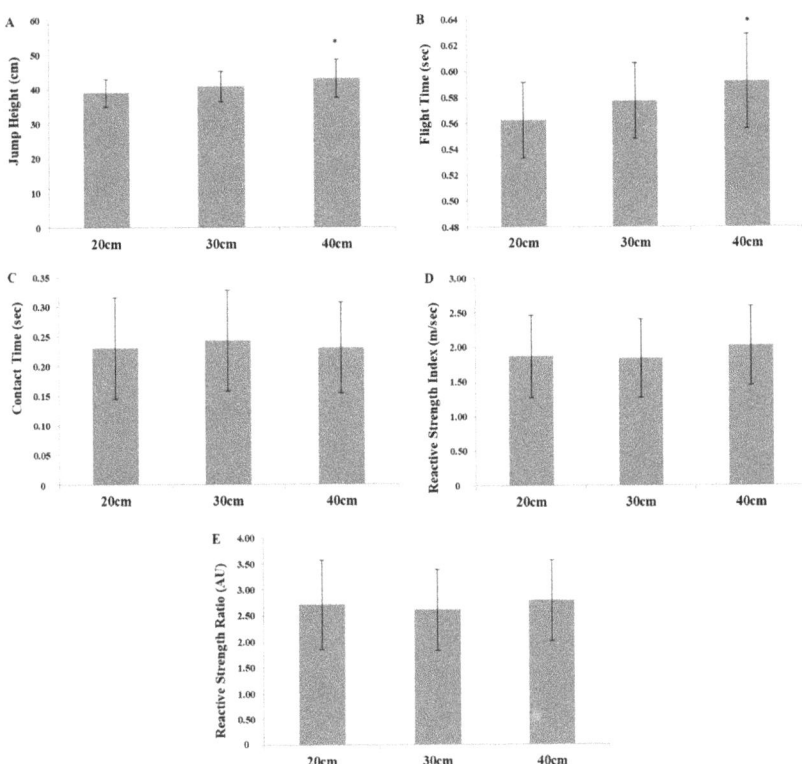

Figure 1. Results from the drop jump test: (**A**) jump height, (**B**) flight time, (**C**) contact time, (**D**) reactive strength index, and (**E**) reactive strength ratio; * $p < 0.05$, significant difference between 40 and 20 cm drop heights.

Table 2. Correlation coefficients between the squat jump and the countermovement jump with weightlifting performance, expressed with Sinclair formula.

	Squat Jump			Countermovement Jump		
	Jump Height	Power	Power per Body Mass	Jump Height	Power	Power per Body Mass
Snatch	0.885 **#	0.753 #	0.890 **#	0.797 *#	0.661 ‡	0.794 *#
Clean and Jerk	0.765 *#	0.634 †	0.780 *#	0.754 #	0.602 ‡	0.762 *#
Total	0.852 *#	0.715 #	0.864 *#	0.808 *#	0.656 ‡	0.813 *#

* $p < 0.05$, ** $p < 0.01$; ‡ large $\leq$ 0.50–0.69; # very large $\leq$ 0.70–0.89.

Table 3. Correlation coefficients between the drop jump from three different drop heights (20, 30, and 40 cm) with weightlifting performance, expressed with Sinclair formula.

	Drop Jump 20 cm			Drop Jump 30 cm			Drop Jump 40 cm		
	Contact Time	RSI	RSR	Contact Time	RSI	RSR	Contact Time	RSI	RSR
Snatch	−0.885 **#	0.866 *#	0.892 **#	−0.899 **#	0.875 **#	0.912 **#	−0.879 **#	0.922 **§	0.920 **#
Clean and Jerk	−0.617 ‡	0.704 #	0.684 ‡	−0.599 ‡	0.673 ‡	0.665 ‡	−0.610 ‡	0.710 #	0.689 ‡
Total	−0.759 *#	0.806 *#	0.804 *#	−0.754 #	0.790 *#	0.801 *#	−0.753 #	0.833 *#	0.819 *#

RSI = Reactive strength index, RSR = reactive strength ratio, * $p < 0.05$, ** $p < 0.01$; ‡ large $\leq$ 0.50–0.69; # very large $\leq$ 0.70–0.89; and § nearly perfect $\geq$ 0.9.

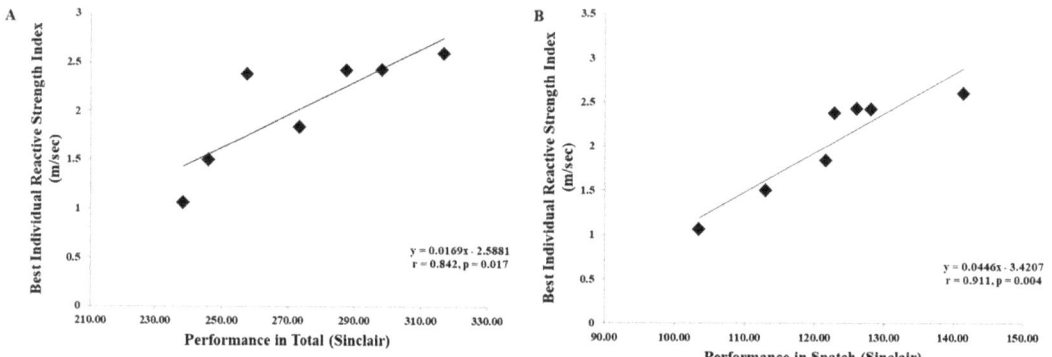

Figure 2. Correlation between the best individual reactive strength index with (**A**) total and (**B**) snatch.

Isometric peak torque was significantly correlated with the snatch (r = 0.796, p = 0.032, very large), almost with the clean and jerk (r = 0.652, p = 0.112, large), and nearly with the total (r = 0.744, p = 0.054, very large). Small to very large correlations were found between the RTD in all time windows and weightlifting performance (Table 4).

Table 4. Correlation coefficients between the rate of torque development with weightlifting performance, expressed with Sinclair formula.

	RTD 20 ms	RTD 40 ms	RTD 60 ms	RTD 80 ms	RTD 100 ms	RTD 120 ms	RTD 150 ms	RTD 200 ms	RTD 250 ms
Snatch	−0.254 ¥	0.315 †	0.718 #	0.725 #	0.726 #	0.751 #	0.766 *#	0.749 #	0.703 #
Clean and Jerk	−0.347 †	0.349 †	0.681 ‡	0.583 ‡	0.660 ‡	0.668 ‡	0.650 ‡	0.651 ‡	0.623 ‡
Total	−0.325 †	0.352 †	0.730 #	0.671 ‡	0.720 #	0.735 #	0.730 #	0.724 #	0.687 ‡

IPT = isometric peak torque, RTD = rate of torque development,* p < 0.05; ¥ small < 0.10–0.29; † moderate ≤ 0.30–0.49; ‡ large ≤ 0.50–0.69 and # very large ≤ 0.70–0.89.

4. Discussion

The purpose of the present study was to investigate the relationship between the RSI during the DJs and the knee extension IPT and RTD with weightlifting performance. The main findings of the study were as follows: (a) the RSI and the contact time calculated from the DJs were significantly correlated with weightlifting performance, (b) individual RSI was significantly positively correlated with the total and the snatch weightlifting performance, and (c) the knee extension IPT and the RTD were moderately to largely correlated with weightlifting performance. These results suggest that the RSI, similar to the CMJ and the SJ, may be a reliable predictor of weightlifting performance, while coaches may consider using the best individual RSI result for predicting weightlifting performance in well-trained male weightlifters. Based also on the current results, a single-joint test, such as the isometric knee extension, may be a moderate predictor of weightlifting performance in well-trained weightlifters.

As expected, weightlifting performance was significantly correlated with all variables of the CMJ and the SJ. Previous studies have shown that performance in the CMJ and the SJ were significantly correlated with weightlifting performance in both male and female weightlifters [6–11,13]. Additionally, a recent meta-analysis showed that performance in the CMJ and the SJ are the best predictors for weightlifting performance [14]. These strong correlations are derived from the biomechanical similarities, and mainly of the lower body triple extension (hip, knee, and ankle extensors), which may be observed in both weightlifting movements and vertical jumping attempts [8,19]. However, whether RSI from the DJ may be correlated with weightlifting performance was unclear. The findings of the present study showed that the contact time, the RSI, and the RSR were the main variables from all DJ heights that were strongly correlated with weightlifting performance. The DJ is a technical demanding vertical jump, in comparison to the CMJ and the SJ, which requires producing a short-time eccentric contraction phase followed by a rapid concentric vertical jump effort [15]. Similarly, during the end of the second pull, in both the snatch and the clean movements, weightlifters drive their bodies under the barbell, emphasizing the strong placement of their lower bodies on the ground. Then, the weightlifters move the barbell overhead (snatch) or on their shoulders (clean), generating a strong whole-body eccentric muscle contraction followed by an abrupt concentric muscle contraction in an attempt to overcome the lifting load and recover in the standing position. Due to these similarities, it might be hypothesized that the RSI and the RSR, as calculated from the DJ, might be strong predictors of weightlifting performance. Therefore, coaches and strength and conditioning professionals may consider using the DJs during training or prior to main competitions for evaluating the athlete's preparedness before the major competitions. Interestingly, lower correlations were found between the RSI and the clean and jerk, which might be attributed to the presence of the jerk in the movement pattern, masking perhaps a stronger correlation outcome. Although the 1-RM strength in the back squat and the front squat or/and in the power snatch and the power clean may be better predictors for competitive performance [14], coaches may consider using a simple, easily executed and practical field test, like the DJ, which provides an index of explosiveness (RSI, RSR) and is also a good predictor of weightlifting performance. However, these results should be viewed with caution since, according to the authors' knowledge, this is the first study that investigated the correlation between the RSI and the RSR with weightlifting performance. More research is required to reach certain conclusions.

Comparison between the different DJ heights showed that the flight time and the jumping height were greater for the 40 cm drop height compared to the 20 cm drop height but not when compared with the 30 cm drop height. In addition, no significant difference was observed for the contact time, the RSI, and the RSR between all conditions evaluated. Therefore, both jumping heights from 30 and 40 cm may be optimal to calculate the RSI and the RSR, although an individual drop height should be preferred. These results are in line with a previous study of 45 college athletes from various sports, which showed that stronger athletes can maintain their reactive strength ability during the DJ compared to their weaker counterparts [33]. Weightlifters who participated in the current study were among the strongest athletes in their body mass category in their country. Moreover, the athletes achieved their best RSI and RSR scores from an optimum drop height of approximately 37 cm. A previous study of 17 national-level power and team sport athletes showed that the optimum drop height was 29.4 ± 16.0 cm, although this was calculated from four different drop heights of 20, 40, 60 and 80 cm [27]. Since, in the current study, six out of seven athletes achieved their best RSI and RSR scores from the 40 cm height, it can be speculated that a 40 cm drop height might be a piece of practical and valuable training information for coaches and strength and conditioning professionals for attempting to increase the power performance of their weightlifters. Still, future studies should focus on the investigation of even higher DJ heights in well-trained weightlifters.

A very large correlation was found between the IPT with the snatch and the total, while the clean and jerk was largely positively correlated with the IPT. Similar to the present findings, a study of sixty-seven male weightlifters under the age of 17 showed significant correlations between the isokinetic knee extension strength at 60, 90, and 180 deg/sec and weightlifting performance (r = 0.597, 0.693, and 0.725, respectively) [23]. However, several studies have shown stronger correlations between weightlifting performance and multi-joint isometric tests such as the isometric mid-thigh pull [6,9,13,21] and the isometric leg press [7,10,11]. The knee extension IPT is a single-joint movement involving only the quadriceps muscles. Consequently, coaches may consider using this particular laboratory test with caution for predicting weightlifting future performance. Additionally, large to very large correlations (ranging from 0.581 to 0.766) were found between the knee extension

RTD in time windows from 0–60 ms to 0–250 ms with the weightlifting performance. Similar results were found in previous studies using the isometric mid-thigh pull and the isometric leg press in trained (r ranging from 0.62 to 0.76) [13], sub-elite (r ranging from 0.580 to 0.767) [21], well-trained (r ranging from 0.446 to 0.655) [10], and elite weightlifters (females; r ranging from 0.69 to 0.80; males; r ranging from 0.660 to 0.733) [7,9]. Thus, the isometric knee extension RTD may also be a valid test for the evaluation of fast force production and for assessing the preparedness of the neuromuscular system in well-trained weightlifters. However, more studies are required to reach safe, relevant conclusions.

This study describes the correlation between the RSI, the knee extension IPT, and the RTD with weightlifting performance in well-trained male weightlifters. The small sample size and the different weight mass categories of the athletes may partially limit the generalization of the results. This particular limitation might be partly counterbalanced by the high level of athletic performance and the long-term training experience of the athletes. Still, weightlifting is an explosive sporting event, where muscle fiber types and neural factors may contribute to performance results; neither fiber type composition nor electromyographic activity were examined in the present study, which might have provided a better understanding of the current results. Further studies should examine the role of the DJ from different drop heights (including heights above 40 cm) as well as the knee extension IPT and the RTD in larger groups of weightlifters and in female weightlifters.

5. Conclusions

The contact time, the RSI and the RSR from the DJ may be strong predictors of weightlifting performance in well-trained weightlifters. These results suggest that coaches may regularly include DJs in their training programs in order to increase lower body power and predict the weightlifting performance of their athletes. Moreover, when athletes approach the competition period and the training load-volume is reduced, then coaches may use DJ scores as an index of the muscular explosiveness and readiness of their athletes before main competitions. Although both the 30 and 40 cm drop heights may effectively be used for all athletes during training, coaches should regularly estimate the optimal individual drop height of each athlete in an attempt to maximize the RSI and the RSR. Additionally, when access to the isometric mid-thigh pull or the isometric leg press performance tests is limited, then the knee extension RTD may be used to predict weightlifting performance and the status of the neuromuscular system of the weightlifter. Therefore, it is suggested that, in line with the CMJ and the SJ power tests, coaches may also effectively use the DJ, the knee extension IPT, and the RTD to predict weightlifting performance in well-trained weightlifters.

Author Contributions: Conceptualization, G.A. and N.Z.; data curation, G.A. and N.Z.; investigation, G.A., M.H. and N.Z.; methodology, G.A. and N.Z.; software, N.Z.; supervision, N.Z.; writing—original draft, G.A., G.T. and N.Z.; writing—review and editing, G.A., M.H., G.T. and N.Z. All authors have read and agreed to the published version of the manuscript.

Funding: This research received no external funding.

Institutional Review Board Statement: The study was conducted according to the guidelines of the Declaration of Helsinki and approved by the National Ethics Committee of Cyprus (protocol code EEBK/EΠ/2020/55, 4 December 2020).

Informed Consent Statement: Informed consent was obtained from all subjects involved in the study.

Data Availability Statement: The data presented in this study are available upon request from the corresponding author.

Acknowledgments: Authors express their gratitude to the athletes who participated in the study.

Conflicts of Interest: The authors declare no conflict of interest.

References

1. Cunanan, A.J.; Hornsby, W.G.; South, M.A.; Ushakova, K.P.; Mizuguchi, S.; Sato, K.; Kyle, C.P.; Stone, M.H. Survey of barbell trajectory and kinematics of the snatch lift from the 2015 world and 2017 pan-American weightlifting championships. *Sports* **2020**, *8*, 118. [CrossRef]
2. Kauhanen, H. A biomechanical analysis of the snatch and clean & jerk techniques of Finish elite and district level weightlifters. *Scand. J. Sports Sci.* **1984**, *6*, 47–56.
3. Storey, A.; Smith, H.K. Unique aspects of competitive weightlifting. *Sports Med.* **2012**, *42*, 769–790. [CrossRef] [PubMed]
4. Blazevich, A.J.; Wilson, C.J.; Alcaraz, P.E.; Rubio-Arias, J.A. Effects of resistance training movement pattern and velocity on isometric muscular rate of force development: A systematic review with meta-analysis and meta-regression. *Sports Med.* **2020**, *50*, 943–963. [CrossRef]
5. Haff, G.G.; Jackson, J.R.; Kawamori, N.; Carlock, J.M.; Hartman, M.J.; Kilgore, J.L.; Morris, R.T.; Ramsey, M.W.; Sands, W.A.; Stone, M.H. Force-time curve characteristics and hormonal alterations during an eleven-week training period in elite women weightlifters. *J. Strength Cond. Res.* **2008**, *22*, 433–446. [CrossRef]
6. Joffe, S.A.; Tallent, J. Neuromuscular predictors of competition performance in advanced international female weightlifters: A cross-sectional and longitudinal analysis. *J. Sports Sci.* **2020**, *38*, 985–993. [CrossRef]
7. Zaras, N.; Stasinaki, A.N.; Spiliopoulou, P.; Arnaoutis, G.; Hadjicharalambous, M.; Terzis, G. Rate of force development, muscle architecture, and performance in elite weightlifters. *Int. J. Sports Physiol. Perform.* **2020**, *16*, 216–223. [CrossRef]
8. Carlock, J.M.; Smith, S.L.; Hartman, M.J.; Morris, R.T.; Ciroslan, D.A.; Pierce, K.C.; Newton, R.U.; Harman, E.A.; Sands, W.A.; Stone, M.H. The relationship between vertical jump power estimates and weightlifting ability: A field-test approach. *J. Strength Cond. Res.* **2004**, *18*, 534–539.
9. Haff, G.G.; Carlock, J.M.; Hartman, M.J.; Kilgore, J.L. Force-time curve characteristics of dynamic and isometric muscle actions of elite women olympic weightlifters. *J. Strength Cond. Res.* **2005**, *19*, 741.
10. Kelekian, G.K.; Zaras, N.; Stasinaki, A.N.; Spiliopoulou, P.; Karampatsos, G.; Bogdanis, G.; Terzis, G. Preconditioning strategies before maximum clean performance in female weightlifters. *J. Strength Cond. Res.* **2022**, *36*, 2318–2321. [CrossRef]
11. Zaras, N.; Stasinaki, A.N.; Spiliopoulou, P.; Hadjicharalambous, M.; Terzis, G. Lean body mass, muscle architecture, and performance in well-trained female weightlifters. *Sports* **2020**, *8*, 67. [CrossRef] [PubMed]
12. Vizcaya, F.J.; Viana, O.; del Olmo, M.F.; Acero, R.M. Could the deep squat jump predict weightlifting performance? *J. Strength Cond. Res.* **2009**, *23*, 729–734. [CrossRef] [PubMed]
13. Hornsby, W.G.; Gentles, J.A.; MacDonald, C.J.; Mizuguchi, S.; Ramsey, M.W.; Stone, M.H. Maximum strength, rate of force development, jump height, and peak power alterations in weightlifters across five months of training. *Sports* **2017**, *5*, 78. [CrossRef] [PubMed]
14. Joffe, S.A.; Price, P.; Chavda, S.; Shaw, J.; Tallent, J. The relationship of lower-body, multijoint, isometric and dynamic neuromuscular assessment variables with snatch, and clean and jerk performance in competitive weightlifters: A meta-analysis. *Strength Cond. J.* **2023**, *45*, 411–428. [CrossRef]
15. Suchomel, T.J.; Sole, C.J.; Stone, M.H. Comparison of methods that assess lower-body stretch-shortening cycle utilization. *J. Strength Cond. Res.* **2016**, *30*, 547–554. [CrossRef]
16. Flanagan, E.P.; Comyns, T.M. The use of contact time and the reactive strength index to optimize fast stretch-shortening cycle training. *Strength Cond. J.* **2008**, *30*, 32–38. [CrossRef]
17. Kipp, K.; Kiely, M.T.; Giordanelli, M.D.; Malloy, P.J.; Geiser, C.F. Biomechanical determinants of the reactive strength index during drop jumps. *Int. J. Sports Physiol. Perform.* **2018**, *13*, 44–49. [CrossRef]
18. Garhammer, J. Biomechanical profiles of Olympic weightlifters. *J. Appl. Biomech.* **1985**, *1*, 122–130. [CrossRef]
19. Isaka, T.; Okada, J.; Funato, K. Kinematic analysis of the barbell during the snatch movement of elite Asian weight lifters. *J. Appl. Biomech.* **1996**, *12*, 508 516. [CrossRef]
20. Campos, J.; Poletaev, P.; Cuesta, A.; Pablos, C.; Carratalà, V. Kinematical analysis of the snatch in elite male junior weightlifters of different weight categories. *J. Strength Cond. Res.* **2006**, *20*, 843–850.
21. Beckham, G.; Mizuguchi, S.; Carter, C.; Sato, K.; Ramsey, M.; Lamont, H.; Hornsby, G.; Haff, G.; Stone, M. Relationships of isometric mid-thigh pull variables to weightlifting performance. *J. Sports Med. Phys. Fitness* **2013**, *53*, 573–581. [PubMed]
22. Zaras, N.; Stasinaki, A.N.; Spiliopoulou, P.; Mpampoulis, T.; Hadjicharalambous, M.; Terzis, G. Effect of inter-repetition rest vs. traditional strength training on lower body strength, rate of force development, and muscle architecture. *Appl. Sci.* **2021**, *11*, 45. [CrossRef]
23. Ince, I.; Ulupinar, S. Prediction of competition performance via selected strength-power tests in junior weightlifters. *J. Sports Med. Phys. Fitness* **2020**, *60*, 236–243. [CrossRef] [PubMed]
24. Ammar, A.; Chtourou, H.; Trabelsi, K.; Padulo, J.; Turki, M.; El Abed, K.; Hoekelmann, A.; Hakim, A. Temporal specificity of training: Intra-day effects on biochemical responses and Olympic-Weightlifting performances. *J. Sports Sci.* **2015**, *33*, 358–368. [CrossRef]
25. Sayers, S.P.; Harackiewicz, D.V.; Harman, E.A.; Frykman, P.N.; Rosenstein, M.T. Cross-validation of three jump power equations. *Med. Sci. Sports Exerc.* **1999**, *31*, 572–577. [CrossRef] [PubMed]
26. Healy, R.; Kenny, I.C.; Harrison, A.J. Reactive strength index: A poor indicator of reactive strength? *Int. J. Sports Physiol. Perform.* **2018**, *13*, 802–809. [CrossRef] [PubMed]

27. Tsoukos, A.; Veligekas, P.; Brown, L.E.; Terzis, G.; Bogdanis, G.C. Delayed effects of a low-volume, power-type resistance exercise session on explosive performance. *J. Strength Cond. Res.* **2018**, *32*, 643–650. [CrossRef]
28. Elias, L.J.; Bryden, M.P.; Bulman-Fleming, M.B. Footedness is a better predictor than is handedness of emotional lateralization. *Neuropsychologia* **1998**, *36*, 37–43. [CrossRef]
29. Ioannides, C.; Apostolidis, A.; Hadjicharalambous, M.; Zaras, N. Effect of a 6-week plyometric training on power, muscle strength, and rate of force development in young competitive karate athletes. *J. Phys. Educ. Sport* **2020**, *20*, 1740–1746. [CrossRef]
30. Panteli, N.; Hadjicharalambous, M.; Zaras, N. Delayed potentiation effect on sprint, power and agility performance in well-trained soccer players. *J. Sci. Sport Exerc.* **2023**, *5*, 1–9. [CrossRef]
31. Stone, M.H.; Sands, W.A.; Pierce, K.C.; Carlock, J.O.N.; Cardinale, M.; Newton, R.U. Relationship of maximum strength to weightlifting performance. *Med. Sci. Sports Exerc.* **2005**, *37*, 1037–1043. [CrossRef] [PubMed]
32. Hopkins, W.G. Measures of reliability in sports medicine and science. *Sports Med.* **2000**, *30*, 1–15. [CrossRef] [PubMed]
33. Beattie, K.; Carson, B.P.; Lyons, M.; Kenny, I.C. The relationship between maximal strength and reactive strength. *Int. J. Sports Physiol. Perform.* **2017**, *12*, 548–553. [CrossRef] [PubMed]

Disclaimer/Publisher's Note: The statements, opinions and data contained in all publications are solely those of the individual author(s) and contributor(s) and not of MDPI and/or the editor(s). MDPI and/or the editor(s) disclaim responsibility for any injury to people or property resulting from any ideas, methods, instructions or products referred to in the content.

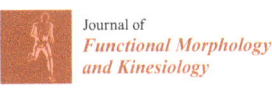

Article

Muscle Strength and Joint Range of Motion of the Spine and Lower Extremities in Female Prepubertal Elite Rhythmic and Artistic Gymnasts

Athanasios Mandroukas, Ioannis Metaxas, Yiannis Michailidis and Thomas Metaxas *

Laboratory of Evaluation of Human Biological Performance, Department of Physical Education and Sport Sciences, Aristotle University of Thessaloniki, 57001 Thessaloniki, Greece; amandrou@phed.auth.gr (A.M.); metaxasi@phed-sr.auth.gr (I.M.); ioannimd@phed.auth.gr (Y.M.)
* Correspondence: tommet@phed.auth.gr

Abstract: The purpose of this study was to investigate and compare the passive joint range of motion (PROM) and muscle strength in prepubertal rhythmic gymnasts (RGs), artistic gymnasts (AGs), and a control group (CG) of the same age. A total of 54 prepubertal girls were divided into three groups: 18 RGs (age 11.14 ± 0.7, height 142.6 ± 5.81, and body mass 31.2 ± 3.63); 18 AGs (age 11.27 ± 0.99, height 139.6 ± 5.85, and body mass 31.7 ± 3.21), and 18 school girls who are defined as CG (age 10.55 ± 0.42, height 145.33 ± 6.95, and body mass 42.1 ± 8.21) participated in the study. All athletes were elites and participated in national competitions. The CG participated only in their school physical education program. Isokinetic peak torques were measured using an isokinetic dynamometer (Cybex II) at 60, 180, and 300°·sec^{-1}. Body mass index was greater in the CG compared to RGs and AGs ($p < 0.001$). PROM in cervical extension in RG was significantly higher compared to the AG and CG ($p < 0.001$). The athlete groups, RG and AG, showed significantly greater PROM in knee flexion ($p < 0.001$), hip flexion ($p < 0.001$), and hip abduction ($p < 0.05$) compared to CG. PROM in hip flexion was different between the left and right leg in RGs. The relative muscle strength of the quadriceps in the RG and AG was significantly greater compared to CG ($p < 0.001$ and $p < 0.01$ respectively). Gymnastics training in prepubertal ages can improve neuromuscular function and increase the relative muscle strength. Therefore, it is essential to note that when evaluating children within the developmental ages, especially those involved in sports, the type of muscle strength to be assessed should be specified.

Keywords: rhythmic gymnastics; artistic gymnastics; muscle strength; range of motion; back; lower extremities

Citation: Mandroukas, A.; Metaxas, I.; Michailidis, Y.; Metaxas, T. Muscle Strength and Joint Range of Motion of the Spine and Lower Extremities in Female Prepubertal Elite Rhythmic and Artistic Gymnasts. *J. Funct. Morphol. Kinesiol.* **2023**, *8*, 153. https://doi.org/10.3390/jfmk8040153

Academic Editor: Diego Minciacchi

Received: 12 September 2023
Revised: 31 October 2023
Accepted: 1 November 2023
Published: 2 November 2023

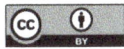

Copyright: © 2023 by the authors. Licensee MDPI, Basel, Switzerland. This article is an open access article distributed under the terms and conditions of the Creative Commons Attribution (CC BY) license (https://creativecommons.org/licenses/by/4.0/).

1. Introduction

Children's physical activity is increasingly characterized by the specialization in a specific sport. Furthermore, the sport requirements and competition have been increased significantly as suggested by the high intensity of the workouts and the frequency of the competitions. With respect to rhythmic gymnastics and artistic gymnastics, the selection of the girls is made from a very young age. Age is an important factor for the selection of athletes in these sports, which require muscle strength, large range of motion, and the combination of these, in order to achieve maximal performance [1,2]. The long and intense training of female athletes can cause, among other things, qualitative changes in the neuromuscular function with favorable conditions for explosive power and vitality [3,4]. At this age the skeleton is soft, and the endurance of the tendons and ligaments is greater than the endurance of the skeleton [5]. As a consequence of improved neuromuscular adaptations, the functional training in rhythmic gymnasts (RGs) and artistic gymnasts (AGs) leads to the correct technique of their particular sports, because, even at these ages, there are changes in the muscle architecture (penal angle), increased coordination, and balance between prime mover or agonist and antagonist muscles [6,7]. The aforementioned are sine qua non to achieve great performances, but, at the same time, they expose the athletes to a great risk of possible repetitive strain injury [8,9].

Rhythmic gymnastics as an artistic sport is highly demanding in the complexity of skills. Exercise in this sport involves coordinating different body parts with the apparatus: the ball, hoop, club, ribbon, and rope. A gymnast might achieve excellent performance when she is able to execute the specific exercises indicating her physical abilities at the best level and showing mastery of the special apparatus movements required by the international Code of Points [10]. Artistic gymnastics is a complex sport consisting of technical skills in the events of floor exercise, the uneven bars, the balance beam, and the vault. Training in both rhythmic and artistic gymnastics requires repetitive and long-lasting workouts in the fundamental elements and the basic positions [11,12] demanding the coordination of handling various apparatus. Muscle strength and power, muscle endurance, as well as large range of motion are required to attain positions not seen very often in sports. Other studies have associated the risk of developing lower back complaints with the specific sports that demand repetitive or high velocity twisting or repetitive bending flexibility, particularly in extension [13,14]. Athletes participating in sports such as rhythmic and artistic gymnastics have been shown to be at increased risk of developing lower back complaints [14–19]. The kind of movements of RGs and AGs require high muscle strength of lower extremities, abdominals, and back muscles. Sufficient muscle strength of the hamstrings and quadriceps is a prerequisite for female athletes to learn proper movement technique and meet the demands of the sport. Conversely, insufficient (decreased) muscle strength can lead to incorrect technique which can negatively affect performance and increase the risk of injury [20]. Furthermore, when there is an imbalance in the relationship between joint range of motion and muscle power, the optimal movement pattern is disrupted and the posture of the spine will be affected, thereby increasing the risk of injury [20,21]. To the best of our knowledge there are few studies examining isokinetic torque and joint passive range of motion (PROM) including RGs compared to AGs and non-exercisers (untrained girls). Thus, the purpose of this study was to examine and compare the joint mobility and muscle strength of the spine and lower extremities in prepubertal elite athletes in rhythmic gymnastics, artistic gymnastics, and untrained participants.

2. Materials and Methods
2.1. Participants

The power analysis was conducted prior to the study being performed, based on previous studies of similar research design [22,23]. An effect size of >0.6, a probability error of 0.05, and a power of 0.95 were used for the 3 groups. Those indicated that 48 participants was the smallest acceptable number of participants to analyze the interaction. The calculations for effect size (ES) and statistical power were performed using G*Power software: Statistical Power Analyzes for Windows, Version 3.1.9.7 according to Cohen's f criteria [24]. This study involved 54 girls, divided into 3 groups: 18 RGs, 18 AGs, and 18 school girls who are defined as the control group (CG) participated in the study. All athletes participated in national competitions. CG participated only in their school's physical education program (2 to 3 40 min weekly classes), which consisted of mainly ball-games, stretching exercises, some calisthenics, and did not take part in any other sport activities in organized form. Basic anthropometric data of the groups are shown in Table 1.

Participants visited the laboratory on two occasions one day apart. The first visit was an orientation session that included anthropometric assessments, measurements of the joint PROM, and also a questionnaire that included their relevant physical and medical profile. In the second visit the participants were tested on the isokinetic dynamometer. After 5 min rest in the supine position, the heart rate (HR) using a monitor (Polar Electro, Sweden) and the blood pressure (BP) using a cuff on the left arm were recorded.

Table 1. Physical characteristics of the participants (means ± SD).

	Rhythmic Gymnasts (RG) (n = 18)	Artistic Gymnasts (AG) (n = 18)	Control Group (CG) (n = 18)
Age (years)	11.14 ± 0.70	11.27 ± 0.99 +	10.55 ± 0.42
Height (cm)	142.6 ± 5.81	139.6 ± 5.85	145.33 ± 6.95 ++
Body mass (kg)	31.2 ± 3.63	31.7 ± 3.21	42.1 ± 8.21 ### +++
Body mass index (Kg/m^2)	15.22 ± 1.76	16.67 ± 1.85	20.06 ± 2.90 ### +++
Years in training (years)	4.03 ± 0.8	4.40 ± 0.5	0
Hours of daily training (hours)	3.83 ± 0.65 *	3.42 ± 0.28	0

* $p < 0.05$ comparison between RGs and AGs, + $p < 0.05$ comparison between the CG and AGs, ++ $p < 0.01$ comparison between the CG and AGs, +++ $p < 0.001$ comparison between the CG and AGs, and ### $p < 0.001$ comparison between the CG and RGs.

Participants reported no musculoskeletal injuries of the lower limbs that would prevent them from performing maximal isokinetic contractions. None of the participants had been doing progressive resistive exercise the previous day before the testing. Participants underwent a though-knee examination before the test. All participants and their parents were informed of the nature, purpose, procedures, potential discomfort, risks, and benefits involved in the study before giving their voluntary written consent for participation. All participants completed a questionnaire that included their relevant medical and physical history. No participant was taking any medication prior to the study that might affect the results of the experiment. This study has been approved by the Institutional Review Board of the Exercise Physiology and Sport Rehabilitation Laboratory, Thessaloniki, Greece (No. 02/2021) and was in accordance with the Declaration of Helsinki.

2.2. Testing Procedures—Measurements of the Joint PROM

Standing height was measured without shoes to the nearest 1.0 cm, using a stadiometer (model 220, Seca, Hamburg, Germany). Body mass was measured to the nearest 0.1 kg using an electronic digital scale (model 770, Seca), with the participants wearing only training shorts. The body mass index (BMI) was calculated as the ratio of body mass in kg to the square of the standing body height in m (kg/m^2).

Joint PROM was tested by two experienced physical therapists that paid special attention in the way the movement began, its stability, as well as the direction of the movement. No warm-up exercises were performed prior to the testing procedures. Both legs were measured and the PROM was recorded. The measurements were taken in a quiet room and all groups were measured for standing height, body mass, and mobility of the spine, hip, and knee joints. Testing procedures were conducted between 11 a.m. and 2 p.m., and the environment temperature was around 22 °C. Participants performed a 5 min warm-up only before muscle strength measurement.

Hip abduction was measured using a Lafayette Gollehon extendable goniometer [25,26], and the rest of the movements were conducted using the Myrin goniometer (Lic Rehab, 17183 Solna, Sweden), which has shown advantages in clinical trials [27] and is reliable [28]. The position of the goniometer was standardized in relation to the anatomical landmarks. All measurements were made on an adjustable bench and were evaluated passively without causing pain at the same time of the day. Three repetitions of the test were carried out for each joint and the highest value was recorded. Joint mobility of the lower extremity was tested in the hip flexion, knee flexion, and hip abduction. In the spine the PROM of the cervical, thoracic, and lumbar spine were examined. Before measuring the articular mobility of the spine in each participant, all the spinous processes from the seventh cervical vertebra (C7) to the first sacral vertebrae (S1) were marked with a red pen. In addition, a straight line in the posterior superior iliac spines and the anterior superior iliac crests was also drawn.

2.2.1. Knee Flexion (Test of the Quadriceps Femoris)

The participant was laid in the prone position on the examination bench. The ankle joint was in plantar flexion just outside the bench. The pelvis was immobilized with a Velcro band to be in constant with the examination bench. The Myrin goniometer was placed 5 cm above the lateral malleolus and adjusted to zero. The examiner used his hand to apply straight equal pressure to the participant's ankle so as to avoid an inward turn of the hip (if the direction of the movement is wrong, the leg extremity that is the ankle joint and the foot would move to the other side of the gluteus maximus muscle). The examiner's pressure was such as to lead the joint through its largest possible orbit without causing pain [29,30]. The other test leader read and took note of the passive joint flexibility, otherwise known as the personal PROM. There were three separate measurements for each participant with small breaks in between. The largest orbit was then recorded.

2.2.2. Hip Flexion—Straight Leg Raising Test (SLR) (Test of the Hamstring Muscles)

The participant was laid in the supine position on the examination bench; the goniometer was strapped to the lateral side of the thigh 5 cm above the patella and was adjusted to zero. Velcro bands immobilized the pelvis and the opposite leg. The examiner moved one of the participant's legs to his shoulder and asked the participant to relax. The examiner, with one hand, stabilized the ankle joint not allowing the internal rotation of the hip and placed the other hand on the participant's straight knee [30,31]. The second examiner recorded the results of any passive movement. Both examiners measured the final orbit of motion.

2.2.3. Hip Abduction (Test of the Adductor Muscles)

With the participant supine on a bench, the Lafayette Gollehon extendable goniometer was placed on a transverse line connecting the anterior superior iliac spines. The fulcrum was adjusted over the iliac spine and the movable arms were strapped to the thighs above the patella. The pelvis was stabilized with a special belt when measuring to keep it still. The hips were in full abduction and knees straight [30].

2.3. Testing Procedures—Mobility of the Spine

2.3.1. Trunk flexion (Stibor Test)

The participant was in the upright position. The identification of the spinous process of the C7 was made after palpation of the 6th and 7th cervical vertebrae. When the head was extended the spinous process of the 6th cervical vertebra could no longer be palpated, whereas the C7 could be palpated. The one end of the metering was placed in the spinous process of C7 and the other on the spinous process of S1. The participant, with stretched knees, hands free, and head relaxed, bends the trunk forward [30,32,33]. In full flexion of the trunk the increased difference was measured (Figure 1).

2.3.2. Cervical Spine

The measurements were performed in 3 planes of movement: flexion—extension, lateral flexion, and axial rotation to both right and left side.

2.3.3. Flexion and Extension of the Cervical Spine

The participant was in a seated position with trunk and head in a straight position. A solid ribbon with Myrin goniometer attached was placed around the head at the point just above the ear. The index of the goniometer pointed to zero. The examiner, giving instructions for the proper movement of the head, stabilized the trunk with once hand while the other hand lightly pressed the participant's head forward. The extension of the head was made from the same starting point, with the trunk stabilized in a similar manner and the goniometer mounted at the same point [27,34].

2.3.4. Lateral Flexion of the Cervical Spine

The participant sat with a straight trunk and head. The stabilizing ribbon was tied around the head, while the Myrin goniometer was placed on the forehead. The index of the goniometer pointed to zero. The examiner stabilized the shoulder with one hand while the other hand lightly pressed the participant's head in the extreme left position (left lateral bending) and then right (right lateral bending). During the lateral bending the participant was instructed to avoid turning the head [27,34].

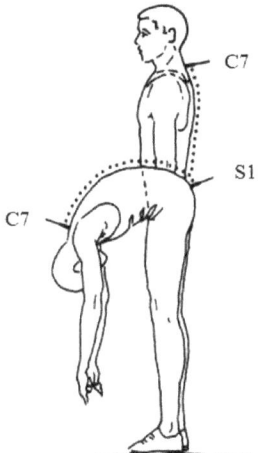

Figure 1. Measurement of the trunk flexion from the upright position (Stibor test). The identification of the seventh cervical vertebra (C7) to the first sacral vertebra (S1).

2.3.5. Rotation of the Cervical Spine

The participant was either seated with a straight trunk and head in the supine position or lying down. The measurement was performed from both starting positions and no differences were found. The adhesive ribbon was placed around the head and the goniometer at the top of it. The index of the goniometer pointed to zero. The examiner stabilized the trunk of the participant and pushed the head slightly to the extreme rotating position [27,34]. The assistant recorded the cervical rotating (left and right) mobility.

2.3.6. Lateral Flexion of the Trunk

The participant was in the upright position with the legs slightly stretched. From this position with the arms stretched and attached to the body, the contact point of the middle finger on the thigh (left and right) was recorded with a pen. After left and right trunk flexion, the contact point of the middle finger on the thigh was re-registered. The distance difference between the two points was measured. During bending the examiner controlled the movement of the participant so as to avoid rotating the torso and pelvis [35,36]. This measurement was performed for the mobility of the thoraco–lumbar junction (Figure 2).

2.3.7. Lumbar Spine (Shober Test)

The participant was in the standing position. The examiner, who was standing behind the participant, identified the posterior superior iliac spines using palpation and marked a straight line corresponding to the height of the spinous process of the 4th sacral vertebra. To secure the neutral position of the pelvis, the upper anterior iliac spines in the anterior part of the body were also marked by the examiner. Then, from the spinous process of the S1 was measured 10 cm upwards, i.e., to the level of the 1st and 2nd lumbar vertebrae (L1–L2). In trunk flexion with knees stretched, the difference will be increased by about 4–5 cm (Figure 3) [30,32,33,37].

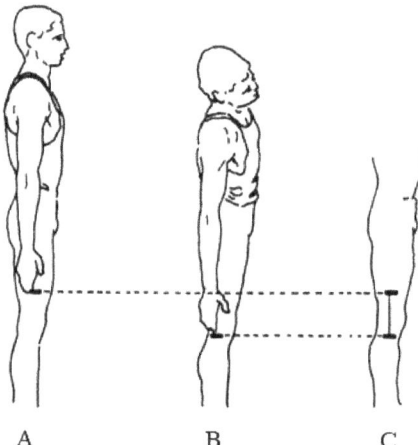

Figure 2. Lateral flexion of the trunk from the upright position. The distance difference between the two points (**A**) and (**B**) was measured (**C**).

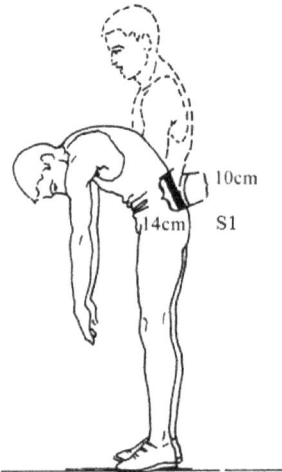

Figure 3. Measurement of the flexion of the lumbar spine (Schober test). From the standing position the distance from the S1 to 10 cm upwards was measured. In trunk flexion in this distance was increased by 4–5 cm.

2.3.8. Thoracic Spine (Ott Test)

The participant was in the standing position. The mobility of the thoracic spine was measured from the spinous process of the C7 and 30 cm downwards. Then, the same distance was measured with the participant in a bending position, where the difference in flexion between positions will be increased by about 3 cm [30,32,38] (Figure 4).

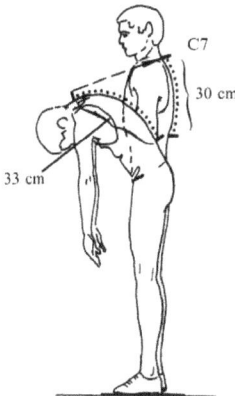

Figure 4. Measurement of the flexion of the thoracic spine (Ott test). The mobility of the thoracic spine was measured from C7 and 30 cm downwards in standing and bending positions. The difference between positions was increased by about 3 cm.

2.4. Concentric Isokinetic Muscle Strength Measurements

Peak torque was measured using a speed controlled isokinetic dynamometer (Cybex II, Lumex Inc., Ronkonkoma, NY, USA), with a specially designed program which included torque comparison adjusted to the weight of the leg. Prior to the testing session, participants followed a standardized warm-up on a cycle ergometer (Monark 839, Varberg, Sweden) for 5 min with low resistance at 60 rev/min, prior to all strength measurements. This exercise was followed by a 5 min partial passive stretching of the knee flexors and extensors according to Mandroukas et al. [22] and the unilateral concentric muscle strength of the dominant leg was measured. The leg used most frequently for kicking the ball was identified as the dominant leg. The factors for the evaluation of strength performance were the absolute peak torque (APT) and the relative peak torque (RPT). APT is defined as the best value from all repetitions and RPT in relative to body mass values, for every type of movement and velocity.

Testing Protocol

For each angular velocity peak isokinetic torque was recorded simultaneously and the torque generated by the limb weight and the dynamometer arm was extracted from the obtained data. The participants were sitting on the chair of the dynamometer with stabilization straps at the trunk, thigh, and tibia to prevent extraneous joint movement. The knee to be tested was positioned at 90° of flexion (0° corresponding to fully extended knee) to align the axis of the dynamometer lever arm with the distal point of the lateral femoral condyle. The length of the lever arm was individually determined, and the resistance pad was placed at 5 cm above the malleoli. The non-tested leg was hanging freely. Knee extension started when the knee was positioned at 90° of flexion, while the knee flexion started when the knee was in full extension (0°). Alignment with an electronic goniometer (Lafayette Instrument Company, Indiana) was used for accuracy of the knee angle positioning and alignment of the joint prior to and during testing sessions. All participants, prior to the commencement of the testing, were familiarized with the isokinetic movements by performing several submaximal contractions under the guidance of the investigators. Participants were instructed to kick the leg as hard and as fast as they could through a complete ROM. Verbal encouragement was given during every trial. Participants were instructed to hold their arms comfortably across their chest to further isolate knee flexion and extension movements. Three repetitions were carried out at each angular velocity, and the best torque value was used. The trial proceeded from the high angular velocity to the low angular velocity. A 30 s rest period between each velocity was given and 60 sec rest period between each velocity measurement. Maximal isokinetic strength was recorded as the torque of the quadriceps and hamstring muscles throughout the whole ROM, at angular velocities of 60, 180, and $300°·s^{-1}$. The concentric strength ratio between the knee flexors and the knee extensors (H:Q ratio) was expressed as the ratio between the peak values at each velocity. The conventional H:Q ratio was calculated by dividing each participant's highest concentric PT leg flexion by the highest concentric PT leg extension.

2.5. Statistical Analysis

Statistical analysis was undertaken using SPSS V.26.0 (SPSS Inc., Chicago, IL, USA). Initially, descriptive statistics were used to calculate means and standard deviations for the testing sessions, for all groups. One-way analysis of variance (ANOVA) and post hoc analysis (Scheffé test) were used to determine which groups in the ANOVA differed from each other. Effect sizes for variance analyses were given as partial eta squared (η_p^2) with values ≥ 0.01, ≥ 0.06, and ≥ 0.14 indicating small, moderate, or large effects, respectively [24]. Also, Cohen's d was evaluated for the t-test as following: d = 0.2 small; d = 0.5 medium; d = 0.8 large; and d = 1.3 very large [24]. The level of statistical significance was set at $p < 0.05$.

3. Results

The RG athletes had a significantly greater ROM in head extension compared to the AG athletes and CG participants ($p < 0.001$, $\eta_p^2 = 0.454$). However, no differences were found among the three groups in left ($\eta_p^2 = 0.050$) and right ($\eta_p^2 = 0.065$) lateral flexion, forward flexion ($\eta_p^2 = 0.011$), and rotation ($\eta_p^2 = 0.072$) (Figure 5).

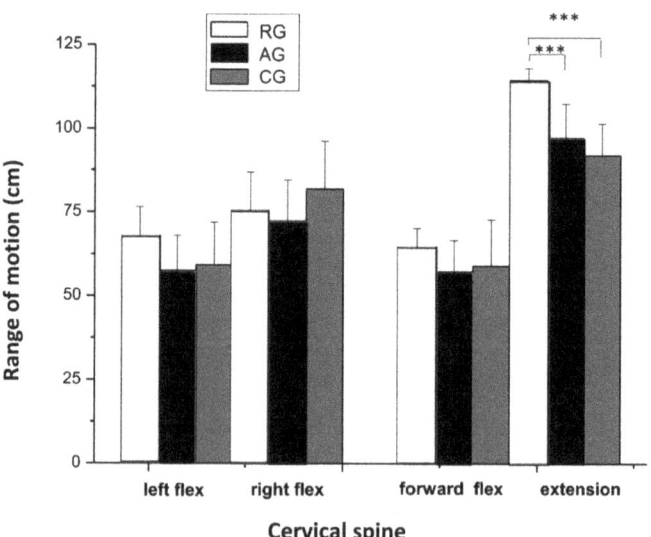

Figure 5. Cervical joint range of motion (means ± SD) during left and right lateral flexion, forward flexion, and extension. RG = rhythmic gymnasts, AG = artistic gymnasts, and CG = control group; *** $p < 0.001$.

The ROM at the lumbar spine was significantly greater ($p < 0.01$, $\eta_p^2 = 0.437$) in the RG athletes compared with AG athletes. No significant differences were found among the three groups in the ROM of the thoracic spine ($\eta_p^2 = 0.064$); the flexion of the trunk from the standing position, from C7 to S1 ($\eta_p^2 = 0.055$); and the lateral bending of the trunk (left–right lateral flexion, $\eta_p^2 = 0.058$) (Figure 6).

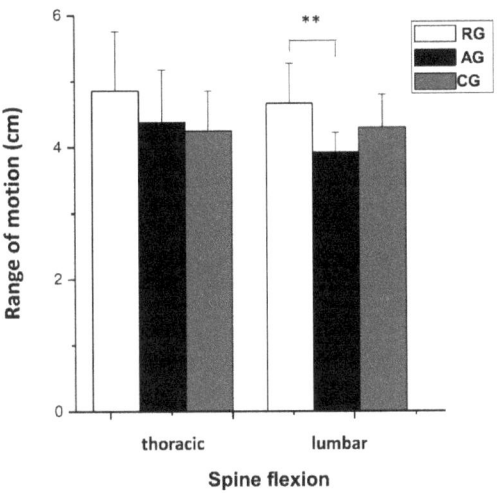

Figure 6. Thoracic and lumbar spine range of motion (means ± SD). RG = rhythmic gymnasts, AG = artistic gymnasts, and CG = control group; ** $p < 0.01$.

The RG group showed significantly greater ROM in knee flexion ($p < 0.001$; right leg: $\eta_p^2 = 0.344$, left leg: $\eta_p^2 = 0.320$), hip flexion ($p < 0.001$; right leg: $\eta_p^2 = 0.913$, left leg: $\eta_p^2 = 0.902$), and hip abduction ($p < 0.05$, right leg: $\eta_p^2 = 0.194$, left leg: $\eta_p^2 = 0.196$) compared to the CG. Also, the ROM was greater in hip flexion ($p < 0.001$) and hip abduction ($p < 0.05$) in the AG group in comparison to the CG. However, no significant differences were found between the RG and AG groups. These results were similar for both the right and left leg (Figure 7).

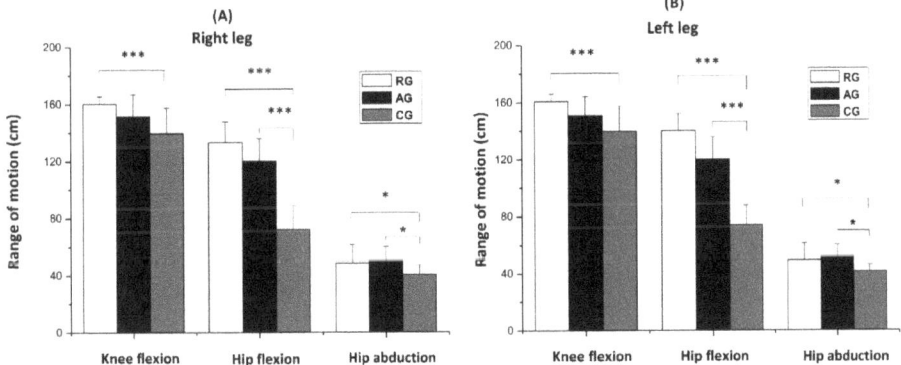

Figure 7. Range of motion (means ± SD) of the knee flexion, hip flexion, and hip abduction of the right leg (**A**) and left leg (**B**). RG = rhythmic gymnasts, AG = artistic gymnasts, and CG = control group; * $p < 0.05$ and *** $p < 0.001$.

Surprisingly, a significant difference was observed in the ROM of hip flexion in the RG group, where the right leg was significantly higher, compared to the left leg ($p < 0.01$, d = 0.5). No significant differences were observed between the left and right leg in hip flexion for the AGs (d = 0.1) and CG (d = 0.1) (Figure 8).

The results of the absolute and relative isokinetic muscle strength between the RGs, AGs, and CG are shown in Table 2. In the absolute isokinetic concentric muscle strength of the quadriceps, the CG had significantly greater strength at $180° \cdot s^{-1}$ ($\eta_p^2 = 0.221$) and

$300°·s^{-1}$ ($\eta_p^2 = 0.238$), compared to the RGs ($p < 0.01$ and $p < 0.05$) and AGs ($p < 0.05$, respectively) groups. No significant differences were found among the three groups, at the slow angular velocity ($60°·s^{-1}$, $\eta_p^2 = 0.058$). However, the relative muscle strength of the quadriceps in the RG and AG groups was significantly greater at $60°·s^{-1}$ compared to the CG ($p < 0.001$ and $p < 0.01$, respectively; $\eta_p^2 = 0.221$) and between the AGs and CG at $180°·s^{-1}$ ($p < 0.05$, $\eta_p^2 = 0.153$). Nevertheless, no significant differences were shown between the RG and CG groups. In knee flexion there were no significant differences in absolute muscle strength between the groups ($60°·s^{-1}$: $\eta_p^2 = 0.019$, $180°·s^{-1}$: $\eta_p^2 = 0.032$, $300°·s^{-1}$: $\eta_p^2 = 0.093$) as well as in the H:Q ratio ($60°·s^{-1}$: $\eta_p^2 = 0.026$, $180°·s^{-1}$: $\eta_p^2 = 0.169$, $300°·s^{-1}$: $\eta_p^2 = 0.028$). However, a significant difference was observed in the relative muscle strength at $60°·s^{-1}$ between RGs and the CG ($p < 0.05$, $\eta_p^2 = 0.184$).

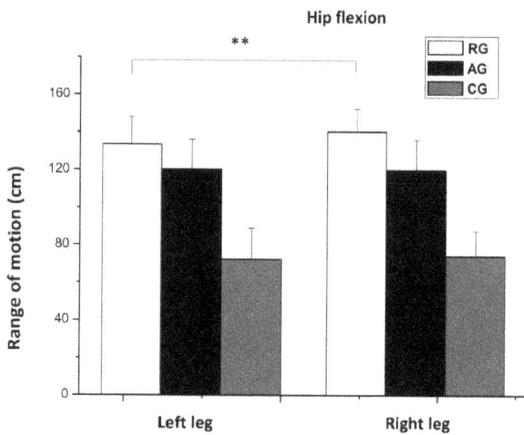

Figure 8. Range of motion (means ± SD) of the hip flexion (hamstring muscles). Comparison between right and left legs among the three groups. RG = rhythmic gymnasts, AG = artistic gymnasts, and CG = control group; ** $p < 0.01$.

Table 2. Quadriceps and Hamstring peak torque values (Nm) and relative body mass values (Nm·kg^{-1}BW) at angular velocities of 60, 180, and $300°·s^{-1}$. Comparison between RGs, AGs, and CG (mean ± SD).

		RG	AG	CG
Quadriceps absolute values (Nm)	$60°·s^{-1}$	82.33 ± 13.3	79.85 ± 11.7	89.89 ± 25.0
	$180°·s^{-1}$	48.28 ± 8.9 ++	53.92 ± 7.9 #	63.11 ± 16.6
	$300°·s^{-1}$	34.28 ± 6.1 +	34.85 ± 4.7 #	44.17 ± 12.2
Hamstring absolute values (Nm)	$60°·s^{-1}$	41.22 ± 7.0	41.31 ± 9.1	44.00 ± 11.7
	$180°·s^{-1}$	26.78 ± 5.1	27.31 ± 7.7	29.56 ± 7.0
	$300°·s^{-1}$	18.00 ± 3.7	17.54 ± 5.9	21.56 ± 7.1
Quadriceps relative to body mass values (Nm·kg^{-1}BW)	$60°·s^{-1}$	2.63 ± 0.25 +++	2.51 ± 0.26 ##	2.14 ± 0.40
	$180°·s^{-1}$	1.55 ± 0.19	1.69 ± 0.14 #	1.50 ± 0.24
	$300°·s^{-1}$	1.09 ± 0.14	1.09 ± 0.66	105 ± 0.19
Hamstring relative to body mass values (Nm·kg^{-1}BW)	$60°·s^{-1}$	1.32 ± 0.19 +	1.29 ± 0.22	1.07 ± 0.30
	$180°·s^{-1}$	0.86 ± 0.19	0.85 ± 0.20	0.71 ± 0.18
	$300°·s^{-1}$	0.58 ± 0.20	0.54 ± 0.16	0.51 ± 0.14
Hamstings:Quadriceps ratio	$60°·s^{-1}$	50.07 ± 5.3	51.73 ± 8.3	48.95 ± 7.5
	$180°·s^{-1}$	55.34 ± 5.7	50.65 ± 9.7	46.84 ± 7.8
	$300°·s^{-1}$	52.51 ± 6.1	50.33 ± 12.5	48.81 ± 7.3

# $p < 0.05$ comparison between AGs and CG, ## $p < 0.01$ comparison between AGs and CG, + $p < 0.05$ comparison between RGs and CG, ++ $p < 0.01$ comparison between RGs and CG, and +++ $p < 0.001$ comparison between RGs and CG.

4. Discussion

The purpose of this study was to examine and compare the joint mobility and muscle strength of the spine and lower extremities in prepubertal elite athletes in rhythmic gymnastics, artistic gymnastics, and untrained subjects of the same age. The results of the study showed that the PROM in cervical extension was notably higher in the RG compared to the AGs and CG. Moreover, both athlete groups, RG and AG, exhibited significantly greater PROM in knee flexion, hip flexion, and hip abduction in comparison to the CG. Additionally, the relative muscle strength of the quadriceps in the RGs and AGs was significantly higher than in the CG.

In agreement with previous studies, the RGs are thinner than average [39] and they have lower BMI than untrained peers [40,41], while the AGs have a mean height score below the 50th percentile [42]. In addition, young AGs appear to have some lower anthropometric characteristics compared to other athletes (e.g., swimmers) and non-athletes [43]. Anthropometric characteristics are significant predictors to performance in rhythmic gymnastics [44] and artistic gymnastics [45].

Generally, the torque–velocity relationship in young populations indicates a similar, adult-like pattern: as the angular velocity increased the peak torque decreased. Quadriceps muscle strength is greater than hamstrings at all angular velocities and in all groups. Several authors have mentioned that in these ages there are no differences between boys and girls. Basa et al. [46] suggested that long-term gymnastic training in prepubertal boys was associated with increased torque of the knee extensors but not of the knee flexors, which is consistent with the findings of our study. Thus, training in gymnastics, artistic and rhythmic, in prepubescent ages may not be associated with increased torque of the knee flexors. Several points of this finding should be taken under consideration. First, muscle strength can be influenced by body size [47] and participants in the CG were taller and heavier than athletes. It is known that individuals with higher body mass have greater absolute strength. This study showed that RGs had greater relative muscle strength because of their lower body mass. There is the possibility that the participants of the three groups under observation were in different levels of sexual maturity (Tanner stage); for example, athletes could be in stage I, whereas the participants of the CG could be in stage II. Moreover, it is well known that elite RGs have an observed delay in pubertal development [48] and skeletal maturation [49]. Second, at this age, physical activities are part of the child's everyday-life activity and so participants in the CG cannot be considered fully sedentary, as is mentioned in another study [50]. All children have taken part in physical education classes at school, which can increase their strength [51]. Finally, in rhythmic gymnastics the high scores in strength tests do not seem to be related to success, as elite RGs do not produce especially high scores in the above tests [52].

RGs were more flexible than both the AGs and the CG. In rhythmic gymnastics, lean body mass and composite measures of joint mobility are significant correlates of attainment [41] and flexibility correlates significantly to performance [53,54]. Some studies have shown that AGs are characterized by a special physical characteristic in comparison to their non-athletic peers or athletes of other sports [55,56]. The selection of the athletes performed by the coaches relates to the demands of the sports (i.e., muscle strength and power and muscle endurance), in order to present mechanical advantages in performing the exercises. Most body exercises in rhythmic gymnastics are based on ballet and are performed by an "en de hors" (turn-out) turn of joints [57]; so, from their early training years they practice performing joints turn-outs, unlike the artistic gymnastics. Probably, in artistic gymnastics a turn-out joint mobility does not help the execution of specific elements. Based on the code, artistic gymnastic elements use less "en de hors" turn of joints in hip abduction. This could be the reason why, in assessing right hip abduction, AGs have higher joint mobility. Spinal mobility was significantly higher for RGs. According to the code in every body group (jumps, balances, turns, and flexibility), elements with back bends obtain a higher evaluation [58]. Back extensions and split leaps with back extensions are common elements in this type of gymnastics, so this emphasis on flexibility and repetitive demand of back extensions places the lumbar spine of the athletes at risk [15]. Increased lumbar lordosis can result in anterior pelvic tilt, which due to repeated loads may lead to spondylolysis [59]. The close relationship between spondylolysis and increased pelvic tilt (i.e., increased lumbosacral angle) has been observed in competitive gymnasts [60]. Therefore, it would be preferable to pay attention to the whole spine or better to its coordination, rather than to the hypermobility of one segment.

Exercises and training programs guided by the rules of evaluation increase mobility in the bending angle of the part of the spine which is already flexible enough and not in the part which shows limited mobility. This refers to the limited mobility of the thoracic spine and the excessive mobility of the lumbar spine. Repetitive hyperextensions in the lumbar spine contribute to overloading the spine. However, it must be pointed out that the spine consists of layers of muscles, some of which have the ability to shorten and others to lengthen [61]. Hence, in terms of muscle strength and mobility, it is hard to find the right way to treat it.

Limitations and Future Directions

This study had several limitations. The biological age was not examined; therefore, there is a possibility that the participants of the three groups under observation were in different levels of sexual maturity (Tanner stage), where the results of the study may have been affected. Also, the participants were prepubertal girls; therefore, the extrapolation of our finding into a general gymnastic should be performed with caution, and care should be taken when applying the study results. Another limitation is that the muscle strength was measured using an isokinetic dynamometer, in the muscle groups of quadriceps and hamstring, and in concentric knee flexion/extension. Therefore, further research should focus on other muscle groups, as well as eccentric strength measurements. Also, future research should include functional strength tests that are related to the sport and important for success in specific gymnastic performance.

5. Conclusions

The present study examined the muscle strength and joint range of motion of the back and lower extremities in prepubertal female RGs, AGs, and a CG. The results of the present study have shown that RGs were more flexible than AGs, which could be a result of their specific sport training and the requirements of the sport. Significant differences were found between left and right leg hip flexion in RGs. This study has also shown that gymnastics training in prepubertal ages, both rhythmic and artistic, can improve neuromuscular function, i.e., technique, and increase relative muscle strength. Therefore, it is essential to note that when evaluating children within the developmental ages, especially those involved in sports, the type of muscle strength to be assessed should be specified.

Author Contributions: Conceptualization, A.M., I.M. and Y.M.; methodology, A.M., I.M., Y.M. and T.M.; software, A.M. and I.M.; validation, A.M., Y.M. and T.M.; formal analysis, A.M. and I.M.; investigation, A.M., I.M., Y.M. and T.M.; resources, A.M., I.M. and Y.M.; data curation, A.M., I.M. and Y.M.; writing—original draft preparation, A.M., I.M. and Y.M.; writing—review and editing, A.M., I.M., Y.M. and T.M.; visualization, A.M. and I.M.; supervision, T.M.; project administration, A.M., I.M. and Y.M. All authors have read and agreed to the published version of the manuscript.

Funding: This research received no external funding.

Institutional Review Board Statement: The study was conducted according to the guidelines of the Declaration of Helsinki and approved by the Institutional Review Board of the Exercise Physiology and Sport Rehabilitation Laboratory, Thessaloniki, Greece (No. 02/2021 approved 30 November 2021).

Informed Consent Statement: Informed consent was obtained from all subjects involved in the study.

Data Availability Statement: The data presented in this study are available on request from the corresponding author. The data are not publicly available due to privacy restrictions.

Acknowledgments: The authors would like to thank all the participants who volunteered to participate in the study.

Conflicts of Interest: The authors declare no conflict of interest.

References

1. Malina, R.M.; Baxter-Jones, A.D.; Armstrong, N.; Beunen, G.P.; Caine, D.; Daly, R.M.; Lewis, R.D.; Rogol, A.D.; Russell, K. Role of intensive training in the growth and maturation of artistic gymnasts. *Sports Med.* **2013**, *43*, 783–802. [CrossRef] [PubMed]
2. Baxter-Jones, A.D.; Helms, P.J. Effects of Training at a Young Age: A Review of the Training of Young Athletes (TOYA) Study. *Pediatr. Exerc. Sci.* **1996**, *8*, 310–327. [CrossRef]
3. Ford, P.; De Ste Croix, M.; Lloyd, R.; Meyers, R.; Moosavi, M.; Oliver, J.; Till, K.; Williams, C. The long-term athlete development model: Physiological evidence and application. *J. Sports Sci.* **2011**, *29*, 389–402. [CrossRef]
4. Bencke, J.; Damsgaard, R.; Saekmose, A.; Jørgensen, P.; Jørgensen, K.; Klausen, K. Anaerobic power and muscle strength characteristics of 11 years old elite and non-elite boys and girls from gymnastics, team handball, tennis and swimming. *Scand. J. Med. Sci. Sports* **2002**, *12*, 171–178. [CrossRef] [PubMed]
5. Bajin, B. Talent identification program for Canadian female gymnasts. In *World Identification Systems for Gymnastic Talent*; Sports Psyche Editions: Montreal, QC, USA, 1987; pp. 34–44.
6. Blimkie, C.J. Resistance training during pre- and early puberty: Efficacy, trainability, mechanisms, and persistence. *Can. J. Sport Sci.* **1992**, *17*, 264–279.
7. Rowland, T.W. *Children's Exercise Physiology*, 2nd ed.; Human Kinetics: Champaign, IL, USA, 2005; pp. 80–84.
8. Kirialanis, P.; Malliou, P.; Beneka, A.; Giannakopoulos, K. Occurrence of acute lower limb injuries in artistic gymnasts in relation to event and exercise phase. *Br. J. Sports Med.* **2003**, *37*, 137–139. [CrossRef]
9. Paxinos, O.; Mitrogiannis, L.; Papavasiliou, A.; Manolarakis, E.; Siempenou, A.; Alexelis, V.; Karavasili, A. Musculoskeletal injuries among elite artistic and rhythmic Greek gymnasts: A ten-year study of 156 elite athletes. *Acta. Orthop. Belg.* **2019**, *85*, 145–149.
10. Giannitsopoulou, E.; Zisi, V.; Kioumourtzoglou, E. Elite performance in rhythmic gymnastics: Do the changes in code of points affect the role of abilities? *J. Hum. Mov. Stud.* **2003**, *45*, 327–346.
11. Cupisti, A.; D'Alessandro, C.; Evangelisti, I.; Piazza, M.; Galetta, F.; Morelli, E. Low back pain in competitive rhythmic gymnasts. *J. Sports Med. Phys. Fitness* **2004**, *44*, 49–53.
12. Russo, L.; Palermi, S.; Dhahbi, W.; Kalinski, S.D.; Bragazzi, N.L.; Padulo, J. Selected components of physical fitness in rhythmic and artistic youth gymnast. *Sport Sci. Health.* **2021**, *17*, 415–421. [CrossRef]
13. Hutchinson, M.R.; Laprade, R.F.; Burnett, Q.M.; Moss, R.; Terpstra, J. Injury surveillance at the USTA Boys' Tennis Championships: A 6-yr study. *Med. Sci. Sports Exerc.* **1995**, *27*, 826–830. [CrossRef] [PubMed]
14. Garrick, J.G.; Requa, R.K. Epidemiology of women's gymnastics injuries. *Am. J. Sports Med.* **1980**, *8*, 261–264. [CrossRef] [PubMed]
15. Hutchinson, M.R. Low back pain in elite rhythmic gymnasts. *Med. Sci. Sports Exerc.* **1999**, *31*, 1686–1688. [CrossRef]
16. Tanchev, P.I.; Dzherov, A.D.; Parushev, A.D.; Dikov, D.M.; Todorov, M.B. Scoliosis in rhythmic gymnasts. *Spine* **2000**, *25*, 1367–1372. [CrossRef] [PubMed]
17. Ciullo, J.V.; Jackson, D.V. Pars interarticularis stress reaction, Spondylolysis, and spondylolisthesis in gymnasts. *Clin. Sports Med.* **1985**, *4*, 95–110. [CrossRef]
18. Hall, S.J. Mechanical contribution to lumbar stress injuries in female gymnasts. *Med. Sci. Sports Exerc.* **1986**, *18*, 599–602. [CrossRef]
19. Jackson, D.W.; Wiltse, L.L.; Cirincoine, R.J. Spondylolysis in the female gymnast. *Clin. Orthop. Relat. Res.* **1976**, *117*, 68–73. [CrossRef]
20. Croisier, J.L.; Forthomme, B.; Namurois, M.H.; Vanderthommen, M.; Crielaard, J.M. Hamstring muscle strain recurrence and strength performance disorders. *Am. J. Sports Med.* **2002**, *30*, 199–203. [CrossRef]
21. Witvrouw, E.; Danneels, L.; Asselman, P.; D'Have, T.; Cambier, D. Muscle flexibility as a risk factor for developing muscle injuries in male professional soccer players. A prospective study. *Am. J. Sports Med.* **2003**, *31*, 41–46. [CrossRef]
22. Mandroukas, A.; Vamvakoudis, E.; Metaxas, T.; Papadopoulos, P.; Kotoglou, K.; Stefanidis, P.; Christoulas, K.; Kyparos, A.; Mandroukas, K. Acute partial passive stretching increases range of motion and muscle strength. *J. Sports Med. Phys. Fitness* **2014**, *54*, 289–297.
23. Van Dillen, L.R.; Bloom, N.J.; Gombatto, S.P.; Susco, T.M. Hip rotation range of motion in people with and without low back pain who participate in rotation-related sports. *Phys. Ther. Sport* **2008**, *9*, 72–81. [CrossRef] [PubMed]
24. Cohen, J. *Statistical Power Analysis for the Behavioral Sciences*, 2nd ed.; Routledge: New York, NY, USA, 2013; pp. 5–17.
25. Pua, Y.H.; Wrigley, T.V.; Cowan, S.M.; Bennell, K.L. Intrarater test-retest reliability of hip range of motion and hip muscle strength measurements in persons with hip osteoarthritis. *Arch. Phys. Med. Rehabil.* **2008**, *89*, 1146–1154. [CrossRef]
26. Tsolakis, C.; Bogdanis, G.C. Acute effects of two different warm-up protocols on flexibility and lower limb explosive performance in male and female high level athletes. *J. Sports Sci. Med.* **2012**, *11*, 669–675. [PubMed]

27. Malmström, E.M.; Karlberg, M.; Melander, A.; Magnusson, M. Zebris versus Myrin: A comparative study between a three-dimensional ultrasound movement analysis and an inclinometer/compass method: Intradevice reliability, concurrent validity, intertester comparison, intratester reliability, and intraindividual variability. *Spine* 2003, *28*, E433–E440. [CrossRef]
28. Antonaci, F.; Ghirmai, S.; Bono, G.; Nappi, G. Current methods for cervical spine movement evaluation: A review. *Clin. Exp. Rheumatol.* 2000, *18*, S-45–S-52.
29. Piva, S.R.; Goodnite, E.A.; Childs, J.D. Strength around the hip and flexibility of soft tissues in individuals with and without patellofemoral pain syndrome. *J. Orthop. Sports. Phys. Ther.* 2005, *35*, 793–801. [CrossRef] [PubMed]
30. Ekstrand, J.; Wiktorsson, M.; Oberg, B.; Gillquist, J. Lower extremity goniometric measurements: A study to determine their reliability. *Arch. Phys. Med. Rehabil.* 1982, *63*, 171–175. [PubMed]
31. de Lucena, G.L.; dos Santos Gomes, C.; Guerra, R.O. Prevalence and associated factors of Osgood-Schlatter syndrome in a population-based sample of Brazilian adolescents. *Am. J. Sports Med.* 2011, *39*, 415–420. [CrossRef]
32. Elena, B.; Ingrid, P.Š.; Šárka, T.; Jan, V. Effects of an exercise program on the dynamic function of the spine in female students in secondary school. *J. Phys. Educ. Sport* 2018, *18*, 831–839. [CrossRef]
33. Bednár, R.; Líška, D.; Gurín, D.; Vnenčaková, J.; Melichová, A.; Koller, T.; Skladaný, Ľ. Low back pain in patients hospitalised with liver cirrhosis—A retrospective study. *BMC Musculoskelet Disord.* 2023, *24*, 310. [CrossRef]
34. American Academy of Orthopaedic Surgeons. *Joint Motion: Method of Measurement and Recording*; American Academy of Orthopaedic Surgeons: Chicago, IL, USA, 1965.
35. Yoshida, A.; Kahanov, L. The effect of kinesio taping on lower trunk range of motions. *Res. Sports Med.* 2007, *15*, 103–112. [CrossRef] [PubMed]
36. Ito, T.; Shirado, O.; Suzuki, H.; Takahashi, M.; Kaneda, K.; Strax, T.E. Lumbar trunk muscle endurance testing: An inexpensive alternative to a machine for evaluation. *Arch. Phys. Med. Rehabil.* 1996, *77*, 75–79. [CrossRef]
37. Rezvani, A.; Ergin, O.; Karacan, I. Validity and reliability of the Metric Measurements in the Assessment of Lumbar Spine Motion in patients with Ankylosing Spondylitis. *Spine* 2012, *37*, E1189–E1196. [CrossRef] [PubMed]
38. Veis, A.; Kanásová, J.; Halmová, N. The level of body posture, the flexibility of backbone and flat feet in competition fitness in 8–11year old girls. *Trends Sport Sci.* 2022, *29*, 5–11. [CrossRef]
39. Georgopoulos, N.A.; Markou, K.B.; Theodoropoulou, A.; Vagenakis, G.A.; Benardot, D.; Leglise, M.; Dimopoulos, J.C.; Vagenakis, A.G. Height velocity and skeletal maturation in elite female rhythmic gymnasts. *J. Clin. Endocrinol. Metab.* 2001, *86*, 5159–5164. [CrossRef] [PubMed]
40. Boros, S. Dietary habits and physical self-concept of elite rhythmic gymnasts. *Biomed. Hum. Kinet.* 2009, *1*, 1–2. [CrossRef]
41. Hume, P.A.; Hopkins, W.G.; Robinson, D.M.; Robinson, S.M.; Hollings, S.C. Predictors of attainment in rhythmic sportive gymnastics. *J. Sports Med. Phys. Fitness* 1993, *33*, 367–377.
42. Georgopoulos, N.A.; Markou, K.B.; Theodoropoulou, A.; Benardot, D.; Leglise, M.; Vagenakis, A.G. Growth retardation in artistic compared with rhythmic elite female gymnasts. *J. Clin. Endocrinol. Metab.* 2002, *87*, 3169–3173. [CrossRef]
43. Siatras, T.; Skaperda, M.; Mameletzi, D. Anthropometric characteristics and delayed growth in young artistic gymnasts. *Med. Probl. Perform. Art.* 2009, *24*, 91–96. [CrossRef]
44. Douda, H.T.; Toubekis, A.G.; Avloniti, A.A.; Tokmakidis, S.P. Physiological and anthropometric determinants of rhythmic gymnastics performance. *Int. J. Sports Physiol. Perform.* 2008, *3*, 41–54. [CrossRef]
45. Claessens, A.L.; Lefevre, J.; Beunen, G.; Malina, R.M. The contribution of anthropometric characteristics to performance in elite female gymnasts. *J. Sports Med. Phys. Fitness* 1999, *39*, 355–360. [PubMed]
46. Bassa, H.; Michailidis, H.; Kotzamanidis, C.; Siatras, T.; Chatzikotoulas, K. Concentric and eccentric isokinetic knee torque in pre-pubeiscent male gymnasts. *J. Hum. Mov. Stud.* 2002, *42*, 213–227.
47. Jaric, S. Role of body size in the relation between muscle strength and movement performance. *Exerc. Sport Sci. Rev.* 2003, *31*, 8–12. [CrossRef]
48. Klentrou, P.; Plyley, M. Onset of puberty, menstrual frequency, and body fat in elite rhythmic gymnasts compared with normal controls. *Br. J. Sports Med.* 2003, *37*, 490–494. [CrossRef]
49. Georgopoulos, N.A.; Markou, K.B.; Theodoropoulou, A.; Paraskevopoulou, P.; Varaki, L.; Kazantzi, Z.; Leglise, M.; Vagenakis, A.G. Growth and pubertal development in elite female rhythmic gymnasts. *J. Clin. Endocrinol. Metab.* 1999, *84*, 4525–4530. [CrossRef] [PubMed]
50. Vamvakoudis, E.; Vrabas, I.S.; Galazoulas, C.; Stefanidis, P.; Metaxas, T.I.; Mandroukas, K. Effects of basketball training on maximal oxygen uptake, muscle strength, and joint mobility in young basketball players. *J. Strength Cond. Res.* 2007, *21*, 930–936. [CrossRef]
51. Stenevi-Lundgren, S.; Daly, R.M.; Lindén, C.; Gärdsell, P.; Karlsson, M.K. Effects of a daily school based physical activity intervention program on muscle development in prepubertal girls. *Eur. J. Appl. Physiol.* 2009, *105*, 533–541. [CrossRef]
52. Batista, A.; Garganta, R.; Ávila-Carvalho, L. Strength in young rhythmic gymnasts. *J. Hum. Sport Exerc.* 2017, *12*, 1162–1175. [CrossRef]
53. Alexander, M. The physiological characteristics of elite rhythmic sportive gymnasts. *J. Hum. Mov. Stud.* 1989, *17*, 49–69.
54. Frenker, R.; Hitzel, N. Predicting attainment in rhythmic sport gymnastics: A three-year longitudinal study. In Proceedings of the First International Olympic Committee Congress on Sports Medicine, Colorado Springs, CO, USA, 29 October–3 November 1989.

55. Garay, A.L.D.; Levine, L.; Carter, J.E.L. *Genetic and Anthropological Studies of Olympic Athletes*; Academic Press: New York, NY, USA, 1974.
56. Sinning, W.E.; Lindberg, G.D. Physical characteristics of college age women gymnasts. *Res. Q.* **1972**, *43*, 226–234. [CrossRef]
57. Jastrjembskaia, N.; Titov, Y. *Rhythmic Gymnastics*; Echo Point Books & Media: Brattleboro, VT, USA, 2016.
58. Fédération Internationale de Gymnastique. 2022–2024 Code of Points: Rhythmic Gymnastics. Available online: https://www.gymnastics.sport/publicdir/rules/files/en_2022-2024%20RG%20Code%20of%20Points.pdf (accessed on 12 May 2022).
59. Mac-Thiong, J.M.; Labelle, H.; Berthonnaud, E.; Betz, R.R.; Roussouly, P. Sagittal spinopelvic balance in normal children and adolescents. *Eur. Spine J.* **2007**, *16*, 227–234. [CrossRef] [PubMed]
60. d'Hemecourt, P.A.; Luke, A. Sport-specific biomechanics of spinal injuries in aesthetic athletes (dancers, gymnasts, and figure skaters). *Clin. Sports Med.* **2012**, *31*, 397–408. [CrossRef] [PubMed]
61. Janda, V. Muscles, Central Nervous Motor Regulation and Back Problems. In *The Neurobiologic Mechanisms in Manipulative Therapy*; Korr, I.M., Ed.; Springer: Boston, MA, USA, 1978; pp. 27–41. [CrossRef]

Disclaimer/Publisher's Note: The statements, opinions and data contained in all publications are solely those of the individual author(s) and contributor(s) and not of MDPI and/or the editor(s). MDPI and/or the editor(s) disclaim responsibility for any injury to people or property resulting from any ideas, methods, instructions or products referred to in the content.

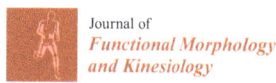

Article

The Reliability of Linear Speed with and without Ball Possession of Pubertal Soccer Players

Nikolaos Manouras, Christos Batatolis, Panagiotis Ioakimidis, Konstantina Karatrantou and Vassilis Gerodimos *

Department of Physical Education and Sports Science, University of Thessaly, 42100 Trikala, Greece
* Correspondence: bgerom@uth.gr

Abstract: Reliable fitness tests with low day-to-day and trial-to-trial variation are a prerequisite for tracking a player's performance or for identifying meaningful changes in training interventions. The present study examined the inter- and intra-session reliability of 30 m linear speed with and without ball possession as well as the reliability of a specific performance index of pubertal soccer players. A total of 40 pubertal (14.87 ± 1.23 years old) male soccer players performed two testing sessions (test–retest) separated by 72 h. Both testing sessions included a protocol consisting of two maximal trials of 30 m linear speed with and without ball possession. A performance index, indicating the difference between the two speed tests, was also calculated using two different equations (delta value and percentage value). The relative and absolute inter-session reliabilities were good/high for all testing variables (ICC = 0.957–0.995; SEM% = 0.62–8.83). There were also good/high relative and absolute intra-session reliabilities observed for all testing variables (ICC = 0.974–0.987; SEM% = 1.26–6.70%). According to the Bland–Altman plots, the differences between test–retest and trials for all observations were within the defined 95% limits of agreement. The reliable testing protocols and performance index for the evaluation of linear speed with and without ball possession, observed in this study, may be used in speed monitoring and training planning of pubertal soccer players.

Keywords: test–retest reproducibility; evaluation; sprint; performance index; dribbling speed; team sports; developmental years

Citation: Manouras, N.; Batatolis, C.; Ioakimidis, P.; Karatrantou, K.; Gerodimos, V. The Reliability of Linear Speed with and without Ball Possession of Pubertal Soccer Players. *J. Funct. Morphol. Kinesiol.* **2023**, *8*, 147. https://doi.org/10.3390/jfmk8040147

Academic Editor: Diego Minciacchi

Received: 13 September 2023
Revised: 7 October 2023
Accepted: 11 October 2023
Published: 16 October 2023

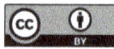

Copyright: © 2023 by the authors. Licensee MDPI, Basel, Switzerland. This article is an open access article distributed under the terms and conditions of the Creative Commons Attribution (CC BY) license (https:// creativecommons.org/licenses/by/ 4.0/).

1. Introduction

Soccer is, mainly, a sport that depends on aerobic metabolism because of its 90 min match duration, but the most crucial actions in a soccer game (i.e., sprinting, jumping, change of direction, and kicking and dribbling a ball) involve the anaerobic metabolic system [1–6]. One of the most important technical skills is sprinting while keeping control of the ball (dribbling the ball), which is considered a hallmark of gifted soccer players [7,8] and decides the outcome of the game [9,10]. According to the official data, each player covers 10,627–12,027 m in a soccer game of which 119–286 m is covered with a ball in possession, depending on the tactical position role of each player [11]. There is also evidence that elite soccer players cover 215–446 m at a top speed of >23 km/h in a soccer game [11]. Therefore, the reliable and valid evaluation of speed with and without a ball in possession in soccer players may be used for physical fitness monitoring (depicting the current physical strengths and weaknesses) and training planning of young soccer players.

Several studies in the scientific literature have examined the validity and the reliability of linear sprint test, using different distances (mainly 5–40 m), in young adults [12] as well as in pre-pubertal and pubertal soccer players [13]. Furthermore, linear sprint tests have shown moderate-to-high intra-session reliability (reliability between trials at the same testing occasion) and inter-session reliability (reliability between the first and the second testing occasions, i.e., test–retest) with ICC values that ranged from 0.57 to 0.98 in young soccer players (using different age groups from U11 to U18) [14–22]. Different factors such as the distance of the sprint, the measured system, the testing protocol, and the time interval between test–retest measurements may affect the reliability of sprint test [16,23–29]; however, future studies are needed to strengthen these findings. Other factors that could affect the reliability of measurement during the developmental years are the age and the maturation stage. Buchheit et al. [14] demonstrated that the age or the maturation stage did not seem to clearly affect the test–retest reliability of linear sprint test in young soccer players from U13 to U18 (although ICC values were different among age groups, the effect size of differences was small). In the same context, Dugdale et al. [17] examined the reliability of 10 m and 20 m linear sprint tests in different age groups of soccer players (U11–U17) and reported lower ICC values in U12 and U17 vs. other age groups; however, the effect size differences were small.

Regarding the reliability of dribbling tests, the greater proportion of studies have examined the reliability of different dribbling agility tests (i.e., Illinois dribbling test, 505 CoD test, UGhent dribbling test, zigzag dribbling test, Bangsbo and Mohr short dribble test, and slalom dribble test) in young soccer players, reporting moderate-to-high reliability [7,9,13,18,20,22,30–32], while few studies have assessed the reliability of the linear dribbling speed [18,22,32]. However, the linear sprint is of crucial importance in soccer because it supports the player in creating a chance to score [33]. This notion has been strengthened by a previous study which determined that scoring players (n = 161) performed linear sprints prior to 45% of all analyzed goals [34]. Previous study [22], which examined the intra-session reliability of linear dribbling speed during a 30 m sprint in 25 young male soccer players aged 15–18 years, reported a high reliability among trials (ICC = 0.88). Similarly, another study [18] that examined the reliability of 20 m linear dribbling speed in young soccer players (10–12 years old) also found a high reliability among trials (Cronbach a = 0.85).

Except for the measurement and evaluation of linear speed with ball possession, which is affected by the level of the player's dribbling technique, a reliable calculation of a specific performance index, which demonstrates the difference between linear speed with and without ball possession, is important especially after the age of 13–14 years, as at that instance the technique is automated. Moreover, the reliable calculation of the difference between the two tests (linear speed with and without ball possession) may be used to provide important information about how much the ball handling technique reduces the soccer player's time required for a sprint, helping soccer coaches to plan training appropriately to eliminate this difference. To the best of our knowledge, no previous study has examined the intra-session and inter-session reliability of such an indicator in pubertal soccer players.

Considering all the above facts, the main objectives of this study were as follows:

(a) To examine the inter-session reliability (reliability between the first and the second testing occasions, i.e., test–retest) as well as the intra-session reliability (reliability between trials at the same testing occasion) of 30 m linear speed with and without ball possession;

(b) To calculate (using two different equations: delta value and percentage value) and examine the intra-session reliability and inter-session reliability of a specific performance index that indicates the difference between the two speed tests (linear speed with and without ball possession) in pubertal soccer players.

2. Materials and Methods

2.1. Participants

Forty pubertal male soccer players (age: 14.87 ± 1.23 years; tanner stage: 3.3 ± 0.46; body height: 169.19 ± 0.38 cm; body mass: 60.61 ± 11.42 kg) who were members of different soccer academies and played at different positions (14 defenders, 16 midfielders, and 10 forwards) volunteered to participate in the current study. All the participants were soccer players from different soccer academies of the region of Thessaly and participated in national soccer championships in the under 16 category. It should be mentioned that the sample of the study was selected through the "Union of Trikala Soccer Academies" from different soccer academies where the soccer players met the appropriate inclusion criteria. The inclusion criteria were that participants should be males, of pubertal age (13.5–16 years old), i.e., in the under 16 category, and healthy with no injury in the upper and lower limbs for at least 6 months before the commencement of the study. The participants should also have more than five years of experience in playing soccer, and they should be training three times per week and should have played at least one official match. Before the testing, the participants and their parents were informed about the evaluation procedure, and they provided their written consent. The study was conducted according to the Declaration of Helsinki and approved by the Ethics Committee of the University of Thessaly.

2.2. Measures

All speed-testing procedures were performed on a natural soccer turf, and the participants wore their soccer footwear during the test. During both testing occasions (test and retest), the participants performed a standardized 25 min warm-up. The first 15 min of the warm-up included 8 min of running exercises (running straight ahead, running with hip out and hip in, running with circling partner, and running with shoulder contact) and 7 min of neuromuscular exercises and sub-maximal speed trials (i.e., skipping, butt kicks, carioca drill, forward and backward running, and submaximal sprints of 20 m). The other 10 min included technical exercises with a ball (running with a ball, team passing, pass and move, and dribble–pass–move) and dynamic stretching (straight leg march, high knees, lunges with torso twists, front swings, side cross swings, and hip in, hip out, and lateral lunges).

Afterward, the participants' 30 m linear speed with and without ball possession was evaluated using a photocell timing system (Newtest 300 series Powertimer, 2000, Oulu, Finland) [35]. The photocell timing system (Newtest) that we used in the present study is widely used in scientific literature to evaluate the speed ability in different populations [36]. According to the manufacturer, the Newtest Powertimer photocell system exhibits a 0.001 s error over a 5 m sprint at a speed of 10.0 m/s [37]. Furthermore, previous studies showed that the Newtest Powertimer photocell system is a reliable instrument for speed measurement [36,37], since it did not show any marked systematic bias, and the random error associated with it was negligible [37].

During the linear speed test without a ball, the participants started from a standing position of 0.3 m behind the starting line. Photocells were positioned at 0 and 30 m along the soccer field. The testing protocol consisted of two maximal trials with a rest period of 3 min between trials. The best recorded sprint time (in seconds) was used for analysis. During the linear speed test with a ball, the ball was placed 0.3 m behind the starting line, and photocells were positioned at 0 and 30 m along the field. The participants were instructed to maintain contact with the ball in every step or every two steps; otherwise, the trial was considered invalid. The testing protocol consisted of two maximal trials with a rest period of 3 min between trials. The best recorded sprint time (in seconds) was used for analysis.

For both testing occasions (test and retest), the performance index was calculated as the difference between the two tests (linear speed without a ball and linear speed with a ball) using two different equations: (a) delta score = (best sprint time with a ball − best sprint time without a ball) and (b) % difference = [(best sprint time with a ball − best sprint time without a ball) ÷ best sprint time without a ball] × 100.

2.3. Design and Procedures

The testing procedures were performed at the start of the competitive season and lasted three days for each participant. During the first day, the participants were familiarized with the testing procedures. Moreover, assessments regarding biological age and anthropometric characteristics (body height and body mass) and the completion of a medical history form were completed on the first day. The assessment of biological age was performed with self-estimation using Tanner's sexual maturation stages and was determined according to pubic hair development [38]. The body mass was also measured to the nearest 0.1 kg using a calibrated physician's scale (Seca model 755; Seca, Hamburg, Germany), while the body height was determined to the nearest 0.1 cm using a telescopic height rod (Seca model 220; Seca, Hamburg, Germany). During the second (test) and third (retest) days, participants' 30 m linear speed with and without ball possession was assessed, with 5 min rest interval between the two tests. The order of testing linear speed with and without ball possession was randomized; however, each participant performed the tests in the same order at both test and retest testing occasions. A computer-generated list of random numbers was used for the allocation of sequence during testing occasions. Both tests (test and retest) were performed in a soccer field, by the same investigator who was also an experienced soccer coach in the developmental ages, at the same time of the day (3–5 p.m.) and under similar environmental conditions (26–28 °C), while the duration between the two tests was 72 h. Participants were asked to follow their normal diet for two days before the study, abstain from intense exercise activity for 48 h before the study, and to have sufficient rest the night before the study.

2.4. Statistical Analysis

All data are presented as mean ± SD and were analyzed using IBM SPSS Statistics v.26 software (IBM Corporation, Armonk, NY, USA). A statistical power analysis (software package GPower 3.0) before the initiation of the study indicated that a total number of 30 participants would yield adequate power (>0.85) and level of significance (<0.05). In the present study, the final sample comprised 40 pubertal soccer players. The normality of data was examined using the Shapiro–Wilk test (all the data followed normal distribution). The inter-session reliability was used to evaluate the reliability between the first and the second testing occasions (test–retest reliability) using the best of the two testing trials, while intra-session reliability was used to examine the reliability between trials on the same testing occasion.

The inter-session and intra-session reliabilities were examined using indicators of both relative (intraclass correlation coefficient—ICC) and absolute reliabilities (standard error of measurement in absolute terms, i.e., SEM, and relative terms, i.e., SEM% and 95% limits of agreement - 95% LOA). We calculated ICC for single measures using a two-way random effect model for absolute agreement for the computation of ICC. The ICC value varies between 0 (indicating no reliability) and 1 (indicating perfect reliability). An ICC value of (a) below 0.5 indicates poor reliability, (b) between 0.5 and 0.75 indicates moderate reliability, (c) between 0.75 and 0.90 indicates good reliability, and (d) above 0.9 indicates high reliability [39]. The SEM quantifies the precision of individual scores on a test and is expressed in the actual units of the original measurement. Furthermore, the SEM may be presented as a percentage value (SEM%) by dividing the mean of the two measurements (test and retest) and multiplying by 100 [40]. A SEM value of (a) below 5% indicates high reliability, (b) above 5% and below 10% generally denotes good reliability, (c) equal to 10% indicates moderate reliability, and (d) above 10% indicates low reliability. The 95% LOA represents the 95% likely range for the difference between the subject's scores in two tests [41]. The range defined by the LOA (upper and lower limits) is regarded as a reference range for changes between pairs of measurements (when the differences between values range within the defined limits of agreement, this generally denotes a good agreement) [41]. The intertrial agreement was also examined graphically by plotting the difference between test and retest as well as the difference between trials on the same testing occasion against their mean, according to the Bland and Altman approach [42]. The Bland–Altman graph expresses good agreement between two measurements, when the differences between measurements for all observations lie within 1.96 SD [42]. The Bland–Altman plots show the measurement error schematically and help to identify the presence of heteroscedasticity (a positive relationship between the degree of measurement error and the magnitude of the measured value). Heteroscedasticity was also tested using a Pearson correlation test to examine whether the absolute intertrial difference (systematic bias) is associated with the magnitude of the measurement. The systematic bias was also calculated as the intertrial difference between test and retest values as well as the difference between trials on the same testing occasion. Finally, paired t-tests were also used to determine possible significant differences in linear speed with and without ball possession between test and retest as well as between trials on the same testing occasion. The level of significance was set at $p < 0.05$.

3. Results
3.1. Inter-Session Reliability

Test and retest values (mean ± SD), as well as relative and absolute reliability indices (ICC, SEM, SEM%, 95% LOA), are presented in Table 1. Non-significant differences between test and retest values were observed ($p > 0.05$). The relative reliability between the test and retest values was high for all testing variables (linear speed with and without ball possession and performance index) with ICC values that ranged from 0.957 to 0.995.

Table 1. Inter-session (test–retest) reliability indices of linear speed with and without ball possession in pubertal soccer players.

Variables	Test	Retest	ICC (95% CI)	SEM	SEM%	95% LOA Lower	95% LOA Upper
Linear speed without ball	4.85 ± 0.43 s	4.89 ± 0.42 s	0.995 (0.960–0.998)	0.03 s	0.62	−0.045	0.13
Linear speed with ball	6.24 ± 0.79 s	6.28 ± 0.78 s	0.982 (0.965–0.990)	0.11 s	1.69	−0.37	0.45
Performance Index							
Delta score	1.39 ± 0.60 s	1.39 ± 0.59 s	0.965 (0.934–0.981)	0.11 s	8.10	−0.43	0.43
Percent value	28.67 ± 12.22%	28.33 ± 12.05%	0.957 (0.919–0.977)	2.52%	8.83	−7	8.45

ICC: intraclass correlation coefficient, 95% CI: 95% confidence interval, 95% LOA: 95% limits of agreement, SEM: standard error of measurement, SEM%: standard error of measurement expressed as a percentage value.

The SEM% values denoted a high reliability for linear speed without ball (SEM% = 0.62) and linear speed with ball (SEM% = 1.69), and the performance index demonstrated higher SEM% values (8.10% expressed as a delta score and 8.83% expressed as a percentage), thereby reporting a good reliability.

Furthermore, the systematic bias was 0.04 s for linear speed with and without ball possession, −0.004 s for the performance index expressed as a delta score, and −0.34% for the performance index expressed as a percentage value. However, it should be mentioned that no presence of heteroscedasticity was observed since the absolute intertrial difference (systematic bias) was not associated with the magnitude of the measurement according to Pearson correlation test ($p = 0.380$–0.989). Thus, all variables were found to be homoscedastic. The Bland–Altman plots graphically present the reliability patterns for the assessment of linear speed with and without ball possession as well as of performance index (Figure 1). According to Bland–Altman plots, the differences between test–retest values for all observations were within the defined 95% LOA in all tested variables. However, it should be noted that the observations in linear speed without ball demonstrated the least dispersion in the Bland–Altman plot (Figure 1A), while the performance index expressed as a percentage value demonstrated the greatest dispersion (Figure 1D).

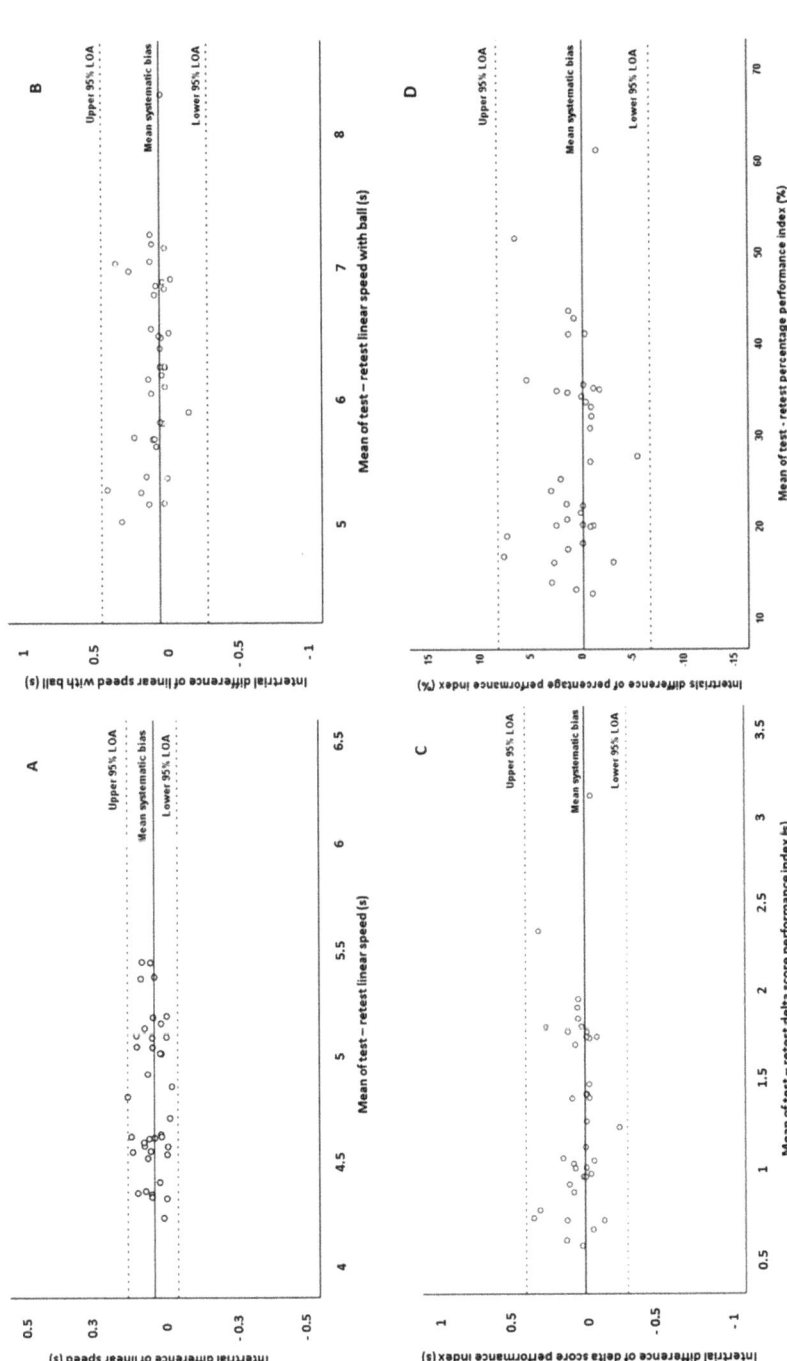

Figure 1. Bland–Altman plots of the linear speed test without ball possession (**A**), linear speed test with ball possession (dribbling) (**B**), performance index expressed as a delta score (**C**), and performance index expressed as a percentage value (**D**) in test and retest measurements. The central solid line characterizes the mean difference between test and retest values (systematic bias), while the upper and lower dashed lines characterize the upper and lower 95% Limits of agreement, LOA (intertrial mean difference of ±1.96 SD of the intertrial difference), respectively.

3.2. Intra-Session Reliability

Test and retest values (mean ± SD), as well as relative and absolute reliability indices (ICC, SEM, SEM%), are presented in Table 2. Non-significant differences between trials for all testing variables were observed ($p > 0.05$). The relative reliability among trials, according to ICC values (ICC = 0.974–0.987), was high for all testing variables. The SEM% values were also denoted a high reliability for linear speed without ball (SEM% = 1.26) and linear speed with ball (SEM% = 1.45), while the performance index demonstrated higher SEM% values (6.17% expressed as a delta score and 6.70% expressed as a percentage), thereby reporting good reliability. Furthermore, the systematic bias was 0.04 s for linear speed without ball, 0.05 s for linear speed with ball possession, 0.02 s for the performance index expressed as a delta score, and 0.21% for the performance index expressed as a percentage value. However, it should be mentioned that no presence of heteroscedasticity was observed since the absolute intertrial difference (systematic bias) was not associated with the magnitude of the measurement according to Pearson correlation test ($p = 0.28$–0.40). Thus, all variables were found to be homoscedastic. The Bland–Altman plots graphically present the intra-session reliability patterns for the assessment of linear speed with and without ball possession as well as of performance index (Figure 2). According to Bland–Altman plots, the differences between trials for all observations were within the defined 95% LOA in all tested variables. However, it should be noted that the observations in linear speed without ball demonstrated the least dispersion in the Bland–Altman plot (Figure 2A), while the performance index expressed as a percentage value demonstrated the greatest dispersion (Figure 2D).

Table 2. Intra-session reliability indices of linear speed linear speed with and without ball possession in pubertal soccer players.

Variables	Trial 1	Trial 2	ICC (95% CI)	SEM	SEM%	95% LOA Lower	95% LOA Upper
Linear speed without ball	4.87 ± 0.44 s	4.90 ± 0.43 s	0.98 (0.957–0.990)	0.06 s	1.26	−0.14	0.20
Linear speed with ball	6.26 ± 0.83 s	6.32 ± 0.77 s	0.987 (0.970–0.993)	0.09 s	1.45	−0.28	0.29
Performance Index							
Delta score	1.40 ± 0.63 s	1.42 ± 0.57 s	0.979 (0.961–0.989)	0.09 s	6.17	−0.24	0.25
Percent value	28.74 ± 12.47%	28.95 ± 11.48%	0.974 (0.951–0.986)	1.93%	6.70	−5.22	5.64

ICC: intraclass correlation coefficient, 95% CI: 95% confidence interval, 95% LOA: 95% limits of agreement, SEM: standard error of measurement, SEM%: standard error of measurement expressed as a percentage value.

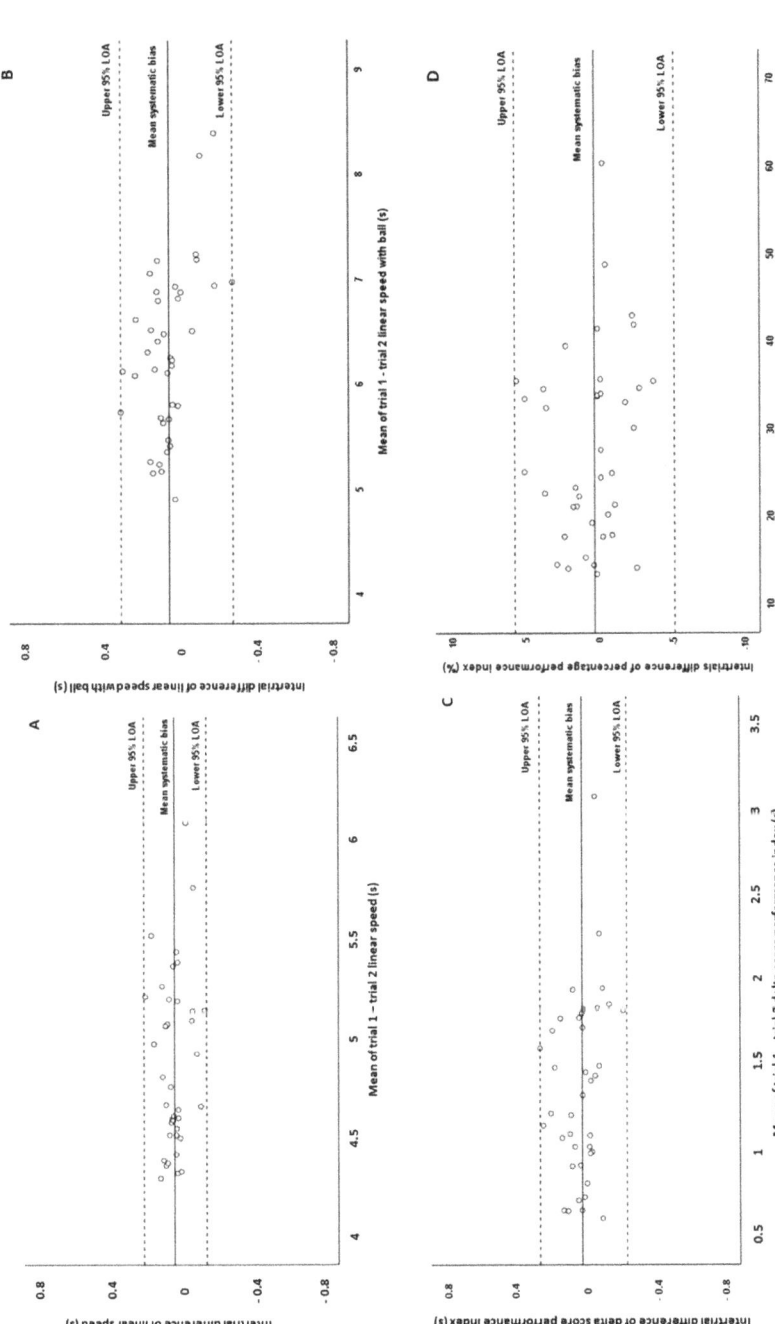

Figure 2. Blanc–Altman plots of the linear speed test without ball possession (**A**), linear speed test with ball possession (dribbling) (**B**), performance index expressed as a delta score (**C**), and performance index expressed as a percentage value (**D**) in test and retest measurements. The central solid line characterizes the mean difference between test and retest values (systematic bias), while the upper and lower dashed lines characterize the upper and lower 95% Limits of agreement, LOA (intertrial mean difference of ±1.96 SD of the intertrial difference), respectively.

4. Discussion

This study examined the inter-session reliability (reliability between the first and the second testing occasions, i.e., test–retest) as well as the intra-session reliability (reliability between trials on the same testing occasion) of linear speed with and without ball possession using different relative and absolute reliability indices (ICC-95% CI, SEM, SEM%, 95% LOA). However, the most important aspect of this study is that it calculated and tested the reliability of a specific performance index, indicating the difference between the two tests (linear speed without and linear speed with ball possession). The main finding is that there are high inter-session and intra-session reliabilities obtained for both linear speed with and without ball possession. Additionally, there are also good/high inter-session and intra-session reliabilities obtained for both performance index methods (delta score and percentage value) used for the calculation of the difference between the two tests. However, it should be mentioned that the relative reliability of the calculated performance index is lower (with greater SEM% values, although acceptably reliable) compared to that observed for absolute scores of linear speed with and without ball possession.

Our results demonstrated a high reliability of the 30 m linear speed test without ball in pubertal soccer players, where the ICC values were 0.98 and 0.995 and the SEM% values were 1.26 and 0.62 for the intra-session reliability and the inter-session reliability, respectively. Previous studies that examined the reliability of linear speed test in young soccer players reported moderate-to-high reliability with a wide range of ICC values that ranged from 0.57 to 0.98 in young soccer players [14–22]. There is evidence that the distance of sprint test may affect the intra-session and inter-session reliabilities (higher reliability with increasing sprinting distance), although further studies are needed to draw more reliable conclusions on this topic. For example, in a previous study, ICC values of 0.87 and 0.97 have been reported for 5 and 20 m, respectively [16]. The testing protocol used could also be an additional factor that could affect the reliability of linear speed. Previous studies that demonstrated a lower reliability of linear speed integrated linear speed testing into complex tests [23] or match simulation protocols [26,28] or required the players to adopt a defined running velocity at the start line [27]. Additionally, previous studies, demonstrating a lower reliability, inferred that the time interval between test–retest measurements (the reliability decreases with the increasing time interval between measurements) [24] as well as the measured system (more consistent results were obtained for timing lights and radar guns compared to global positioning systems where the results vary [25,29]) could affect the reliability of linear speed. In our study, we chose the Newtest Powertimer photocell system that is a reliable instrument for speed measurement [36,37] as well as a small time interval between test and retest measurements (72 h) to strengthen the reliability of the measurement.

Several studies, in the scientific literature, have used different agility tests to evaluate dribbling performance in young soccer players and have reported moderate-to-high reliability [7,9,13,18,20,22,30–32]. On the other hand, limited studies have focused on the reliability of linear speed with ball possession, reporting good-to-high reliability (ICC-r = 0.85–0.98 [18,22,32]; this finding is in agreement with the results of the present study, where the ICC (0.987 for intra-session and 0.982 for intersession) and SEM% (1.45 for intra-session and 1.69 for intersession) values were high. Additionally, in the present study, we observed high ICC values for both intra-session reliability (ICC = 0.974–0.979) and inter-session reliability (ICC = 0.957–0.965) of the performance index that we calculated to indicate the difference between the two tests (linear speed and dribbling speed). However, the SEM% values that we observed for the performance index were higher (SEM% = 6.17–8.83; reporting good reliability) compared to those observed for the absolute values of linear speed with and without ball possession (SEM% = 0.62–1.69; reporting high reliability). Furthermore, the performance index (especially which is expressed as a percentage value) demonstrated the greatest dispersion in the Bland–Altman plots compared to the absolute values of linear speed with and without ball possession. The lower absolute reliability (greater SEM% values) and the greater dispersion in the Bland–Altman plots for the assessment of this parameter may be attributed to the fact that the performance index is a composite of two absolute scores (linear speed with and without ball possession), each possibly varying in the same or a different direction with reassessment, resulting maybe in error propagation. It should be also mentioned that both methods used for the calculation of specific performance index were almost equally reliable (similar ICC and SEM% values), although the performance index expressed as a percentage value showed greater dispersion in the Bland–Altman plots compared to the performance index expressed as a delta value. In the scientific literature, there are no similar references that assessed the reliability of this performance index in young soccer players to compare our results. Nevertheless, the results of this study are in line with previous studies that calculated and examined the reliability of other speed performance indices such as change of direction deficit (CoDD), reporting lower reliability compared to absolute scores of different agility and linear sprint tests [43,44]. However, it should be mentioned that the performance index of our study in more reliable than the CoDD index of previous studies in young soccer players. Thus, the results of this study and previous studies demonstrate that the calculated speed performance indices should be interpreted and used with more caution.

This study has some limitations that could affect its outcomes, and, as a result, their generalization. Firstly, the results of this study are clearly limited to pubertal male soccer players (13.5–16 years old) with previous experience of playing soccer of least five years. Whether these results can be generalized to other age groups (i.e., younger or older age groups), sex (females where the scientific literature is limited), or training status individuals (i.e., soccer players with less training experience in soccer) is unknown and could be examined in future studies. Moreover, the results of the present study are limited to the testing protocol (30 m linear speed with and without ball possession) as well as to the measured system (photocell timing system) used. We did not measure intermediate distances (i.e., 5, 10, 15, and 20 m) or other speed/agility test categories (i.e., change in direction and repeated sprint) with and without ball possession in order to examine their intra-session and inter-session reliabilities. Future studies could also examine and compare the reliability of these measurements using different measured systems (i.e., photocell timing system vs. radar guns vs. global positioning systems). The sample size (although it yielded adequate power as mentioned in the methods section) may be an additional limitation of this study. A larger sample could further strengthen the results of the present study. Finally, the main objective of this study was to examine the reliability of a new variable (performance index) in pubertal soccer players; however, this study did not assess other metrics, such as sensitivity, homogeneity, validity, etc. Future studies could examine, apart from reliability, and the other metrics associated with this variable (performance index) in different groups of soccer players.

5. Conclusions

In conclusion, both 30 m linear speed tests with and without ball possession showed high intra-session and inter-session reliabilities in pubertal male soccer players. Furthermore, the performance index (difference between the two tests), which we calculated using two different equations (delta score and percentage value), is also reliable for the evaluation of pubertal male soccer players. Reliable testing protocols for the evaluation of linear speed with and without ball possession may be used, by coaches and physical conditioning trainers, in speed monitoring and training planning of pubertal soccer players. The performance index, which we calculated in the present study (using two different equations), may be used to provide significant information about how much the ball handling technique reduces the soccer player's time required for a sprint. Therefore, in this way, soccer coaches can design, implement, and guide appropriate training programs to eliminate this difference (sprint time of linear speed test with and without ball possession), aiming to improve dribbling technique using specialized soccer exercises.

Author Contributions: Conceptualization, N.M., K.K. and V.G.; methodology, N.M., C.B. and P.I.; investigation, N.M., C.B. and P.I.; data curation, N.M., K.K. and V.G.; writing—original draft preparation, N.M.; writing—review and editing, K.K. and V.G.; supervision, V.G. All authors have read and agreed to the published version of the manuscript.

Funding: This research received no external funding.

Institutional Review Board Statement: The study was conducted in accordance with the Declaration of Helsinki and approved by the Ethics Committee of The University of Thessaly (protocol code: 1340; date of approval: 4 April 2021).

Informed Consent Statement: Informed consent was obtained from all participants and their parents involved in the study.

Data Availability Statement: Data are unavailable due to privacy or ethical restrictions.

Acknowledgments: We wish to thank our participants for their involvement in the present study.

Conflicts of Interest: The authors declare no conflict of interest.

References

1. Bangsbo, J.; Mohr, M.; Krustrup, P. Physical and metabolic demands of training and match-play in the elite football player. *J. Sports Sci.* **2006**, *24*, 665–674. [CrossRef] [PubMed]
2. Ekblom, B. Applied physiology of soccer. *Sports Med.* **1986**, *3*, 50–60. [CrossRef] [PubMed]
3. Hoff, J.; Helgerud, J. Endurance and strength training for soccer players: Physiological considerations. *Sports Med.* **2004**, *34*, 165–180. [CrossRef] [PubMed]
4. Manouras, N.; Papanikolaou, Z.; Karatrantou, K.; Kouvarakis, P.; Gerodimos, V. The efficacy of vertical vs. horizontal plyometric training on speed, jumping performance and agility in soccer players. *Int. J. Sports Sci. Coach.* **2016**, *11*, 702–709. [CrossRef]
5. Reilly, T.; Williams, A.M.; Franks, A. A multidisciplinary approach to talent identification in soccer. *J. Sports Sci.* **2000**, *18*, 695–702. [CrossRef]
6. Stølen, T.; Chamari, K.; Castagna, C.; Wisløff, U. Physiology of soccer: An update. *Sports Med.* **2005**, *35*, 501–536. [CrossRef]
7. Bekris, E.; Gissis, I.; Kounalakis, S. The dribbling agility test as a potential tool for evaluating the dribbling skill in young soccer players. *Res. Sports Med.* **2018**, *26*, 425–435. [CrossRef]
8. Sawczuk, T.; Jones, B.L.; Scantlebury, S.; Weakley, J.; Read, D.; Costello, N.B.; Darrall-Jones, J.D.; Stokes, K.; Till, K. Between-Day Reliability and Usefulness of a Fitness Testing Battery in Youth Sport Athletes: Reference Data for Practitioners. *Meas. Phys. Educ. Exerc. Sci.* **2018**, *22*, 11–18. [CrossRef]
9. Hachana, Y.; Chaabene, H.; Ben Rajeb, G.; Khlifa, R.; Aouadi, R.; Chamari, K.; Gabbett, T.J. Validity and reliability of new agility test among elite and subelite under 14-soccer players. *PLoS ONE* **2014**, *9*, e95773. [CrossRef]
10. Huijgen, B.C.; Elferink-Gemser, M.T.; Post, W.; Visscher, C. Soccer skill development in professionals. *Int. J. Sports Med.* **2009**, *30*, 585–591. [CrossRef]
11. Di Salvo, V.; Baron, R.; Tschan, H.; Calderon Montero, F.J.; Bachl, N.; Pigozzi, F. Performance characteristics according to playing position in elite soccer. *Int. J. Sports Med.* **2007**, *28*, 222–227. [CrossRef]
12. Altmann, S.; Ringhof, S.; Neumann, R.; Woll, A.; Rumpf, M.C. Validity and reliability of speed tests used in soccer: A systematic review. *PLoS ONE* **2019**, *14*, e0220982. [CrossRef]
13. Paul, D.J.; Nassis, G.P. Physical Fitness Testing in Youth Soccer: Issues and Considerations Regarding Reliability, Validity and Sensitivity. *Pediatr. Exerc. Sci.* **2015**, *27*, 301–313. [CrossRef] [PubMed]
14. Buchheit, M.; Mendez-Villanueva, A. Reliability and stability of anthropometric and performance measures in highly-trained young soccer players: Effect of age and maturation. *J. Sports Sci.* **2013**, *31*, 1332–1343. [CrossRef] [PubMed]
15. Christou, M.; Smilios, I.; Sotiropoulos, K.; Volaklis, K.; Pilianidis, T.; Tokmakidis, S.P. Effects of resistance training on the physical capacities of adolescent soccer players. *J. Strength Cond. Res.* **2006**, *20*, 783–791. [CrossRef]
16. Comfort, P.; Stewart, A.; Bloom, L.; Clarkson, B. Relationships between strength, sprint and jump performance in well-trained youth soccer players. *J. Strength Cond. Res.* **2014**, *28*, 173–177. [CrossRef]
17. Dugdale, J.H.; Arthur, C.A.; Sanders, D.; Hunter, A.M. Reliability and validity of field-based fitness tests in youth soccer players. *Eur. J. Sport Sci.* **2019**, *19*, 745–756. [CrossRef]
18. Kovacevic, Z.; Zuvela, F.; Kuvacic, G. Metric Characteristics of Tests Assessing Speed and Agility in Youth Soccer Players. *Sport Mont.* **2018**, *16*, 9–14. [CrossRef]
19. Krolo, A.; Gilic, B.; Foretic, N.; Pojskic, H.; Hammami, R.; Spasic, M.; Uljevic, O.; Versic, S.; Sekulic, D. Agility Testing in Youth Football (Soccer) Players; Evaluating Reliability, Validity, and Correlates of Newly Developed Testing Protocols. *Int. J. Environ. Res. Public Health* **2020**, *17*, 294. [CrossRef]
20. Makhlouf, I.; Tayech, A.; Mejri, M.A.; Haddad, M.; Behm, D.G.; Granacher, U.; Chaouachi, A. Reliability and validity of a modified Illinois change-of-direction test with ball dribbling speed in young soccer players. *Biol. Sport* **2022**, *39*, 295–306. [CrossRef]

21. Pardos-Mainer, E.; Casajús, J.A.; Gonzalo-Skok, O. Reliability and sensitivity of jumping, linear sprinting and change of direction ability tests in adolescent female football players. *Sci. Med. Football* **2019**, *3*, 183–190. [CrossRef]
22. Wilson, R.S.; Smith, N.M.A.; Ramos, S.P.; Giuliano-Caetano, F.; Aparecido Rinaldo, M.; Santiago, P.R.P.; Cunha, S.A.; Moura, F.A. Dribbling speed along curved paths predicts attacking performance in match-realistic one vs. one soccer games. *J. Sports Sci.* **2019**, *37*, 1072–1079. [CrossRef] [PubMed]
23. Bullock, W.; Panchuk, D.; Broatch, J.; Christian, R.; Stepto, N.K. An integrative test of agility, speed and skill in soccer: Effects of exercise. *J. Sci. Med. Sport* **2012**, *15*, 431–436. [CrossRef] [PubMed]
24. Haugen, T.A.; Tønnessen, E.; Seiler, S. Speed and countermovement-jump characteristics of elite female soccer players, 1995–2010. *Int. J. Sports Physiol. Perform.* **2012**, *7*, 340–349. [CrossRef]
25. Meylan, C.; Trewin, J.; McKean, K. Quantifying Explosive Actions in International Women's Soccer. *Int. J. Sports Physiol. Perform.* **2017**, *12*, 310–315. [CrossRef]
26. Small, K.; McNaughton, L.R.; Greig, M.; Lohkamp, M.; Lovell, R. Soccer fatigue, sprinting and hamstring injury risk. *Int. J. Sports Med.* **2009**, *30*, 573–578. [CrossRef]
27. Sonderegger, K.; Tschopp, M.; Taube, W. The Challenge of Evaluating the Intensity of Short Actions in Soccer: A New Methodological Approach Using Percentage Acceleration. *PLoS ONE* **2016**, *11*, e0166534. [CrossRef]
28. Williams, J.D.; Abt, G.; Kilding, A.E. Ball-Sport Endurance and Sprint Test (BEAST90): Validity and reliability of a 90-minute soccer performance test. *J. Strength Cond. Res.* **2010**, *24*, 3209–3218. [CrossRef]
29. Yanci, J.; Calleja-Gonzalez, J.; Camara, J.; Mejuto, G.; San Roman, J.; Los Arcos, A. Validity and reliability of a global positioning system to assess 20 m sprint performance in soccer players. *Proc. Inst. Mech. Eng.* **2017**, *231*, 68–71. [CrossRef]
30. Pojskic, H.; Aslin, E.; Krolo, A.; Jukic, I.; Uljevic, O.; Spasic, M.; Sekulic, D. Importance of Reactive Agility and Change of Direction Speed in Differentiating Performance Levels in Junior Soccer Players: Reliability and Validity of Newly Developed Soccer-Specific Tests. *Front. Physiol.* **2018**, *9*, 506. [CrossRef]
31. Duncan, M.; Richardson, D.; Morris, R.; Eyre, E.; Clarke, N. Test-retest reliability of soccer dribbling tests in children. *J. Motor Learn. Develop.* **2021**, *9*, 526–532. [CrossRef]
32. Padrón-Cabo, A.; Rey, E.; Kalén, A.; Costa, P.B. Effects of Training with an Agility Ladder on Sprint, Agility, and Dribbling Performance in Youth Soccer Players. *J. Hum. Kinet.* **2020**, *73*, 219–228. [CrossRef]
33. Haugen, T.; Tønnessen, E.; Hisdal, J.; Seiler, S. The role and development of sprinting speed in soccer. *Int. J. Sports Physiol. Perform.* **2014**, *9*, 432–441. [CrossRef]
34. Faude, O.; Koch, T.; Meyer, T. Straight sprinting is the most frequent action in goal situations in professional football. *J. Sports Sci.* **2012**, *30*, 625–631. [CrossRef]
35. Karsten, B.; Larumbe-Zabala, E.; Kandemir, G.; Hazir, T.; Klose, A.; Naclerio, F. The effects of a 6-week strength training on critical velocity, anaerobic running distance, 30-m sprint and yo-yo intermittent running test performances in male soccer players. *PLoS ONE* **2016**, *11*, e0151448. [CrossRef] [PubMed]
36. Shalfawi, S.A.I.; Tønnessen, E.; Enoksen, E.; Ingebrigtsen, J. Assessing day-to-day reliability of the Newtest 2000 sprint timing system. *Servian J. Sports Sci.* **2011**, *5*, 107–113.
37. Enoksen, E.; Tønnessen, E.; Shalfawi, S. Validity and reliability of the Newtest Powertimer 300-series testing system. *J. Sports Sci.* **2009**, *27*, 77–84. [CrossRef] [PubMed]
38. Tanner, J.M.; Whitehouse, R.H. Clinical longitudinal standards for height, weight, height velocity, weight velocity, and stages of puberty. *Arch. Dis. Child.* **1976**, *51*, 170–179. [CrossRef]
39. Koo, T.K.; Li, M.Y. A Guideline of Selecting and Reporting Intraclass Correlation Coefficients for Reliability Research. *J. Chiropr. Med.* **2016**, *15*, 155–163. [CrossRef]
40. Svensson, E.; Waling, K.; Häger-Ross, C. Grip strength in children: Test-retest reliability using Grippit. *Acta Paediatr.* **2008**, *97*, 1226–1231. [CrossRef]
41. Atkinson, G.; Nevill, A.M. Statistical methods for assessing measurement error (reliability) in variables relevant to sports medicine. *Sports Med.* **1998**, *26*, 217–238. [CrossRef] [PubMed]
42. Bland, J.M.; Altman, D.G. Statistical methods for assessing agreement between two methods of clinical measurement. *Lancet* **1986**, *1*, 307–310. [CrossRef]
43. Sammoud, S.; Bouguezzi, R.; Negra, Y.; Chaabene, H. The Reliability and Sensitivity of Change of Direction Deficit and Its Association with Linear Sprint Speed in Prepubertal Male Soccer Players. *J. Funct. Morphol. Kinesiol.* **2021**, *6*, 41. [CrossRef] [PubMed]
44. Taylor, J.M.; Cunningham, L.; Hood, P.; Thorne, B.; Irvin, G.; Weston, M. The reliability of a modified 505 test and change-of-direction deficit time in elite youth football players. *Sci. Med. Football* **2019**, *2*, 157–162. [CrossRef]

Disclaimer/Publisher's Note: The statements, opinions and data contained in all publications are solely those of the individual author(s) and contributor(s) and not of MDPI and/or the editor(s). MDPI and/or the editor(s) disclaim responsibility for any injury to people or property resulting from any ideas, methods, instructions or products referred to in the content.

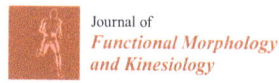

Article

A Novel Metric "Exercise Cardiac Load" Proposed to Track and Predict the Deterioration of the Autonomic Nervous System in Division I Football Athletes

S. Howard Wittels [1,2,3,4], Eric Renaghan [5], Michael Joseph Wishon [4], Harrison L. Wittels [4], Stephanie Chong [4], Eva Danielle Wittels [4], Stephanie Hendricks [4], Dustin Hecocks [4], Kyle Bellamy [6], Joe Girardi [6], Stephen Lee [7], Tri Vo [8], Samantha M. McDonald [4,9,*] and Luis A. Feigenbaum [5,6]

1. Department of Anesthesiology, Mount Sinai Medical Center, Miami, FL 33140, USA; shwittels@gmail.com
2. Department of Anesthesiology, Wertheim School of Medicine, Florida International University, Miami, FL 33199, USA
3. Miami Beach Anesthesiology Associates, Miami, FL 33140, USA
4. Tiger Tech Solutions, Inc., Miami, FL 33140, USA; joe@tigertech.solutions (M.J.W.); hl@tigertech.solutions (H.L.W.); schong591@gmail.com (S.C.); evadanielle@gmail.com (E.D.W.); steph.hendricks@gmail.com (S.H.); dustin@tigertech.solutions (D.H.)
5. Department of Athletics, Sports Science, University of Miami, Miami, FL 33146, USA; eric.renaghan@miami.edu (E.R.); lfeigenbaum@med.miami.edu (L.A.F.)
6. Department of Physical Therapy, Miller School of Medicine, University of Miami, Miami, FL 33146, USA; k.bellamy1@umiami.edu (K.B.); j.girardi@miami.edu (J.G.)
7. United States Army Research Laboratory, Adelphi, MD 20783, USA; stephen.j.lee28.civ@mail.mil
8. Navy Medical Center—San Diego, San Diego, CA 92134, USA; huu@g.clemson.edu
9. School of Kinesiology and Recreation, Illinois State University, Normal, IL 61761, USA
* Correspondence: smmcdo4@ilstu.edu; Tel.: +1-309-438-5008

Abstract: Current metrics like baseline heart rate (HR) and HR recovery fail in predicting overtraining (OT), a syndrome manifesting from a deteriorating autonomic nervous system (ANS). Preventing OT requires tracking the influence of internal physiological loads induced by exercise training programs on the ANS. Therefore, this study evaluated the predictability of a novel, exercise cardiac load metric on the deterioration of the ANS. Twenty male American football players, with an average age of 21.3 years and body mass indices ranging from 23.7 to 39.2 kg/m^2 were included in this study. Subjects participated in 40 strength- and power-focused exercise sessions over 8 weeks and wore armband monitors (Warfighter Monitor, Tiger Tech Solutions) equipped with electrocardiography capabilities. Exercise cardiac load was the product of average training HR and duration. Baseline HR, HR variability (HRV), average HR, and peak HR were also measured. HR recovery was measured on the following day. HRV indices assessed included the standard deviation of NN intervals (SDNN) and root mean square of successive RR interval differences (rMSSD) Linear regression models assessed the relationships between each cardiac metric and HR recovery, with statistical significance set at $\alpha < 0.05$. Subjects were predominantly non-Hispanic black (70%) and aged 21.3 ($\pm$1.4) years. Adjusted models showed that exercise cardiac load elicited the strongest negative association with HR recovery for previous day ($\beta = -0.18 \pm 0.03$; $p < 0.0000$), one-week ($\beta = -0.20 \pm 0.03$; $p < 0.0000$) and two-week ($\beta = -0.26 \pm 0.03$; $p < 0.0000$) training periods compared to average HR (βetas: -0.09 to -0.02; $p < 0.0000$) and peak HR (βetas: -0.13 to -0.23; $p < 0.0000$). Statistically significant relationships were also found for baseline HR ($p < 0.0000$), SDNN ($p < 0.0000$) and rMSSD ($p < 0.0000$). Exercise cardiac load appears to best predict ANS deterioration across one- to two-week training periods, showing a capability for tracking an athlete's physiological tolerance and ANS response. Importantly, this information may increase the effectiveness of exercise training programs, enhance performance, and prevent OT.

Keywords: exercise training; overtraining; sports; strength and conditioning; autonomic nervous system; football players

Citation: Wittels, S.H.; Renaghan, E.; Wishon, M.J.; Wittels, H.L.; Chong, S.; Wittels, E.D.; Hendricks, S.; Hecocks, D.; Bellamy, K.; Girardi, J.; et al. A Novel Metric "Exercise Cardiac Load" Proposed to Track and Predict the Deterioration of the Autonomic Nervous System in Division I Football Athletes. *J. Funct. Morphol. Kinesiol.* **2023**, *8*, 143. https://doi.org/10.3390/jfmk8040143

Academic Editor: Diego Minciacchi

Received: 15 August 2023
Revised: 8 September 2023
Accepted: 20 September 2023
Published: 7 October 2023

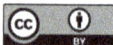

Copyright: © 2023 by the authors. Licensee MDPI, Basel, Switzerland. This article is an open access article distributed under the terms and conditions of the Creative Commons Attribution (CC BY) license (https://creativecommons.org/licenses/by/4.0/).

1. Introduction

Overtraining (OT) manifests from a deteriorating autonomic nervous system (ANS) due to an imbalance between training load and recovery [1]. Among its many functions, the ANS regulates the activity of the cardiac system in response to changes in physiological stimuli (e.g., O_2 demand during exercise) [2,3]. Thus, any deficiencies in the ANS may impair cardiac function, subsequently reducing exercise capacity and sports performance [4]. The absence of observable, external warning signs specific to OT presents significant challenges. Upon reaching OT, an athlete requires an extensive period of rest for full recovery [5]. Therefore, identifying metrics that accurately assess the physiological tolerance of athletes is critical for optimizing exercise training, enhancing performance, and avoiding OT.

Currently, the measures of cardiac function like baseline heart rate (HR) and heart rate variability (HRV) are used as reliable indicators of OT, as athletes often exhibit abnormal values when in OT [5,6]. A significant limitation of these metrics is their inability to predict early ANS deterioration, leaving athletes and coaches no opportunities for avoiding OT. Moreover, a large proportion of studies previously narrowed their focus to evaluating HR recovery, a metric representing the ANS response, to a single bout of high intense exercise training [7]. HR recovery responses were typically monitored in the acute period up to 72 h post-exercise [8]. OT, however, occurs consequent to repeated bouts of high intensity exercise training coupled with inadequate recovery [1]. Thus, these studies provided limited information about tracking the ANS response to chronic high intensity exercise training and the potential prevention of OT. Another significant limitation of current research is the absence of metrics accurately quantifying the physiological load endured by cardiac muscles during exercise training. Current metrics merely quantify the intensity of an exercise training session, providing an incomplete estimation of the total physiological load [9]. Additionally, determining the level of intensity relies on using maximum HR and HR-reserve. These methods are highly variable and falsely imply a universal maximum HR of 220 beats per min and equivalent age-related declines in cardiac function across all populations [10]. Consequently, these measures likely provide inaccurate, indirect estimates of the physiological load.

Lastly, an increasing number of studies use HRV metrics. HRV is a systemic metric that constantly measures the interplay between the parasympathetic and sympathetic nervous systems [11]. HRV, defined as the time variation between each heartbeat, is sensitive to many non-specific changes in physiological stimuli including respiration, hormonal reactions, metabolic processes, stress, and recovery [11] Thus, fluctuations in HRV are difficult to discern, leading to inconclusive evidence on the direction and magnitude of its response and adaptation to exercise training [12]. These significant limitations highlight the need for a metric that accurately measures the physiological load on the cardiac muscles and physiological tolerance of each athlete. With this metric, coaches may be able to monitor the physiological impact of short- and long-term exposures to high intensity exercise training and determine the appropriate amount of recovery time. This information may lead to more effectively designed exercise training programs, specific to each athlete, enhancing their performance and preventing OT.

Therefore, the purpose of this study was to evaluate a novel metric that directly quantified the physiological load placed on the cardiac muscle ("exercise cardiac load" herein) during daily and weekly strength- and power-focused exercise training in Division I collegiate football athletes. Existing exercise cardiac metrics including baseline HR, average HR, peak HR, and select HRV indices (SDNN and rMSSD) were analyzed for comparative purposes. We hypothesized that the exercise cardiac load quantified for both daily and weekly training sessions would better predict ANS deterioration than existing cardiac metrics. Specifically, we anticipated that exercise cardiac load would exhibit a strong, positive association with baseline HR and HR recovery 24 h post-exercise training, reflecting reduced ANS recovery and function, respectively. Additionally, we hypothesized a stronger association for cumulative exposures to high exercise cardiac loads compared to acute exposures.

2. Materials and Methods

2.1. Study Design

This study employed a prospective study design among sample of Division I collegiate male American football players. All cardiac measures including exercise cardiac load, average training heart rate, average peak training HR, baseline HR, HRV, and specifically SDNN and rMSSD were measured on all study subjects throughout the 8-week summer football training program. The training cardiac metrics represented the physiological load placed on the cardiac muscles during "active" training. Baseline HR and HRV metrics presented the 24 h *recovery* of the ANS. HR recovery reflected the *function* of the ANS 24 h post training.

2.2. Subjects

Subjects were recruited from a Division I collegiate football team located in the southeastern state of Florida, United States. The athletes were participating in an 8-week, summer football training program. The prospective participants were recruited from a pre-selected group of athletes the coaches identified as "starters", which were athletes that competed in nearly every regulation game and for most of its duration. Importantly, no exclusion criteria for study participation were imposed. The athletes were, on average, 21.3 years of age, classified as obese with body mass indices ranging from 23.7 to 39.2 kg/m^2. The sample was predominantly non-Hispanic black. Prior to any measurements, the athletes were informed of the benefits and risks of the study and conflicts of interests of all the authors. All athletes participating voluntarily consented to the study. All study protocols followed the ethical principles defined in the declaration of Helsinki and were approved by the university's Institutional Review Board (IRB #20191223).

2.3. Methodology

2.3.1. Summer Football Training Program

The summer training program ran from the beginning of May to the end of June 2022. This program lasted 9 total weeks with two, 4-week training blocks separated by 1 week of rest. All exercise sessions occurred in the morning between 0600 and 0900. Athletes completed 40 total sessions: 5 consecutive sessions per week. The duration of the sessions averaged 163.5 ($\pm$30.8) min and ranged from 90.0 to 240.9 min (~1.5 to 4.0 h). The training load varied daily and between each athlete. All athletes, regardless of position, were exposed to the same strength and power-focused resistance training, speed training (i.e., short-distance sprints), and agility training regimens. Given the prospective nature of this study, no changes in the training programs were made.

2.3.2. Cardiac Measurement

Participants were fitted with armband monitors equipped with temperature, electrocardiography (ECG), photoplethysmography (PPG), and inertial measurement unit (IMU) capabilities (Warfighter Monitor^{TM} (WFM), Tiger Tech Solutions Inc., Miami, FL, USA). The WFM armbands were previously validated in several diverse subpopulations [13]. Monitors were placed on the posterior aspect of the left upper arm, secured with an elastic band, and worn at the start and throughout each training session. Although the WFM device collected several biometric parameters, only HR and HRV-related variables were analyzed.

2.3.3. Physiological Load Metrics of All Training Sessions

The physiological load of each training session was estimated using several cardiac metrics including exercise cardiac load, average HR, and peak HR.

Exercise Cardiac Load

Exercise cardiac load quantified the physiological load endured by the cardiac muscle while "actively training". An "active training" state was defined as a sustained HR ≥ 85 beats per min (bpm). Thus, exercise cardiac load was the product of the athlete's average HR and duration (min) of each session and was calculated as follows:

Exercise Cardiac Load(total heartbeats) = Average HR(bpm) * Session Duration(min)

The exercise cardiac load was normalized with the largest exercise cardiac load measured from any athlete during the 8-week training program and multiplied by 100.

Average and Peak HR during Training

Average training HR was calculated by averaging all the HR values measuring above 85 bpm collected during each training session. Periods where HR values ≤ 85 bpm were defined as "non-active" and represented periods when athletes were not actively training. *Peak training HR* was defined as the highest HR value achieved during each training session.

2.3.4. The Measures of 24 h ANS Recovery and Function

Several cardiac metrics that measured 24 h post training were used as indicators of ANS recovery and function including baseline HR, HRV indices, and HR recovery. Baseline HR and HR recovery are considered the "gold standard" measure of ANS recovery and response, respectively. HRV is shown to correlate well with baseline HR and HR recovery.

24 h Baseline HR

A 24 h baseline HR represented ANS recovery. Baseline HR was measured in the early morning and followed at least four min of inactivity, per established protocols [14]. Specifically, baseline HR was measured prior to the start (0600–0700) of the following day's exercise training session. Each athlete was required to remain nearly motionless in a seated position for a period of 5 min to collect a "resting" baseline HR.

24 h Heart Rate Variability

HRV is defined as the time variation between heartbeats [15]. The metrics used to evaluate HRV included the standard deviation of NN intervals (SDNN) and the root mean square of successive differences (rMSSD), described in detail elsewhere [16]. These metrics were calculated during a 5 min interval where the athletes were seated nearly motionless prior to the start of each training session.

24 h HR Recovery

HR recovery was measured during the next-day's exercise training session to track ANS function following acute bouts of exercise. HR recovery was defined as the reduction in HR during 30 s rest intervals representing localized parasympathetic activation. HR recovery was measured within the first 30 s of rest as, during this period, HR exhibits the greatest rate of change [17]. HR recovery was quantified for all rest intervals occurring throughout the training session and then averaged.

Importantly, baseline HR and HR recovery were measured 24 h following a training session. As such, baseline HR and HR recovery were not measured following one or more rest days. Including rest days would likely dilute the association and not accurately represent the acute and chronic influence of the physiological training load on ANS recovery and function (see Figure 1).

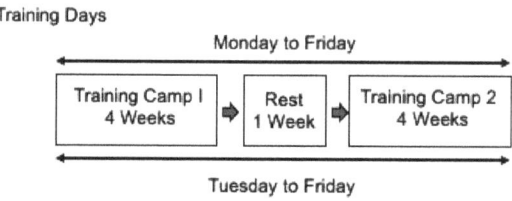

Figure 1. A Schematic of the 8-Week Summer Football Training Camp.

2.4. Statistical Analyses

This study sought to understand the associations between the cardiac metrics of daily and weekly training sessions and the ANS recovery and function. For daily sessions, the cardiac metrics, representing physiological load, were averaged across the 8 training weeks. Exercise cardiac load, average training HR, and peak training HR served as the independent variables. For weekly sessions, one- and two-week averages of exercise cardiac load, average training HR and peak HR served as the independent variables. The one- and two-week averages represented the physiological loads of the previous 5 and 10 training sessions, respectively. Similar calculations were performed for baseline HR, SDNN, and rMSSD, and these metrics also served as independent variables. Next-day HR recovery served as the primary outcome variable. Associations were quantified using two-tailed, linear regression models and were performed separately for each metric. For all models, β coefficients and standard errors were estimated, and the a priori threshold for statistical significance was set at $\alpha = 0.05$. Statistical analyses were performed in MATLAB, version 2021b (MathWorks, Natick, MA, USA).

3. Results

Table 1 displays the cardiac and ANS recovery of the athletes during the 8-week summer training program. The average number and duration of the sessions completed were 40 and 163.5 (± 30.6) min, respectfully. The athletes, on average, elicited a baseline HR of 62.6 (± 6.9) bpm, ranging between 46.3 and 80.5 bpm. During the conditioning sessions, athletes exhibited an average HR of 133.3 (± 8.4) bpm, ranging between 111.4 and 164.1 bpm and a peak HR of 167.1 (± 9.7) bpm, ranging between 140.3 and 194.4 bpm. The average exercise cardiac load to which the athletes were exposed was 19,776.6 (± 3837.8) heartbeats, ranging between 10,016.1 and 30,507.8 heartbeats per session. HR recovery following the exercise cardiac load of the previous conditioning session was, on average, 27.7 (± 6.2) bpm, ranging between 11.2 and 47.4 bpm. Lastly, the SDNN and rMSSD indices of athlete HRV were on average, 80.5 (± 18.9) milliseconds, ranging between 40.0 and 119.9 milliseconds; and 62.6 (± 17.3) milliseconds, ranging between 18.0 and 102.2 milliseconds, respectively.

Adjusted linear regression and correlation coefficients representing the associations between several cardiac metrics and next-day HR recovery are presented in Table 2. For baseline HR, a statistically significant negative association with next-day recovery was observed with an increasing magnitude (β range: -0.42 to -0.23; $p < 0.0000$) in the slope of this relationship for both daily and weekly exposures to exercise training. Statistically significant negative associations were also observed for average HR (β range: -0.09 to -0.02; $p < 0.0000$) and peak HR (β range: -0.23 to -0.13; $p < 0.0000$) and next-day HR recovery, albeit lower in magnitude compared to baseline HR. These associations were shown across both daily and weekly exposures to training sessions with a progressive increase in magnitude of the slope observed only for peak HR. Interestingly, exercise cardiac load (total heart beats occurring during a single training session) exhibited the strongest, statistically significant negative association with next-day HR recovery following a 2-week exposure to training sessions, with longer exposures resulting in greater decreases in next-day HR recovery. Like peak HR, the magnitude of the relationship between exercise cardiac load and next-day HR recovery progressively increased across both daily and weekly exposures to exercise training (β range: -0.26 to -0.28; $p < 0.0000$). Graphical representations of these relationships appear in Figure 2A–D.

Table 1. Cardiac Metrics and ANS Recovery During a Summer 8-Week Football Training Program in Division I Collegiate Athletes.

	Summer Football Training Program					
	8 Weeks	1st Week	4th Week	8th Week	1st, 4-Week Block	2nd, 4-Week Block
Cardiac Metrics						
Average HR (bpm)	133.3 (8.4)	132.8 (5.7)	133.6 (11.1)	129.9 (6.9)	134.6 (8.8)	132.0 (7.6)
Peak HR (bpm)	167.1 (9.7)	167.3 (7.3)	165.4 (11.0)	164.9 (9.8)	167.6 (9.6)	166.6 (9.7)
Cardiac Load (total heart beats)	19,776.6 (3837.8)	19,358.7 (2840.9)	19,322.1 (4372.2)	18,067.5 (3756.2)	19,550.9 (3476.6)	20,008.4 (4170.7)
SDNN (ms)	80.5 (18.9)	84.5 (14.2)	72.3 (15.8)	77.5 (17.4)	76.5 (17.4)	84.7 (17.4)
rMSSD (ms)	62.6 (17.3)	68.3 (15.5)	51.1 (12.6)	53.3 (15.5)	58.3 (15.5)	64.3 (15.5)
ANS Recovery						
HR Recovery (bpm)	27.7 (6.2)	28.4 (4.8)	26.0 (6.3)	28.4 (6.6)	27.2 (5.7)	28.2 (6.7)
Baseline HR (bpm)	62.6 (6.9)	64.6 (6.6)	62.6 (7.1)	61.3 (5.9)	63.5 (6.7)	61.8 (6.9)

Table 2. Adjusted Linear Associations Between Cardiac Metrics and ANS Deterioration in Division I Collegiate Football Athletes.

	Slope (β)	SE	Adjusted R^2	*p*-Value
Cardiac Metrics				
Baseline HR (bpm)				
Previous Day	−0.23	0.04	0.43	<0.0000
1-Week	−0.34	0.05	0.55	<0.0000
2-Week	−0.42	0.05	0.62	<0.0000
Average HR (bpm)				
Previous Day	−0.09	0.04	0.23	<0.0000
1-Week	−0.09	0.05	0.23	<0.0000
2-Week	−0.02	0.06	0.13	<0.0000
Peak HR (bpm)				
Previous Day	−0.13	0.03	0.35	<0.0000
1-Week	−0.20	0.04	0.46	<0.0000
2-Week	−0.23	0.04	0.49	<0.0000
Cardiac Load (total heart beats)				
Previous Day	−0.18	0.03	0.61	<0.0000
1-Week	−0.20	0.03	0.69	<0.0000
2-Week	−0.26	0.03	0.71	<0.0000
SDNN (ms)				
Previous Day	0.06	0.01	0.38	<0.0000
1-Week	0.09	0.01	0.51	<0.0000
2-Week	0.09	0.01	0.61	<0.0000
rMSSD (ms)				
Previous Day	0.04	0.01	0.30	<0.0000
1-Week	0.07	0.01	0.46	<0.0000
2-Week	0.09	0.01	0.53	<0.0000

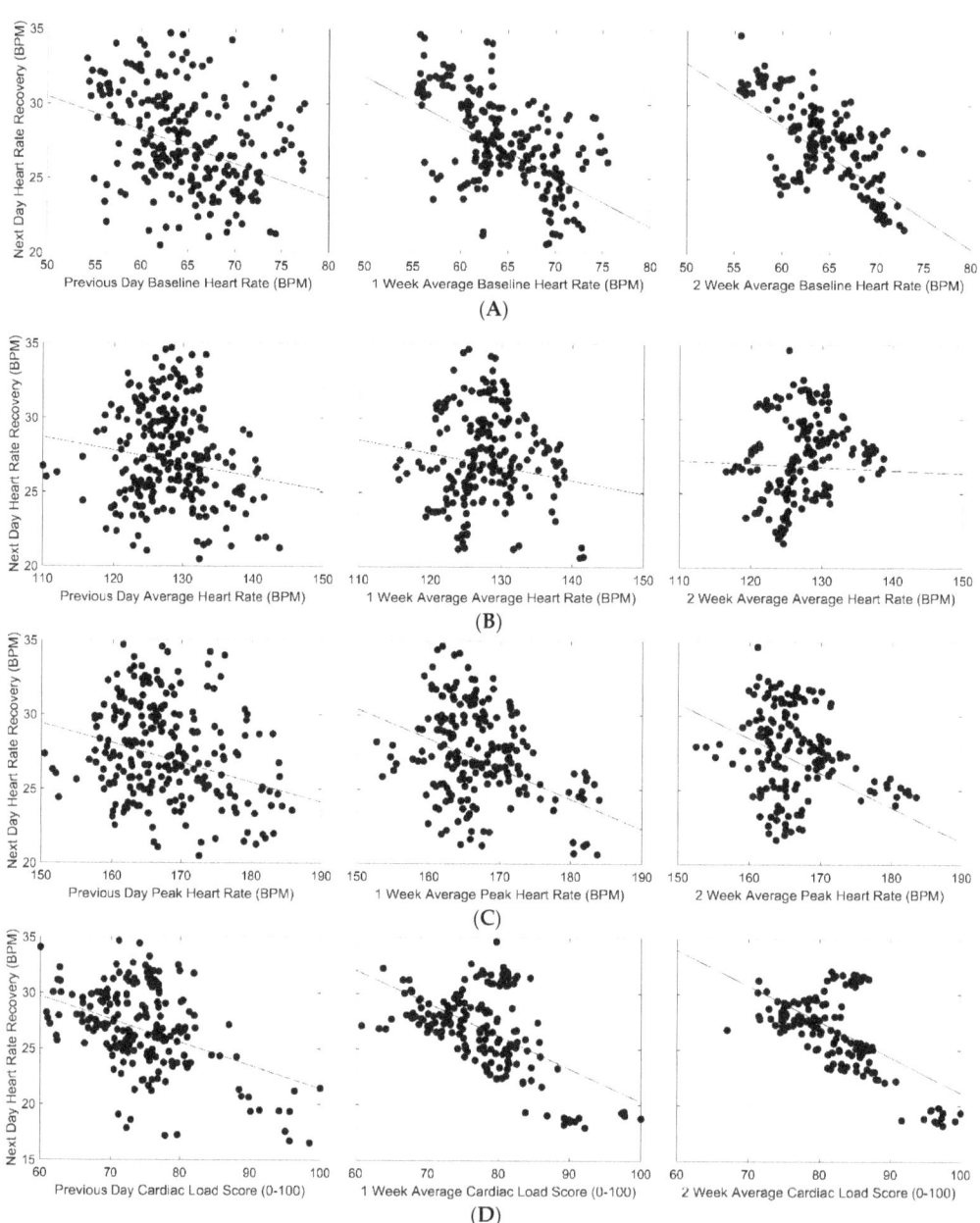

Figure 2. (**A**) Linear Associations Between Previous Day, 1- and 2-Week Baseline HR, and Next-Day HR Recovery. (**B**) Linear Associations Between Previous Day, 1- and 2-Week Average HR, and Next-Day HR Recovery. (**C**) Linear Associations Between Previous Day, 1- and 2-Week Peak HR, and Next-Day HR Recovery. (**D**) Linear Associations Between Previous Day, 1- and 2-Week Exercise Cardiac Load, and Next-Day HR Recovery.

The associations between HRV, represented by SDNN and rMSSD indices, and next-day HR recovery are also shown in Table 2. Statistically significant positive associations between both the indices of HRV and next-day HR recovery were observed. Additionally, increasing magnitudes in the slopes were observed across both daily and weekly exposures to training (β = 0.06, 0.09, 0.10 and 0.04, 0.07, 0.09; p < 0.0000, respectively). Interestingly, compared to baseline HR, peak HR, and cardiac load, the magnitudes of the slopes for SDNN and rMSSD were smaller and in opposing directions. Graphical representations of these associations are displayed in Figure 3.

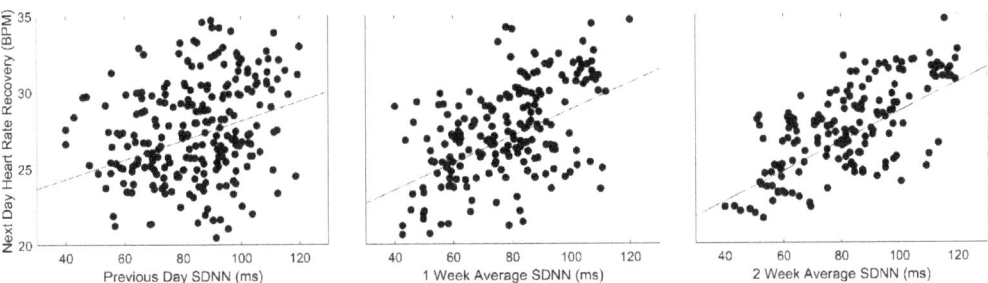

Figure 3. Linear Associations Between Previous Day, 1- and 2-Week Heart Rate Variability, and Next-Day HR Recovery. rMSSD (top) and SDNN (bottom).

4. Discussion

The purpose of this study was to evaluate the associations between daily and weekly exposures to high intensity, training sessions and the response of the ANS in a sample of Division I football athletes. The major findings of this study were (1) the exercise cardiac load metric exhibited stronger, negative relationships with next-day HR recovery compared to average and peak training HRs, (2) progressive increases in the relationships for exercise cardiac load and peak HR were observed across both daily and weekly exposures to training sessions, and (3) positive associations were observed for HRV metrics; although statistically significant, the strengths of the relationships for SDNN and rMSSD were smaller in comparison to all cardiac metrics.

A novel aspect of this study was that the exercise cardiac load metric introduced in this study exhibited stronger relationships with next-day HR recovery than the other cardiac training metrics. This finding suggests that for high intensity training sessions, exercise cardiac load best predicts ANS deterioration. The exercise cardiac load metric differs considerably from other cardiac training metrics used in this study and others [18,19]. Exercise cardiac load measures the total number of heartbeats occurring in an "active state", directly quantifying the physiological load endured by the cardiac muscle. Conversely, other metrics like average training HR, peak training HR, HR reserve, etc., simply quantify exercise intensity at a glimpse, which identifies the level of effort at which an athlete is actively working [9,20]. Consequently, these metrics only partially quantify the physiological load endured by the cardiac muscle during exercise training [21]. Moreover, exercise intensity, usually expressed as a percentage of cardiac capacity (e.g., %HR maximum, % peak HR, %HR reserve) is calculated using flawed equations and assumptions. For example, without consistent empirical support, these equations assume that all individuals elicit a 220-bpm maximum cardiac rate that linearly declines with age and that resting HR is accurately approximated in a non-rested state [10]. These significant limitations likely explain the lower magnitudes observed in this study for the average HR and peak HR associations with next-day HR recovery. Interestingly, in this study, exercise cardiac load elicited a lower magnitude of the association with next-day HR recovery compared to baseline HR. Importantly, this observation does not suggest that baseline HR is a better metric for predicting ANS deterioration. Unlike exercise cardiac load, baseline HR is primarily used for determining, at a given point in time, whether an athlete reached an OT state. As such, baseline HR is not capable of predicting ANS deterioration but rather serves as a useful criterion for diagnosing OT [20]. Taken together, the exercise cardiac load directly assesses the physiological load induced on cardiac muscles, potentially providing the accurate tracking of each athlete's physiological tolerance and predictions of ANS deterioration and OT.

Another unique finding of this study was the observation of progressively increasing strength of the relationships between exercise cardiac load and next-day HR recovery across longer-term exposures to high intensity training sessions. This finding supports the existing literature that consistently shows that ANS deterioration occurs consequent to repeated exposures of high intensity exercise training followed by inadequate recovery [22]. In this study, the football athletes participated in 5 consecutive days of high intensity sessions of considerably long duration (90.0 to 240.9 min). At the end of each week, athletes were given a 48 h recovery period. Interestingly, in additional analyses (data not shown), the relationship between exercise cardiac load and next-day HR recovery weakened when comparing the HR recovery on Monday of the following week to the cardiac load of the previous Friday's session. This observation might suggest that a 48 h period allows for, in this sample of athletes, sufficient recovery time. However, the increased strength of the negative association between exercise cardiac load and next-day HR recovery from the one-week to two-week cumulative exposure contradicts this notion. In fact, the latter observation highlights the exacerbated ANS deterioration consequent to insufficient recovery. Moreover, this observation emphasizes the utility of tracking the physiological load endured by the cardiac muscle and the response of the ANS. For coaches, this information may identify the athlete's physiological tolerance, subsequently indicating requisite modifications to their training program to potentially avert further ANS deterioration and prevent OT.

Notably, this study observed statistically significant, positive associations between HRV indices and next-day HR recovery. This finding suggests that increases in HRV indices following daily and/or weekly exposures to high intense training loads may indicate a sufficient recovery of the ANS. While this finding is supported by some scientific studies, others refute the ability of HRV indices to accurately reflect the ANS response [6,12]. In support, studies previously showed that increases in HRV indices were positively associated with ANS recovery following acute and chronic bouts of endurance exercise training. Conversely, others reported that these same trends led to functional overreaching [23], a state immediately preceding overtraining. Another study demonstrated that declines in HRV, a suggested indicator of ANS deterioration, found among functionally overreaching athletes were associated with improved performance [24]. The inconclusive evidence is likely attributable to the increased complexity of HRV in addition to its high sensitivity to non-specific changes in physiological stimuli. Thus, until a more concrete understanding of the responses and adaptations of HRV to exercise training is reached, its use in tracking and predicting ANS deterioration may be inappropriate. Of interest, compared to the exercise cardiac load metric evaluated in this study, the magnitudes of the associations for SDNN and rMSSD appeared smaller (β range: -0.26 to -0.18 vs. 0.04 to 0.09, respectively). This finding may further support the use of the exercise cardiac load metric for tracking and predicting ANS deterioration in athletes.

Strengths and Limitations

This study possesses a few strengths and weaknesses warranting attention. First and foremost, this study introduced a novel metric that directly assessed the physiological load placed on the cardiac muscles, which was strongly associated with ANS deterioration. As such, the exercise cardiac load metric may provide sport coaches with an accurate and practical tool for identifying each athlete's physiological tolerance, predicting ANS deterioration, and potentially preventing OT. Second, this study employed a prospective study design in a natural sport setting, likely allowing for a better translation of these findings to similar types of sports. Third, this study assessed the physiological loads of high intensity training, which are scarcely evaluated in the current literature, with a large proportion of studies focusing on endurance exercise training. Given that many contact sports implement training programs, these findings significantly contribute to the scientific literature, as it reaches an understudied area in sports. Fourth, this study evaluated the influence of daily and weekly exposures of high intensity training, providing important information on the longitudinal impact of this type of training on ANS deterioration. The current study is not without its limitations. First, the study sample only included 20 university-aged, adult males competing on a singular football team, potentially reducing the generalizability of the findings. Second, this study did not include female athletes, further restricting the generalizability of this study. Lastly, extraneous factors potentially affecting the ANS including nutritional status and sleep were not measured.

5. Conclusions

Collectively, the observations of this study demonstrated several concepts regarding the physiological load of exercise and the response of the ANS, specifically for sports implementing training programs. First, our study introduces a novel metric that strongly predicts the potential deterioration of the ANS induced by exercise training and outperforms existing cardiac metrics like baseline HR and HR recovery. Second, repeated exposures to high intensity training with minimal recovery exacerbates the deterioration of ANS, highlighting the need for a longitudinal tracking of the cardiac loads in exercise training programs. Additionally, our study suggests a potential misuse of HRV consequent to its increased complexity and sensitive nature. For future studies aiming to further understand the influence of exercise training on the response of the ANS, the use of exercise cardiac load as described in this study or similarly designed metrics in addition to including several longitudinal timepoints are strongly encouraged. Moreover, future studies should include samples of female athletes and athletes of similar sports.

6. Practical Implications

The ECL metric is a novel, practical, and simple measure of an athlete's physiological tolerance to exercise training. This metric allows coaches to track the influence of acute and cumulative exercise training on the ANS of each athlete to (1) prevent declines in sport performance, functional overreaching, and overtraining; (2) individualize programs that train athletes within their physiological reserve; and (3) optimize training programs and sport performance.

Author Contributions: The authors each contributed to the development of this manuscript in the following ways, Conceptualization, S.H.W., E.R., H.L.W., M.J.W., S.L., K.B., J.G. and L.A.F.; methodology, S.C., E.D.W., S.H., K.B., J.G. and D.H.; software, S.H.W., H.L.W. and M.J.W.; validation, S.H.W., H.L.W. and M.J.W.; formal analysis, M.J.W., H.L.W. and S.M.M.; investigation, S.C., E.D.W., S.H., K.B., J.G. and D.H.; resources, S.H.W., H.L.W., K.B., J.G., T.V. and E.R.; data curation, M.J.W.; writing—original draft preparation, S.M.M.; writing—review and editing, S.M.M., H.L.W. and M.J.W.; visualization, S.M.M., H.L.W. and M.J.W.; supervision, S.H.W., H.L.W. and M.J.W.; project administration, H.L.W., S.C., K.B., J.G. and L.A.F.; funding acquisition, S.H.W and H.L.W. All authors have read and agreed to the published version of the manuscript.

Funding: This research received no external funding.

Institutional Review Board Statement: The study was conducted in accordance with the Declaration of Helsinki and approved by the Institutional Review Board of University of Miami (IRB# 20191223 and 22 June 2020) for studies involving humans.

Informed Consent Statement: Informed consent was obtained from all subjects involved in the study.

Data Availability Statement: Data presented in the current paper are available upon request.

Conflicts of Interest: The following authors are paid employees of Tiger Tech Solutions Inc., owner of the Warfighter Monitor (WFM) used in this study: S.H.W., M.J.W., H.L.W., S.C., E.D.W., S.H., D.H. and S.M.M. Authors K.B., S.L., L.A.F, T.V. and E.R. have no conflicts of interest to disclose.

References

1. Kellmann, M.; Bertollo, M.; Bosquet, L.; Brink, M.; Coutts, A.J.; Duffield, R.; Erlacher, D.; Halson, S.L.; Hecksteden, A.; Heidari, J.; et al. Recovery and Performance in Sport: Consensus Statement. *Int. J. Sports Physiol. Perform.* **2018**, *13*, 240–245. [CrossRef] [PubMed]
2. Freeman, J.V.; Dewey, F.E.; Hadley, D.M.; Myers, J.; Froelicher, V.F. Autonomic Nervous System Interaction with the Cardiovascular System During Exercise. *Prog. Cardiovasc. Dis.* **2006**, *48*, 342–362. [CrossRef]
3. Schüttler, D.; Hamm, W.; Bauer, A.; Brunner, S. Routine Heart Rate-Based and Novel ECG-Based Biomarkers of Autonomic Nervous System in Sports Medicine. *Dtsch. Z. Sportmed.* **2020**, *71*, 141–150. [CrossRef]
4. Kreher, J.B.; Schwartz, J.B. Overtraining Syndrome: A Practical Guide. *Sports Health* **2012**, *4*, 128–138. [CrossRef] [PubMed]
5. Djordjevic, D.; Stanojević, D.; Tosic, J. Heart Rate Modulations in Overtraining Syndrome. *Serb. J. Exp. Clin. Res.* **2013**, *14*, 125–133.
6. Bellenger, C.R.; Fuller, J.T.; Thomson, R.L.; Davison, K.; Robertson, E.Y.; Buckley, J.D. Monitoring Athletic Training Status through Autonomic Heart Rate Regulation: A Systematic Review and Meta-Analysis. *Sports Med.* **2016**, *46*, 1461–1486. [CrossRef]
7. Kliszczewicz, B.; Williamson, C.; Bechke, E.; McKenzie, M.; Hoffstetter, W. Autonomic Response to a Short and Long Bout of High-Intensity Functional Training. *J. Sports Sci.* **2018**, *36*, 1872–1879. [CrossRef]
8. Bosquet, L.; Merkari, S.; Arvisais, D.; Aubert, A.E. Is Heart Rate a Convenient Tool to Monitor Over-Reaching? A Systematic Review of the Literature. *Br. J. Sports Med.* **2008**, *42*, 709. [CrossRef]
9. Weltman, A.; Snead, D.; Seip, R.; Schurrer, R.; Weltman, J.; Rutt, R.; Rogol, A. Percentages of Maximal Heart Rate, Heart Rate Reserve and VO$_2$max for Determining Endurance Training Intensity in Male Runners. *Int. J. Sports Med.* **2008**, *11*, 218–222. [CrossRef]
10. Robergs, R.; Landwehr, R. The Surprising History of the "HRmax=220-Age" Equation. *Int. J. Online Eng.* **2002**, *5*, 1–10.
11. Lundstrom, C.J.F.; Nicholas, A.; Biltz, G. Practices and Applications of Heart Rate Variability Monitoring in Endurance Athletes. *Int. J. Sports Med.* **2023**, *44*, 9–19. [CrossRef]
12. Thamm, A.; Freitag, N.; Figueiredo, P.; Doma, K.; Rottensteiner, C.; Bloch, W.; Schumann, M. Can Heart Rate Variability Determine Recovery Following Distinct Strength Loadings? A Randomized Cross-Over Trial. *Int. J. Environ. Res. Public. Health* **2019**, *16*, 4353. [CrossRef]
13. Peck, J.; Wishon, M.J.; Wittels, H.; Lee, S.J.; Hendricks, S.; Davila, H.; Wittels, S.H. Single Limb Electrocardiogram Using Vector Mapping: Evaluation and Validation of a Novel Medical Device. *J. Electrocardiol.* **2021**, *67*, 136–141. [CrossRef]
14. Speed, C.; Arneil, T.; Harle, R.; Wilson, A.; Karthikesalingam, A.; McConnell, M.; Phillips, J. Measure by Measure: Resting Heart Rate across the 24-Hour Cycle. *PLoS Digit. Health* **2023**, *2*, e0000236. [CrossRef]
15. Sacha, J.; Pluta, W. Different Methods of Heart Rate Variability Analysis Reveal Different Correlations of Heart Rate Variability Spectrum with Average Heart Rate. *J. Electrocardiol.* **2005**, *38*, 47–53. [CrossRef] [PubMed]
16. Bourdillon, N.; Yazdani, S.; Vesin, J.-M.; Schmitt, L.; Millet, G.P. RMSSD Is More Sensitive to Artifacts Than Frequency-Domain Parameters: Implication in Athletes' Monitoring. *J. Sports Sci. Med.* **2022**, *21*, 260–266. [CrossRef] [PubMed]
17. Nandi, P.S.; Spodick, D.H. Recovery from Exercise at Varying Work Loads. Time Course of Responses of Heart Rate and Systolic Intervals. *Br. Heart J.* **1977**, *39*, 958–966. [CrossRef]
18. Da Cunha, F.A.; de Tarso Veras Farinatti, P.; Midgley, A.W. Methodological and Practical Application Issues in Exercise Prescription Using the Heart Rate Reserve and Oxygen Uptake Reserve Methods. *J. Sci. Med. Sport* **2011**, *14*, 46–57. [CrossRef]
19. Esco, M.R.; Chamberlain, N.; Flatt, A.A.; Snarr, R.L.; Bishop, P.A.; Williford, H.N. Cross-Validation of Age-Predicted Maximal Heart Rate Equations among Female Collegiate Athletes. *J. Strength. Cond. Res.* **2015**, *29*, 3053–3059. [CrossRef]
20. Coates, A.M.; Hammond, S.; Burr, J.F. Investigating the Use of Pre-Training Measures of Autonomic Regulation for Assessing Functional Overreaching in Endurance Athletes. *Eur. J. Sport. Sci.* **2018**, *18*, 965–974. [CrossRef]
21. Mann, T.; Lamberts, R.P.; Lambert, M.I. Methods of Prescribing Relative Exercise Intensity: Physiological and Practical Considerations. *Sports Med.* **2013**, *43*, 613–625. [CrossRef] [PubMed]
22. Lehmann, M.; Foster, C.; Gastmann, U.; Keizer, H.; Steinacker, J.M. Definition, Types, Symptoms, Findings, Underlying Mechanisms, and Frequency of Overtraining and Overtraining Syndrome. In *Overload, Performance Incompetence, and Regeneration in Sport*; Lehmann, M., Foster, C., Gastmann, U., Keizer, H., Steinacker, J.M., Eds.; Springer US: Boston, MA, USA, 1999; pp. 1–6. [CrossRef]
23. Le Meur, Y.; Pichon, A.; Schaal, K.; Schmitt, L.; Louis, J.; Gueneron, J.; Vidal, P.P.; Hausswirth, C. Evidence of Parasympathetic Hyperactivity in Functionally Overreached Athletes. *Med. Sci. Sports Exerc.* **2013**, *45*, 2061–2071. [CrossRef] [PubMed]
24. Thiel, C.; Vogt, L.; Bürklein, M.; Rosenhagen, A.; Hübscher, M.; Banzer, W. Functional Overreaching during Preparation Training of Elite Tennis Professionals. *J. Hum. Kinet.* **2011**, *28*, 79–89. [CrossRef] [PubMed]

Disclaimer/Publisher's Note: The statements, opinions and data contained in all publications are solely those of the individual author(s) and contributor(s) and not of MDPI and/or the editor(s). MDPI and/or the editor(s) disclaim responsibility for any injury to people or property resulting from any ideas, methods, instructions or products referred to in the content.

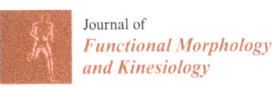

Article

Examination of Countermovement Jump Performance Changes in Collegiate Female Volleyball in Fatigued Conditions

Paul T. Donahue *, Ayden K. McInnis, Madelyn K. Williams and Josey White

School of Kinesiology and Nutrition, University of Southern Mississippi, Hattiesburg, MS 39406, USA; madelyn.k.williams@usm.edu (M.K.W.); josey.white@usm.edu (J.W.)
* Correspondence: paul.donahue@usm.edu

Abstract: The purpose of this investigation was to examine changes in countermovement vertical jump performance after a single sport-specific training session in a sample of collegiate female volleyball athletes. Eleven NCAA Division I volleyball athletes performed countermovement vertical jumps with and without an arm swing prior to and immediately after a sport-specific training session. Each participant completed two jumps in each condition using a portable force platform. Paired samples t-tests were performed within each jump condition. When using an arm swing, mean braking force was the only variable to display a statistically significant change ($p < 0.05$). In the no-arm-swing condition, mean propulsive force, propulsive net impulse, jump height and reactive strength index modified all statistically increased ($p < 0.05$). Time to takeoff was statistically reduced ($p < 0.05$). Additionally, a single-subject analysis was performed across all eleven participants resulting in general trends seen in the no-arm-swing condition, whereas the arm-swing condition displayed inconsistent findings across participants.

Keywords: countermovement jump; athlete monitoring; force–time curve

1. Introduction

The sport of volleyball emphasizes having a strong ability to jump as it is a critical component of the technical skills needed to compete (blocking and hitting) [1–3]. Vertical jump testing has become a common assessment of neuromuscular fatigue in athletic populations [4,5]. This is in part due to the ease of testing protocols and insight obtained from specific variables that relate directly to neuromuscular function. Jump assessments have been performed using a multitude of methodologies making jump height and peak power common variables of interest [6]. This has created conflicting findings throughout the literature regarding changes in jump performance in states of neuromuscular fatigue for a variety of reasons.

First, several protocols have been used when performing vertical jump assessments. The most common difference between these protocols is the utilization of an arm swing (AS) movement. Previous investigations have shown that, when using an arm swing, jump performance will typically be greater, as evidenced by larger jump heights being achieved [7–11]. It was been proposed that, when using an AS during vertical jump assessments, individuals may use a different movement strategy [7]. While the AS may provide a level of ecological validity to the testing, any fatigue an individual may be experiencing can be masked by changing the relative usage of the arms to create upward momentum. Second, the device being used to assess jump performance can have a large impact on our ability to determine the level of fatigue. When using traditional field-testing devices (Vertec), jump height is the only variable that can be collected. As mentioned previously, the usage of an AS can mask changes in jump strategy to maintain jump height. When using these traditional devices, an AS jump is required to determine jump height. Similarly, when using jump mats, only jump height can be assessed. Though either an AS

Citation: Donahue, P.T.; McInnis, A.K.; Williams, M.K.; White, J. Examination of Countermovement Jump Performance Changes in Collegiate Female Volleyball in Fatigued Conditions. *J. Funct. Morphol. Kinesiol.* **2023**, *8*, 137. https://doi.org/10.3390/jfmk8030137

Academic Editor: Diego Minciacchi

Received: 3 August 2023
Revised: 12 September 2023
Accepted: 14 September 2023
Published: 17 September 2023

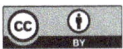

Copyright: © 2023 by the authors. Licensee MDPI, Basel, Switzerland. This article is an open access article distributed under the terms and conditions of the Creative Commons Attribution (CC BY) license (https://creativecommons.org/licenses/by/4.0/).

or no arm swing (NAS) methodology can be used, underlying strategies that determine jump height and offer a more thorough analysis cannot be assessed.

Cormack et al. reported [12] reductions in jump performance immediately post-match that were maintained for 24 post-match from pre-match in Australian rules football athletes. Specifically, flight time was reduced by approximately 3%, and relative mean force was reduced by approximately 2%. In contrast, Hoffman et al. [13] found peak power and force were maintained pre- to post-match in soccer athletes. Interestingly, Johnston et al. [14] reported no changes in peak force while reductions in peak power were present over a competition period. This reduction in power with no reduction in force points to a change in movement velocity rather than force outputs in a fatigued state [14]. More recently it has been reported that no changes were seen in male volleyball athletes from pre- to post-sport-specific training sessions [15]. Thus, this investigation sought to examine the changes in vertical jump assessments using both AS and NAS conditions in a sample of female collegiate volleyball athletes with pre- and post-sport-specific training.

2. Materials and Methods

This investigation employed a cross-sectional study design to assess changes in CMJ performance before and after a sport-specific volleyball training session. Testing took place during the spring training period and was a part of the regular athlete monitoring program that all athletes participated in as a part of their sports participation. The training session was approximately 2 h in duration. During the training session, six participants wore inertial sensors (Vert, Mayfonk Athletic, Fort Lauderdale, FL, USA) to measure jump counts. The average jump count for the six participants during the session was 103.66 with a range of 81 to 165 jumps.

2.1. Subjects

Eleven NCAA Division I female indoor volleyball athletes (age: 19.77 ± 1.09 years; height: 178.56 ± 7.81 cm; body mass: 72.42 ± 7.81 kg) participated in this study. A post-hoc power analysis was performed using G*Power (version 3.1.9.7). This calculation was completed using the jump height from the no-arm-swing condition (NAS) with an effect size of 1.76. Observed power was calculated as 0.99. All participants were cleared to partake in team-related activities by the sports medicine staff and were free of injury at the time of testing and during the 4 weeks before testing taking place. This study was conducted according to the guidelines of the Declaration of Helsinki and was approved by the University of Southern Mississippi institutional review board (20-478). Each participant provided informed written consent prior to testing.

2.2. Procedures

Participants performed all jumping trials after performing a warm-up directed by the team's strength and conditioning staff. Warm-ups took approximately 10 min to complete and consisted of dynamic lower body movements as well as submaximal vertical jumps. All trials were completed using a self-selected countermovement depth and foot position. Verbal instructions were given before initiation of each trial to "jump as high as possible".

During the NAS trials, a dowel (polyvinyl chloride, <1.0 kg) was placed across the upper back in a manner similar to the position of a barbell during the back squat exercise [1,2]. Participants were instructed to maintain contact between the dowel and the upper back during the duration of the trial. During arm swing (AS) trials, participants were instructed to begin each trial with both arms raised above their head. They were then allowed to swing their arms in any manner they desired to obtain the greatest jump height. All trials were collected using a portable force platform (AMTI, Accupower, Watertown, MA, USA) sampling at 1000 Hz. Each trial began with participants having one second of quiet standing before being given a "3, 2, 1, Go" countdown. During the quiet standing phase, body mass was calculated from the vertical ground reaction force. A 30-s rest period was given between trials. NAS trials were performed before AS trials during both testing sessions.

2.3. Data Analysis

Raw vertical ground reaction force data was then exported and analyzed using a customized Excel spreadsheet (v.2308, Microsoft, Redmond, WA, USA) [1,2,16]. The spreadsheet was modeled using methods previously reported by Chavda et al. [17]. CMJ phase definitions followed those suggested by McMahon et al. [18]. Briefly, the phases of interest for this investigation were defined as the braking and propulsive phases. Braking was defined as the point at which vertical ground reaction force surpassed the calculated body mass during one second of quiet stance prior to the trial initiation until the instant the center of mass velocity reaches zero. The propulsive phase was defined as the end of the braking phase to the point of takeoff. The center of mass velocity was calculated by finding the center of mass acceleration for each sample by subtracting the calculated body mass from the vertical force data. Then, integration of acceleration data with respect to time using the trapezoidal rule, beginning 30 ms before movement initiation as recommended by Owen et al. [19], provided the center of mass velocity. Integration of the center of mass velocity data with respect to time provided the center of mass displacement. As for variable calculations, time to takeoff was calculated as the duration from movement initiation to the point of takeoff. Reactive strength index modified was calculated as jump height divided by time to takeoff [20]. Finally, all force variables are presented as net force (measured force − body mass).

2.4. Statistical Analysis

Mean data for the two trials in each condition were used in the statistical analysis. Reliability analysis for each variable used both intraclass correlation coefficient (ICC) and coefficient of variation (CV) from the pre-testing data. ICC was calculated using a two-way random approach. Reliability was deemed acceptable with ICC values greater than 0.80 and CV values of less than 10%. To compare conditions, a paired samples t-test was conducted for each variable. Significance for all tests was a priori set at $p < 0.05$. Effect sizes were calculated as Hedge's g and interpreted using the criteria of trivial (<0.2), small (0.2–0.6), moderate (0.61–1.20), large (1.21–2.0), very large (2.0–4.0) and nearly perfect ($\geq$4.0) [21]. All statistical analyses were performed using SPSS (v28.0, SPSS Inc., Chicago, IL, USA).

Additionally, single-subject analyses were performed on each variable of interest to determine if the changes seen were outside the individual variability exhibited during the pretest. Variability was assessed using pretest CV values [22].

3. Results

All variables demonstrated acceptable levels of reliability (Table 1). Data are reported as means $\pm$ SD and displayed in Table 2. In the AS condition, only mean braking force displayed a significant increase from pre to post ($p = 0.047$, $g = 0.66$). In the NAS condition, mean propulsive force increased from pre to post ($p = 0.002$, $g = 1.18$) coinciding with an increase in propulsive net impulse ($p = 0.038$, $g = 0.70$). Jump height significantly improved pre to post ($p = 0.001$, $g = 1.70$). Additionally, time to takeoff was significantly reduced ($p = 0.015$, $g = 0.85$). Finally, RSIm was significantly improved ($p = 0.001$, $g = 1.47$).

When using the single subject analysis, each variable displayed an individual response, where both positive and negative changes were seen as well as no change. In the AS condition, seven participants showed an increase in mean braking force with two having a reduction and two with no change. Three participants showed a reduction in braking duration, while two had an increase in duration and six had no change. Braking net impulse was increased in six individuals, with decreases in two individuals and no change was shown in three. Propulsive mean force was increased in four, reduced in four, and showed no change in three. Propulsive duration increased in four, reduced in three, and no change was seen in four. Propulsive net impulse was increased in four participants, reduced in four, and showed no change in three. Five participants displayed an increase in countermovement depth, with one reducing depth and five having no change. Jump height was increased in six, decreased in four, and no change was seen in one participant.

Time to takeoff was reduced in five individuals, increased in four and no change was seen in two. Lastly, RSIm was increased in five participants, reduced in two individuals and no change was seen in four.

Table 1. Intraclass Correlation Coefficient (ICC) and Coefficient of Variations (CV).

	ICC (95% CI)	CV (95% CI)
Arm Swing		
Braking Mean Force	0.91 (0.77–0.96)	3.71 (1.49–5.93)
Braking Duration	0.94 (0.86–0.97)	5.22 (2.01–8.42)
Braking Impulse	0.84 (0.61–0.93)	5.77 (2.75–8.79)
Propulsive Mean Force	0.99 (0.97–0.99)	1.81 (0.76–2.86)
Propulsive Duration	0.86 (0.64–0.95)	2.12 (1.03–3.22)
Propulsive Net Impulse	0.97 (0.89–0.99)	1.84 (0.37–3.30)
Countermovement Depth	0.88 (0.61–0.96)	3.26 (2.09–4.42)
Time To Takeoff	0.94 (0.87–0.98)	1.08 (0.55–1.61)
Jump Height	0.97 (0.93–0.99)	1.97 (1.14–2.80)
RSIm	0.95 (0.90–0.98)	2.39 (1.30–3.48)
No Arm Swing		
Braking Mean Force	0.91 (0.78–0.96)	6.38 (2.92–9.81)
Braking Duration	0.93 (0.86–0.97)	5.89 (3.22–8.56)
Braking Impulse	0.84 (0.61–0.93)	4.16 (3.03–9.76)
Propulsive Mean Force	0.91 (0.80–0.96)	2.79 (1.53–4.05)
Propulsive Duration	0.88 (0.80–0.95)	2.90 (1.66–4.14)
Propulsive Net Impulse	0.93 (0.85–0.97)	1.62 (0.44–2.80)
Countermovement Depth	0.88 (0.61–0.96)	3.56 (2.03–5.08)
Time To Takeoff	0.94 (0.87–0.98)	2.17 (1.03–3.30)
Jump Height	0.97 (0.93–0.99)	2.74 (0.87–4.61)
RSIm	0.95 (0.90–0.98)	4.10 (2.16–6.04)

Table 2. Changes from Pre to Post Testing (mean ± SD).

	Arm Swing Condition				
	Pre	Post	p	g	%Δ
Mean Braking Force (N)	496.93 ± 145.62	**536.29 ± 170.51**	**0.047**	0.656	7.9
Braking Duration (ms)	201.41 ± 39.39	196.86 ± 56.70	0.704	0.114	2.6
Braking Net Impulse (N*s)	96.46 ± 24.03	100.31 ± 28.52	0.386	0.263	4.0
Mean Propulsive Force (N)	624.42 ± 119.76	630.52 ± 119.91	0.413	0.248	1.0
Propulsive Duration (ms)	336.59 ± 23.21	339.91 ± 35.86	0.573	0.169	1.0
Propulsive Net Impulse (N*s)	210.27 ± 35.16	213.19 ± 28.73	0.554	0.178	1.4
Countermovement Depth (cm)	39.51 ± 5.66	41.08 ± 7.11	0.103	0.521	4.0
Jump Height (cm)	33.84 ± 4.74	34.19 ± 4.46	0.545	0.182	1.0
Time to Takeoff (ms)	992.13 ± 99.26	971.95 ± 89.05	0.321	0.303	2.0
RSImod	0.34 ± 0.05	0.35 ± 0.05	0.133	0.475	2.9
	No Arm Swing Condition				
	Pre	Post	p	g	%Δ
Mean Braking Force (N)	527.45 ± 155.94	570.61 ± 149.25	0.097	0.551	8.2
Braking Duration (ms)	189.23 ± 34.28	170.73 ± 42.92	0.099	0.527	9.8
Braking Net Impulse (N*s)	95.89 ± 20.73	92.54 ± 19.63	0.548	0.188	3.5
Mean Propulsive Force (N)	619.03 ± 100.74	**668.30 ± 116.16**	**0.002**	1.179	8.0
Propulsive Duration (ms)	319.23 ± 36.23	317.41 ± 24.14	0.764	0.089	0.6
Propulsive Net Impulse (N*s)	197.81 ± 33.04	**213.19 ± 38.67**	**0.038**	0.695	7.8
Countermovement Depth (cm)	35.90 ± 6.39	35.58 ± 6.16	0.421	0.244	0.9
Jump Height (cm)	28.95 ± 4.97	**31.27 ± 5.00**	**0.001**	1.700	8.0
Time to Takeoff (ms)	873.09 ± 103.28	**831.95 ± 99.83**	**0.015**	0.852	4.7
RSImod	0.33 ± 0.06	**0.38 ± 0.07**	**0.001**	1.466	15.2

Bold values represent statistically significant differences between time points. RSImod = reactive strength index modified.

During the NAS condition, six participants showed an increase in mean braking force. Two displayed a reduction and three had no change during post-testing. Five individuals displayed a reduction in braking duration. One increased duration and five had no change. Five participants saw an increase in braking impulse, four had a reduction and two had no change. Nine participants increased propulsive mean force with two experiencing no change (Figure 1). Six individuals saw a reduction in propulsive duration with three increasing duration. Two participants had no change in propulsive duration (Figure 2). Propulsive net impulse was increased in 10 participants and no change was seen in one (Figure 3). Countermovement depth was reduced in three participants, increased in two, and had no change in six. Jump height increased in ten participants and one had no change. Time to takeoff was reduced in seven individuals, increased in two individuals, and showed no change in two individuals. Lastly, RSIm was increased in nine individuals and no change was seen in two.

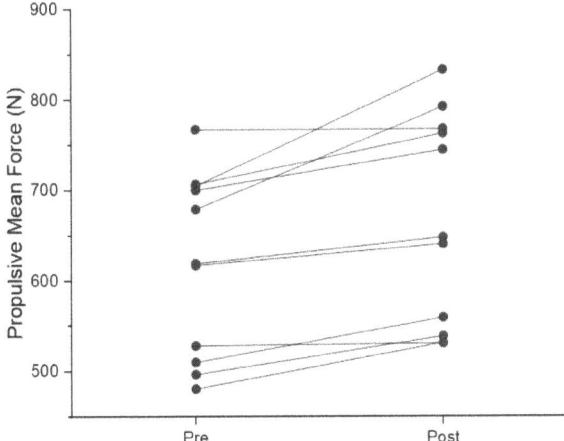

Figure 1. Individual change in propulsive mean force during NAS condition.

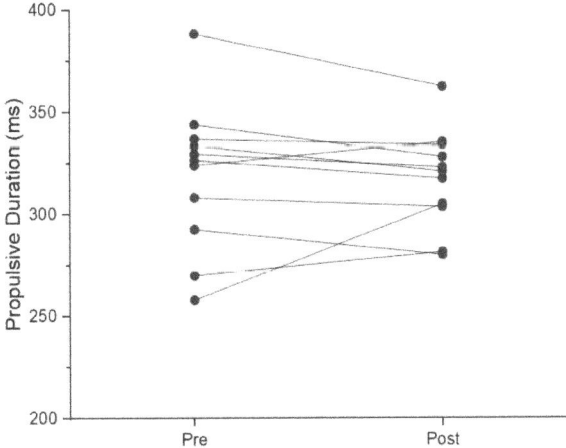

Figure 2. Individual change in propulsive duration during NAS condition.

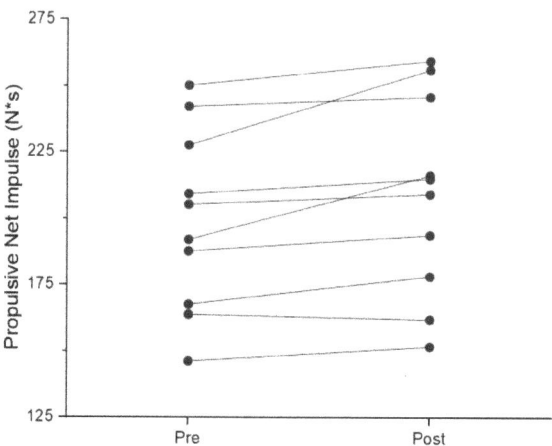

Figure 3. Individual change in propulsive net impulse during NAS condition.

4. Discussion

The main findings of this investigation were that, in the NAS condition, jump performance saw more changes from pre- to post-practice than the number of changes seen in the AS condition. These findings both support previous investigations, where no change was seen in the CMJ performance of volleyball athletes after fatiguing tasks, and are in contrast to the greater body of literature on changes in CMJ performance as a result of fatigue [12,14,23,24]. In a review of changes in physical performance testing post-competition, CMJ jump height was reduced between 1.6 and 6 cm [23]. Within this review, a variety of sports were used, and testing occurred at a variety of time intervals post-competition. While the general trend of a reduction in jump height was seen, no controls for the type of CMJ or how the CMJ was measured were used in the review [23]. Thus, a wide range of reductions in jump height and effect sizes (0.22–1.22) were seen [23]. Gathercole et al. [4] previously displayed that different forms of vertical jump testing in a fatigued state provided different results. Under the same fatigue conditions, countermovement jump performance displayed different findings than squat jumps in terms of fatigue sensitivity [4]. This illustrates similar findings to the present investigation where the NAS condition displayed changes in jump height that were not seen in the AS condition. Not only is it important to select which vertical jump assessment is used, but other methodological considerations, such as arm swing utilization, also need to be accounted for.

Previous investigations have used either the AS or NAS jump test based on a variety of factors. If using the Vertec device to assess jump performance then an AS has to be employed, whereas if using linear transducers, force plates, or jump mats, either methodology can be used. This creates potential issues in the literature as it has been shown that within-subject outputs and jump strategies can shift based on the use of an AS [7–9,25]. Hoffman et al. found [13] there to be no differences pre- and post-competition when completing a NAS testing protocol in collegiate female soccer athletes, whereas McLellan et al. [26] found there to be a decrease in peak force in post-match testing of rugby league athletes using an AS. This lack of consistency in findings throughout the literature can be explained through a variety of factors concerning methodologies. The findings in the current study point to the need for consistency in the literature as a change from pre- to post-testing differed based on the jump condition used. This is the first investigation, to the author's knowledge, that used both AS and NAS conditions to assess the changes to jump performance in a fatigued state. Previous investigations that have used multiple forms of vertical jump have manipulated the countermovement itself by using the squat jump (SJ) or depth jumps [4]. Gathercole et al. [4] found that the CMJ task was best in assessing immediate and prolonged neuromuscular fatigue in the jumping task used. Interestingly, CMJ performance was diminished during the immediate post-exercise condition using a NAS methodology where performance was improved in the current study [4]. The results of the current study, however, support the findings of Moreno-Perez et al. [27] who found an increase in jump height post competition in semi-professional basketball athletes. This coincided with an increase in the dorsiflexion range of motion. Additionally, in a sample of snowboard athletes, a small increase in jump height post excise was observed [28]. This increase in jump height occurred with a decrease in propulsive mean force and an increase in propulsive time as well as time to takeoff [28]. This is in line with the current study, where an increase in propulsive mean force increased and time to takeoff decreased, suggesting a change in movement strategy during the immediate fatigued state.

As has been stated in many of the previous investigations centered on jump testing to assess neuromuscular fatigue, the source of the fatigue (exercise, sport-specific training, competition) and the athletes themselves, play a critical role in the findings of this study. Cooper et al. [24] found there to be a significant reduction in jump height, force, and power in a sample of recreationally trained individuals after completing a fatiguing task of continuous vertical jumps. However, Robineau et al. [29] found there to be no statistical reduction in CMJ height after a simulated soccer game in eight amateur soccer athletes. Moreover, Cortis et al. [30] found an increase non-statistically significant increase in jump height in a sample of 10 senior male soccer athletes after a match. This demonstrates that sample demographics and the method by which fatigue is induced can impact findings related the vertical jump performance. In a similar study to the current investigation, professional male volleyball athletes displayed no differences in any CMJ metric after a sport-specific training session [15]. However, the authors failed to report whether individuals were allowed to use an AS. Though the exact methods used were not disclosed, the results are similar to the present investigation. As volleyball is a sport that relies heavily on vertical jump ability, changes in jump performance may be limited. With volleyball athletes needing to complete the vertical jump task in fatigued states during training and competition, post-testing may not produce significant changes. Based on the previous findings and those of the current investigation, future investigations should examine the changes in CMJ metrics over consecutive days of training and competition [15].

The use of the single-subject analysis in this study provides additional valuable information that has not previously been reported. A general trend was seen across all participants during the NAS that was not seen during the AS condition. An example of this can be seen in the increase in propulsive mean force, where nine of the eleven subjects saw an increase in the NAS condition. During the AS condition, propulsive mean force increased in four participants, reduced in four, and had no change in three. This is important for several reasons. First, of the four individuals displaying an increase in AS propulsive mean force, two had an increase in propulsive net impulse during the AS condition; both of these individuals also showed increased propulsive duration. The other two participants that saw an increase in propulsive mean force and had reductions in propulsive duration resulting either in no change or a reduction in propulsive net impulse. This indicates a potential change in the strategy being used that is masked at the group level by individuals having the opposite strategy shift occur (reduce force and increase duration). Thus, practitioners interested in changes in performance as a result of competition and practice should use single-subject analysis rather than group means, as individuals can respond to similar exercises and stresses differently.

This study is not without limitations. First, the sample size used for this investigation is small. This is due to the roster size during the spring training period (offseason) in which new members of the team and injured athletes were not taking part in training as they would during the competitive season. However, though the sample size is small, previous investigations have used similar sample sizes [15,29–31] Secondly, this investigation was conducted using a cross-sectional design and results from this study may not be transferable across all training sessions. The training load based on individual jump counts is similar to what has been previously reported in professional volleyball athletes [32]. Based on the previous investigations that have examined pre- and post-changes based on a fatiguing exercise session or game scenario, we feel that the outcomes of this investigation provide a unique examination of jump performance change on both the group and individual levels [13,15,26].

5. Conclusions

In conclusion, CMJ performance post-sport-specific training appears to be influenced by the jump testing methodology used. This is important for practitioners to consider when selecting a methodology to assess neuromuscular fatigue in their athletes. As both the NAS and AS conditions displayed changes on the individual level, practitioners using both methodologies appear suited for assessing neuromuscular fatigue. Practitioners should also consider examining individual changes in addition to group changes as every variable in the current study is subject to a level of individual change.

Author Contributions: Conceptualization, P.T.D. and A.K.M.; methodology, P.T.D., M.K.W. and J.W.; investigation, P.T.D., M.K.W. and J.W.; writing—original draft preparation, P.T.D. and A.K.M. writing—review and editing, P.T.D. and A.K.M. All authors have read and agreed to the published version of the manuscript.

Funding: This research received no external funding.

Institutional Review Board Statement: The study was conducted in accordance with the Declaration of Helsinki and approved by the Institutional Review Board (or Ethics Committee) of University of Southern Mississippi (21–256 and 07/27/2021) for studies involving humans.

Informed Consent Statement: Informed consent was obtained from all subjects involved in the study.

Data Availability Statement: The data presented in this study are available on request from the corresponding author.

Conflicts of Interest: Authors declare no conflict of interest.

References

1. Legg, L.; Rush, M.; Rush, J.; McCoy, S.; Garner, J.C.; Donahue, P.T. Association Between Body Composition and Vertical Jump Performance in Female Collegiate Volleyball Athletes. *Int. J. Kinesiol. Sports Sci.* **2021**, *9*, 43–48. [CrossRef]
2. Rush, M.E.; Littlefield, T.; McInnis, A.K.; Donahue, P.T. Positional Comparison of Jump Performance in NCAA Division I Female Volleyball Athletes. *Int. J. Kinesiol. Sports Sci.* **2022**, *10*, 1–6. [CrossRef]
3. Marques, M.C.; Van Den Tillaar, R.; Vescovi, J.D.; González-Badillo, J.J. Changes in Strength and Power Performance in Elite Senior Female Professional Volleyball Players during the In-Season: A Case Study. *J. Strength Cond. Res.* **2008**, *22*. [CrossRef]
4. Gathercole, R.J.; Sporer, B.C.; Stellingwerff, T.; Sleivert, G.G. Comparison of the Capacity of Different Jump and Sprint Field Tests to Detect Neuromuscular Fatigue. *J. Strength Cond. Res.* **2015**, *29*, 2522–2531. [CrossRef]
5. Claudino, J.G.; Cronin, J.; Mezêncio, B.; McMaster, D.T.; McGuigan, M.; Tricoli, V.; Amadio, A.C.; Serrão, J.C. The Countermovement Jump to Monitor Neuromuscular Status: A Meta-Analysis. *J. Sci. Med. Sport* **2017**, *20*, 397–402. [CrossRef]
6. Gathercole, R.; Sporer, B.; Stellingwerff, T.; Sleivert, G. Alternative Countermovement-Jump Analysis to Quantify Acute Neuromuscular Fatigue. *Int. J. Sports Physiol. Perform.* **2015**, *10*, 84–92. [CrossRef]
7. Heishman, A.; Brown, B.; Daub, B.; Miller, R.; Freitas, E.; Bemben, M. The Influence of Countermovement Jump Protocol on Reactive Strength Index Modified and Flight Time: Contraction Time in Collegiate Basketball Players. *Sports* **2019**, *7*, 37. [CrossRef]
8. Hara, M.; Shibayama, A.; Takeshita, D.; Hay, D.C.; Fukashiro, S. A Comparison of the Mechanical Effect of Arm Swing and Countermovement on the Lower Extremities in Vertical Jumping. *Hum. Mov. Sci.* **2008**, *27*, 636–648. [CrossRef]
9. Harman, E.A.; Rosenstein, M.T.; Frykman, P.N.; Rosenstein, R.M. The Effects of Arms and Countermovement on Vertical Jumping. *Med. Sci. Sports Exerc.* **1990**, *22*, 825. [CrossRef]
10. Lees, A.; Vanrenterghem, J.; Clercq, D.D. Understanding How an Arm Swing Enhances Performance in the Vertical Jump. *Biomech.* **2004**, *37*, 1929–1940. [CrossRef]
11. Feltner, M.E.; Bishop, E.J.; Perez, C.M. Segmental and Kinetic Contributions in Vertical Jumps Performed with and without an Arm Swing. *Res. Q. Exerc. Sport* **2004**, *75*, 216–230. [CrossRef]
12. Cormack, S.J.; Newton, R.U.; McGuigan, M.R. Neuromuscular and Endocrine Responses of Elite Players to an Australian Rules Football Match. *Int. J. Sports Physiol. Perform.* **2008**, *3*, 359–374. [CrossRef] [PubMed]

13. Hoffman, J.R.; Nusse, V.; Kang, J. The Effect of an Intercollegiate Soccer Game on Maximal Power Performance. *Can. J. Appl. Physiol.* **2003**, *28*, 807–817. [CrossRef]
14. Johnston, R.D.; Gibson, N.V.; Twist, C.; Gabbett, T.J.; MacNay, S.A.; MacFarlane, N.G. Physiological Responses to an Intensified Period of Rugby League Competition. *J. Strength Cond. Res.* **2013**, *27*, 643. [CrossRef]
15. Cabarkapa, D.V.; Cabarkapa, D.; Whiting, S.M.; Fry, A.C. Fatigue-Induced Neuromuscular Performance Changes in Professional Male Volleyball Players. *Sports* **2023**, *11*, 120. [CrossRef]
16. Donahue, P.T.; Rush, M.; McInnis, A.K.; Littlefield, T. Phase Specific Comparisons of High and Low Vertical Jump Performance in Collegiate Female Athletes. *J. Sci. Sport Exerc.* **2022**. [CrossRef]
17. Chavda, S.; Bromley, T.; Jarvis, P.; Williams, S.; Bishop, C.; Turner, A.N.; Lake, J.P.; Mundy, P.D. Force-Time Characteristics of the Countermovement Jump: Analyzing the Curve in Excel. *Strength Cond. J.* **2018**, *20*, 67–77. [CrossRef]
18. McMahon, J.J.; Suchomel, T.J.; Lake, J.P.; Comfort, P. Understanding the Key Phases of the Countermovement Jump Force-Time Curve. *Strength Cond. J.* **2018**, *40*, 96–106. [CrossRef]
19. Owen, N.J.; Watkins, J.; Kilduff, L.P.; Bevan, H.R.; Bennett, M.A. Development of a Criterion Method to Determine Peak Mechanical Power Output in a Countermovement. *J. Strength Cond. Res.* **2014**, *28*, 1552–1558. [CrossRef]
20. Ebben, W.P.; Petushek, E.J. Using the Reactive Strength Index Modified to Evaluate Plyometric Performance. *J. Strength Cond. Res.* **2010**, *24*, 1983–1987. [CrossRef]
21. Hopkins, W.G. A Scale of Magnitudes for Effect Statistics. Available online: http://www.sportsci.org/resource/stats/effectmag.html (accessed on 8 January 2019).
22. Donahue, P.T.; Peel, S.A.; McInnis, A.K.; Littlefield, T.; Calci, C.; Gabriel, M.; Rush, M. Changes in Strength and Jump Performance over a 10 Week Competitive Period in Male Collegiate Golfers. *J. Trainology* **2022**, *11*, 22–27. [CrossRef]
23. Doeven, S.H.; Brink, M.S.; Kosse, S.J.; Lemmink, K.A.P.M. Postmatch Recovery of Physical Performance and Biochemical Markers in Team Ball Sports: A Systematic Review. *BMJ Open Sport Exerc. Med.* **2018**, *4*, e000264. [CrossRef] [PubMed]
24. Cooper, C.N.; Dabbs, N.C.; Davis, J.; Sauls, N.M. Effects of Lower-Body Muscular Fatigue on Vertical Jump and Balance Performance. *J. Strength Cond. Res.* **2020**, *34*, 2903. [CrossRef] [PubMed]
25. Vaverka, F.; Jandačka, D.; Zahradník, D.; Uchytil, J.; Farana, R.; Supej, M.; Vodičar, J. Effect of an Arm Swing on Countermovement Vertical Jump Performance in Elite Volleyball Players. *J. Hum. Kinet.* **2016**, *53*, 41–50. [CrossRef] [PubMed]
26. McLellan, C.P.; Lovell, D.I.; Gass, G.C. Markers of Postmatch Fatigue in Professional Rugby League Players. *J. Strength Cond. Res.* **2011**, *25*, 1030. [CrossRef]
27. Moreno-Pérez, V.; Del Coso, J.; Raya-González, J.; Nakamura, F.Y.; Castillo, D. Effects of Basketball Match-Play on Ankle Dorsiflexion Range of Motion and Vertical Jump Performance in Semi-Professional Players. *J. Sports Med. Phys. Fit.* **2020**, *60*, 110–118. [CrossRef]
28. Gathercole, R.J.; Stellingwerff, T.; Sporer, B.C. Effect of Acute Fatigue and Training Adaptation on Countermovement Jump Performance in Elite Snowboard Cross Athletes. *J. Strength Cond. Res.* **2015**, *29*, 37. [CrossRef]
29. Robineau, J.; Jouaux, T.; Lacroix, M.; Babault, N. Neuromuscular Fatigue Induced by a 90-Minute Soccer Game Modeling. *J. Strength Cond. Res.* **2012**, *26*, 555. [CrossRef]
30. Cortis, C.; Tessitore, A.; Lupo, C.; Perroni, F.; Pesce, C.; Capranica, L. Changes in Jump, Sprint, and Coordinative Performances After a Senior Soccer Match. *J. Strength Cond. Res.* **2013**, *27*, 2989. [CrossRef]
31. Cortis, C.; Tessitore, A.; Lupo, C.; Pesce, C.; Fossile, E.; Figura, F.; Capranica, L. Inter-Limb Coordination, Strength, Jump, and Sprint Performances Following a Youth Men's Basketball Game. *J. Strength Cond. Res.* **2011**, *25*, 135. [CrossRef]
32. Skazalski, C.; Whiteley, R.; Bahr, R. High Jump Demands in Professional Volleyball—Large Variability Exists between Players and Player Positions. *Scand. J. Med. Sci. Sports* **2018**, *28*, 2293–2298. [CrossRef] [PubMed]

Disclaimer/Publisher's Note: The statements, opinions and data contained in all publications are solely those of the individual author(s) and contributor(s) and not of MDPI and/or the editor(s). MDPI and/or the editor(s) disclaim responsibility for any injury to people or property resulting from any ideas, methods, instructions or products referred to in the content.

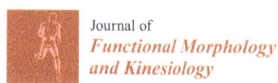

Article

Exercise Cardiac Load and Autonomic Nervous System Recovery during In-Season Training: The Impact on Speed Deterioration in American Football Athletes

Eric Renaghan [1], Harrison L. Wittels [2], Luis A. Feigenbaum [1,3], Michael Joseph Wishon [2], Stephanie Chong [2], Eva Danielle Wittels [2], Stephanie Hendricks [2], Dustin Hecocks [2], Kyle Bellamy [4], Joe Girardi [3], Stephen Lee [5], Tri Vo [6], Samantha M. McDonald [2,7,*] and S. Howard Wittels [2,8,9,10]

[1] Department of Athletics, Sports Science, University of Miami, Miami, FL 33146, USA; eric.renaghan@miami.edu (E.R.); lfeigenbaum@med.miami.edu (L.A.F.)
[2] Tiger Tech Solutions, Inc., Miami, FL 33156, USA; hl@tigertech.solutions (H.L.W.); joe@tigertech.solutions (M.J.W.); schong591@gmail.com (S.C.); evadanielle@gmail.com (E.D.W.); steph.hendricks@gmail.com (S.H.); dustin@tigertech.solutions (D.H.); shwittels@gmail.com (S.H.W.)
[3] Department of Physical Therapy, Miller School of Medicine, University of Miami, Miami, FL 33146, USA; j.girardi@miami.edu
[4] Department of Athletics, Nutrition, University of Miami, Miami, FL 33146, USA; k.bellamy1@umiami.edu
[5] United States Army Research Laboratory, Adelphi, MD 20783, USA; stephen.j.lee28.civ@mail.mil
[6] Navy Medical Center-San Diego, San Diego, CA 92134, USA; huuv@g.clemson.edu
[7] School of Kinesiology and Recreation, Illinois State University, Normal, IL 61761, USA
[8] Department of Anesthesiology, Mount Sinai Medical Center, Miami, FL 33140, USA
[9] Department of Anesthesiology, Wertheim School of Medicine, Florida International University, Miami, FL 33199, USA
[10] Miami Beach Anesthesiology Associates, Miami, FL 33140, USA
* Correspondence: smmcdo4@ilstu.edu; Tel.: +1-309-438-5008

Citation: Renaghan, E.; Wittels, H.L.; Feigenbaum, L.A.; Wishon, M.J.; Chong, S.; Wittels, E.D.; Hendricks, S.; Hecocks, D.; Bellamy, K.; Girardi, J.; et al. Exercise Cardiac Load and Autonomic Nervous System Recovery during In-Season Training: The Impact on Speed Deterioration in American Football Athletes. *J. Funct. Morphol. Kinesiol.* **2023**, *8*, 134. https://doi.org/10.3390/jfmk8030134

Academic Editor: Diego Minciacchi

Received: 16 July 2023
Revised: 15 August 2023
Accepted: 28 August 2023
Published: 12 September 2023

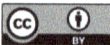

Copyright: © 2023 by the authors. Licensee MDPI, Basel, Switzerland. This article is an open access article distributed under the terms and conditions of the Creative Commons Attribution (CC BY) license (https:// creativecommons.org/licenses/by/ 4.0/).

Abstract: Fully restoring autonomic nervous system (ANS) function is paramount for peak sports performance. Training programs failing to provide sufficient recovery, especially during the in-season, may negatively affect performance. This study aimed to evaluate the influence of the physiological workload of collegiate football training on ANS recovery and function during the in-season. Football athletes recruited from a D1 college in the southeastern US were prospectively followed during their 13-week "in-season". Athletes wore armband monitors equipped with ECG and inertial movement capabilities that measured exercise cardiac load (ECL; total heartbeats) and maximum running speed during and baseline heart rate (HR), HR variability (HRV) 24 h post-training. These metrics represented physiological load (ECL = HR·Duration), ANS function, and recovery, respectively. Linear regression models evaluated the associations between ECL, baseline HR, HRV, and maximum running speed. Athletes (n = 30) were 20.2 ± 1.5 years, mostly non-Hispanic Black (80.0%). Negative associations were observed between acute and cumulative exposures of ECLs and running speed ($\beta = -0.11 \pm 0.00$, $p < 0.0000$ and $\beta = -0.15 \pm 0.04$, $p < 0.0000$, respectively). Similarly, negative associations were found between baseline HR and running speed ($\beta = -0.45 \pm 0.12$, 95% CI: -0.70, -0.19; $p = 0.001$). HRV metrics were positively associated with running speed: (SDNN: $\beta = 0.32 \pm 0.09$, $p < 0.03$ and rMSSD: $\beta = 0.35 \pm 0.11$, $p < 0.02$). Our study demonstrated that exposure to high ECLs, both acutely and cumulatively, may negatively influence maximum running speed, which may manifest in a deteriorating ANS. Further research should continue identifying optimal training: recovery ratios during off-, pre-, and in-season phases.

Keywords: exercise training; overtraining; sports; strength and conditioning; collegiate

1. Introduction

Optimal sports performance requires complete recovery of the autonomic nervous system (ANS) [1]. The ANS regulates many physiological processes involved in athletic performance such as skeletal muscle contraction, cardiac function, and vascular compliance [2]. As such, the functionality of the ANS affects performance metrics such as speed, agility, reaction time, force production, and power output [3,4]. For sports such as collegiate football, the repeated powerful movements profoundly impact the ANS, often leading to prolonged sympathetic nervous system dominance [5,6]. Full recovery of the ANS is paramount for peak sports performance during competitions [5]. Failing to provide adequate recovery, especially during in-season, invites negative consequences such as non-functional overtraining, and decrements in sports performance, all signs of a deteriorating ANS [7,8].

The window of recovery following competitions varies for each sport and depends on its duration, intensity, etc. For contact sports such as collegiate football, athletes endure, for nearly four hours, heightened levels of adrenaline, maximal force production, and power output [5]. These prolonged competitions result in augmented physical and mental fatigue, skeletal muscle damage, energy depletion, and muscular soreness. As such, football athletes may require at least 72 h for full recovery [5,9–13]. Sport performance researchers recommend markedly reducing training volume and limiting high-intensity training during the in-season allowing for sufficient post-competition recovery [14]. While strong evidence supports the necessity of recovery, reports suggest that many coaches fear reducing training volume as it may detrain athletes, resulting in poor performance [6]. Interestingly, studies show detraining occurs during the in-season however, most significantly among "reserve" or "bench" players, the athletes who are minimally exposed to competitive play [6]. The trepidation of detraining likely leads to coaches training athletes at higher volumes and intensities. Consequently, studies also show that higher training loads during the in-season predispose athletes to injury (e.g., ligament tears or muscle strains), likely a result of a deteriorating ANS [15].

A significant limitation of the former research, however, is the limited number of studies on collegiate football, a sport played by nearly 25% of all NCAA athletes [16]. Studies examining the influence of training volume during the in-season in contact sports primarily focused on soccer and rugby athletes [17,18]. Comparatively, collegiate football differs considerably as competitions are 50 to 60% longer and pose a greater risk for severe injuries. This risk is likely exacerbated if training regimens do not account for supramaximal efforts performed during football competitions, however, this remains unclear [6]. Therefore, this study aimed to evaluate the influence of the physiological demand imposed upon collegiate football athletes during the in-season and the recovery and function of the ANS. Specifically, we examined the association between the exercise cardiac load (total heartbeats) endured during the preceding week's training sessions and ANS recovery and function among collegiate football athletes. We hypothesized that the sustained, hyperbolic cardiac load endured among competing athletes would compound the impact of the weekly training sessions on the ANS throughout the in-season. Specifically, we anticipated observing a negative association between 24-h baseline heart rate (HR) and maximum running speed and a positive association between heart rate variability (HRV) and maximum speed, each representing ANS recovery and function, respectively.

2. Materials and Methods

2.1. Study Design

The current study employed a 13-week, prospective study design among a sample of Division I collegiate male football athletes during their "in-season" training. The physiological load of weekly training was estimated using an exercise cardiac load metric. ANS recovery was measured using baseline HR and HRV and ANS function was estimated via the athletes' top speed reached during weekly trainings.

2.2. Subjects

Subjects were recruited from a Division I collegiate football team located in the southeastern region of the State of Florida. The athletes were participating in their routine

13-week "in-season" training program. Practice sessions included aerobic, speed, strength, agility, and power-focused exercises. While each training session varied daily and weekly, the athletes consistently engaged in moderate-vigorous intensity exercise lasting between 120 to 180 min every, Tuesday, Wednesday, Thursday, Friday, and Sunday (Figure 1). The prospective participants were recruited from a pre-selected group of athletes the coaches identified as "starters", which were athletes that competed in nearly every regulation game and for most of its duration. Starters were recruited as they endured a greater physiological load during a given week consequent to participating in weekly competitions. Additionally, due to the wide variability in movement patterns across player positions, only starting athletes playing "heavy running" positions including cornerback, running back, tight end, and wide receiver were included in the primary analyses. Prior to any measurements, the athletes were informed of the benefits and risks of the study and the conflicts of interest of all authors. All athletes participating voluntarily consented to the study. All study protocols followed the ethical principles defined in the Declaration of Helsinki and were approved by the university's Institutional Review Board (IRB #20191223).

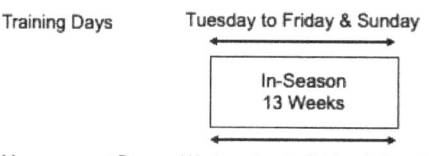

Figure 1. Schematic of 13-week In-Season Collegiate Football Training Program.

2.3. Methodology

2.3.1. Cardiac and ANS Measurement

Thirty participants were fitted with armband monitors equipped with temperature, electrocardiography (ECG), photoplethysmography (PPG), and inertial measurement unit (IMU) capabilities (Warfighter Monitor (WFM), Tiger Tech Solutions Inc., Miami, FL, USA). The WFM armbands were previously validated in several diverse subpopulations [19]. Monitors were placed on the posterior aspect of the left upper arm, secured with an elastic band, and worn at the start and throughout each training session (n = 128). Although the WFM device collected several biometric parameters, only cardiac function and IMU data were analyzed.

2.3.2. Exercise Cardiac Load during In-Season Weekly Training

Exercise cardiac load (ECL) represented the physiological load athletes endured during each training session. ECL was the product of the athlete's average HR (bpm) and duration (minutes) of weekly training sessions. Both HR and duration are strong contributors to physiological load during exercise [14]. Only HRs sustained at ≥85 bpm were calculated for average HR as this threshold was considered "active training". ECL was normalized with the largest ECL measured, from any athlete, during the in-season and multiplied by 100 for purposes of correlation.

$$ECL\ (total\ heartbeats) = Average\ HR(\text{bpm}) \times Session\ Duration\ (\text{minutes})$$

2.3.3. ANS Recovery

Next-day baseline HR represented ANS recovery. Baseline HR was measured in the early morning and following at least 4 min of inactivity, per established protocols [20]. Specifically, baseline HR was measured prior to the start (0600–0700) of the following day's exercise training session. Each athlete was required to remain nearly motionless in a seated position for a period of 5 min to collect a "resting" baseline HR.

The HRV metrics used included the standard deviation of NN intervals (SDNN) and the root mean square of successive differences (rMSSD). HRV was measured during the same 5-min interval as baseline HR. Further details on these metrics are described elsewhere [21].

2.3.4. Maximum Running Speed

Maximum running speed served as the outcome variable and was defined as the fastest recorded speed in miles per hour (mph) by an athlete during a single training session. Speed was calculated using a nine-degree-of-freedom inertial measurement unit (9-DOF IMU) on the WFM. The 9-DOF IMU provides a three-axis accelerometer, gyroscope, and magnetometer. Utilizing the magnetometer and the accelerometer the normal vector (z-axis) was identified and gravity was removed to give us the remaining accelerometer data which contains the two-dimensional, x- and y-plane of accelerations. Utilizing the gyroscope, the x and y accelerometer values were forced to zero during non-movement periods. Further, with the gyroscope, the dominant movement direction within the x and y planes was identified. We then, integrated the accelerometer data with a starting value of zero along the dominant direction in the x-y plane to quantify velocity. To calculate absolute speed, the directional component was removed [22,23].

2.4. Statistical Analyses

The current study evaluated the associations between ECL, HRV, baseline HR of both acute and cumulative exposures to in-season training, and its influence on maximum running speed. For acute training, (e.g., daily sessions) ECLs, HRV, and baseline HR values were averaged across daily sessions for each of the 13 weeks of in-season training. For the cumulative exposures, ECL was averaged over one training week. Maximum running speed served as the primary outcome variable. Associations were quantified using linear regression models and were performed separately for each metric. The normality of the conditional distributions was assessed via the Kolmogorov-Smirnov test and was deemed normally distributed. For all models, β coefficients and standard errors were estimated, and the *a priori* threshold for statistical significance was set at α = 0.05. Statistical analyses were performed in MATLAB, version 2021b (MathWorks, Natick, MA, USA).

3. Results

The descriptive characteristics of the sample of D1 collegiate football athletes are presented in Table 1. Of all the starters (n = 30), 16.7%, 23.3%, 13.3%, and 20.0% were cornerbacks, running backs, tight ends, and wide receivers, respectively. Athletes were, on average, 20.2 ± 1.5 years of age, predominantly non-Hispanic Black 80.0%, and had an average body mass index of 27.6 ± 2.3 kg/m^2 and ranging from 23.7 to 32.5 kg/m^2.

Table 1. Descriptive Characteristics of Starting Football Athletes (n = 30).

	Mean (SD)	Median (Min, Max)
Age (years)	20.2 (1.5)	20.0 (18.0, 23.0)
Anthropometrics		
Weight (kg)	94.38 (9.7)	92.97 (77.1, 112.5)
Height (m)	1.85 (0.06)	1.84 (1.75, 1.86)
Body Mass Index (kg/m^2)	27.6 (2.3)	27.5 (23.7, 32.5)
Race/Ethnicity (%)		
NH White	6.7	
NH Black	80.0	
Other	0.0	
Hispanic	13.3	
Football Position (%)		
Cornerback	16.7	
Defensive Back	3.3	
Linebacker	16.7	
Running Back	23.3	

Table 1. Cont.

	Mean (SD)	Median (Min, Max)
Safety	6.7	
Tight End	13.3	
Wide Receiver	20.0	

NH = non-Hispanic; SD = standard deviation; min = minimum; max = maximum; kg = kilogram; m = meter.

Table 2 shows the weekly average and 50th percentiles for the average exercise cardiac load of in-season training sessions and the recovery and function of the athletes' ANS. The acute and cumulative ECL of in-season training were 21,800.0 ± 4600.0 and 108,700.0 ± 22,800.0 total heartbeats, respectively. On average, the next-day baseline HR was 60.9 ± 8.6 bpm and ranged from 48.8 to 112.2 bpm. The average maximum running speed achieved across 25 weeks of in-season training was 17.3 ± 1.4 mph and ranged from 15.0 to 22.0 mph.

Table 2. Average Training Load, ANS Recovery and ANS Function Among Starting Football Athletes.

	Mean (SD)	Median (Min, Max)
Exercise Cardiac Load *		
Daily (acute exposure)	21.8 (4.6)	23.7 (8.4, 34.8)
Weekly (cumulative exposure)	108.7 (22.8)	114.9 (43.9, 159.8)
ANS Recovery		
Baseline HR (bpm)	60.9 (8.6)	59.8 (48.8, 112.2)
SDNN (bpm)	81.3 (2.0)	81.2 (77.4, 84.2)
rMSSD (bpm)	70.1 (1.7)	70.1 (66.2, 73.4)
ANS Function		
Maximum Running Speed (mph)	17.3 (1.4)	17.2 (15.0, 22.0)

Expressed in the total number of heartbeats; bpm = beats per minute. * average training HR·session duration.

The correlation coefficients for the associations between exercise cardiac load, ANS recovery, and maximum running speed during in-season training are presented in Table 3. Statistically significant, negative associations between both acute and cumulative exposure to exercise cardiac loads and maximum running speed achieved during in-season training (acute: $\beta = -0.11 \pm 0.00$, 95% CI: $-0.12, -0.10$; $p < 0.0000$; cumulative: $\beta = -0.15 \pm 0.04$, 95% CI: 0.00, 0.72; $p < 0.0000$). Strong statistically significant correlations were also found between ANS recovery metrics and maximum running speed. Specifically, baseline HR was negatively associated with maximum speed ($\beta = -0.45 \pm 0.12$, 95% CI: $-0.70, -0.19$; $p = 0.001$). Both metrics of HRV, rMSSD and SDNN, were significantly and positively associated with maximum running speed: ($\beta = 0.32 \pm 0.09$, 95% CI: 0.14, 0.50; $p < 0.03$ and $\beta = 0.35 \pm 0.11$, 95% CI: 0.13, 0.57; $p < 0.02$).

Table 3. Adjusted Regression Coefficients for the Association Between ECL and ANS Recovery and Function (Maximum Running Speed [mph]).

	β (SE)	95% CI	Adjusted R^2	p-Value
Exercise Cardiac Load *				
Daily (acute exposure)	−0.11 (0.00)	[−0.12, −0.10]	0.64	0.0000
Weekly (cumulative exposure)	−0.15 (0.04)	[−0.00, 0.72]	0.73	0.0000
ANS Recovery				
Baseline HR (bpm)	−0.45 (0.12)	[−0.70, −0.19]	0.56	0.0011
SDNN (ms)	0.32 (0.09)	[0.14, 0.50]	0.55	0.0287
rMSSD (ms)	0.35 (0.11)	[0.13, 0.57]	0.52	0.0151

CI = confidence intervals; bpm = beats per min; ms = milliseconds; mph = miles per hour. * average training HR·session duration.

4. Discussion

The purpose of this study was to examine the association between ECL endured across 13 weeks of in-season training and ANS recovery and function among D1 football players. We hypothesized that higher ECLs endured across weekly in-season training would elicit a negative influence on maximum running speed. The major findings of this study were that among "starters", (1) both acute and cumulative exposures to high exercise cardiac loads were negatively associated with maximum running speed achieved during in-season training, (2) deteriorating maximum running speed was strongly associated with higher baseline HRs, and (3) HRV (rMSSD and SDNN) were positively associated with maximum running speed.

One novel aspect of this study was the strong, negative associations observed between both acute and cumulative exposures to high ECLs and maximum running speed during 13 weeks of in-season training. Specifically, for athletes in "heavy-running" positions (e.g., wide receiver and tight end), acute and cumulative exposures to high ECLs during in-season training negatively impacted their performance with linear, progressive reductions in maximum running speed. In collegiate football, short sprints at near maximal or maximal speed are critical to a team's offense and defense, significantly influencing their overall game performance and outcome. Similar to the current study, several studies previously documented decrements in sports performance consequent to excessive acute and chronic exercise training loads. However, most were reported among adult rugby and soccer players in European countries. These sports represent a small fraction of collegiate athletes in the United States as opposed to collegiate football, which accounts for 25% of all NCAA athletes [16]. Moreover, the outcomes of these studies were more focused on soft-tissue injuries, training, and game absenteeism, and less so on performance-based outcomes (e.g., speed, power) [18]. The negative impact on performance-based outcomes is critical to detect as it likely precedes an injury that significantly disrupts physical movement (e.g., muscle strain/tear, ligament strain), requiring passive recovery and rehabilitation [24]. With that, the strong relationship between ECL and maximum running speed observed in this study highlights the potential utility of ECL as a monitoring tool for optimizing performance. ECL quantifies the physiological tolerance of each athlete, using the total exercise load endured by the cardiac muscle during training (HR x duration). Using that physiological feedback provides coaches with a non-invasive measure to program more effective pre- and in-season training regimens and possibly prevent significant decrements in sports performance, non-functional overreaching, and overtraining.

Interestingly, the current study also demonstrated a strong negative association between next-day baseline HR and maximum running speed. That is, athletes exhibiting higher next-day baseline HRs, on average, showed larger decrements in their maximum running speed. This observation possibly suggests that deteriorating speed may manifest from insufficient recovery of the ANS. Given the paralleling negative association between ECL and maximum running speed reported in the current study, the suboptimal recovery of the ANS could be consequent to acute and cumulative exposures to high ECLs. Established evidence demonstrates the negative neurophysiological consequences of high training loads and insufficient recovery. For example, studies show excessive training partially impairs neural signaling (e.g., firing rate) [12], mitochondrial function [13], glucose tolerance [10], skeletal muscle repair [11], etc., all of which require at least 48–72 h or more for full recovery [9]. Without sufficient recovery, ANS function may begin deteriorating and negatively affect the contractile properties of skeletal muscle (e.g., shortening velocity) and performance outcomes such as maximum running speed. Monitoring the relationships between ECL, ANS recovery/function, and performance is likely most critical during the in-season as in addition to exercise training, athletes perform supraphysiological efforts during 3- to 4-h-long competitions. The reductions in maximum running speed observed in this study are the antithetical outcome to the primary goal of in-season training, which is achieving peak athletic performance. For this purpose, sports performance experts recommend substantially decreasing volume and intensity variation in weekly training to focus on maintaining the athletes' level of fitness and refining sport-specific movement patterns [6,25]. The decrements in performance in this study may highlight the suboptimal translation of recommendations to the real-world sports realm.

Analogous to our baseline HR finding, rMSSD and SDNN were positively associated with maximum running speed. That is, on average, athletes running at lower maximum speeds likely exhibited lower HRV, an indication of insufficient ANS recovery 24 h post-training. Several studies previously documented lower HRV, including rMSSD and SDNN, immediate and short-term post-intense exercise (0–12 h). However, HRV typically returned to baseline values within 24 h [26–28]. The discrepancies between the current study and others are potentially attributed to different types of sports (e.g., running and cycling vs. strength and power), duration and frequency of high-intensity training, and sufficient rest intervals between and within sessions. The lower HRV observed *in tandem* with lower maximum running speeds observed in this study aligns with the nature of the off-, pre-, and in-season training programs and the negative association found between baseline HR and maximum running speed. Football practices, across all seasons, were typically long in duration (~2 to 4 h), occurred 5 to 6 times per week, and included several high-intensity training sessions. As such, the nature of these sessions, specifically during the in-season, likely explains our HRV findings. Additionally, the negative association between next-day baseline HR and maximum running speed further confirms this observation. In healthy populations, baseline HR is inversely associated with HRV such that higher baseline HRs correlate with lower HRV. In the current study, this relationship is also observed [29]. For example, in Figures 2 and 3, at the same maximum running speed (e.g., 12.0 mph), higher baseline HRs and lower HRV values are observed, both indicating some degree of ANS dysfunction.

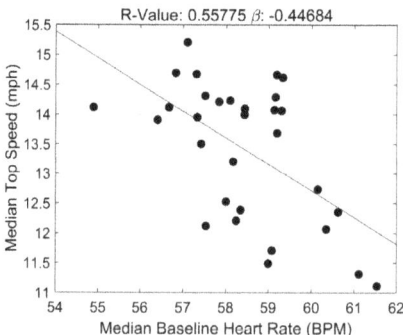

Figure 2. Correlation Between Next-Day Baseline HR and Maximum Running Speed in D1 Football Athletes.

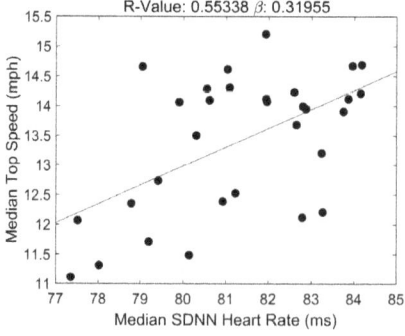

Figure 3. Correlation Between HRV (SDNN) and Maximum Running Speed in D1 Football Athletes.

It should be acknowledged, however, that although the metrics referenced in this paper (speed, baseline HR, etc.) correlate, they should not be viewed as surrogates for one another. For instance, while the findings for both metrics of ANS recovery (RMSSD, SDNN, baseline HR) were consistent, each metric provides different physiological information [30]. This is important as athletes exhibit high inter-individual variability in their physiological response and tolerance to training [31]. As such, it is strongly recommended that coaches utilize a holistic approach to monitoring and evaluating their athletes in an effort to prevent deterioration and maximize performance.

4.1. Strengths and Limitations

There are several strengths of the current study. First, this study employed a prospective design in a natural setting, which allowed for stronger evidential conclusions and unique insight into collegiate football training and its potential consequences on athletic performance. Second, the ECL metric more accurately measured the total physiological (internal) workload endured by athletes during training as opposed to other methods quantifying workload using sets, repetitions resistance loads, etc. As such, ECL may be a more effective tool for monitoring athletic performance and preventing ANS deterioration. Third, maximum running speed was measured objectively using a device measuring inertial movement. This likely provided a more accurate measure of maximum speed compared to other metrics such as field-based testing and global positioning systems. This study also has a few limitations. First, our sample only included collegiate football players from one D1 university in a single geographical location, limiting the generalizability of our findings. Second, maximum running speed, ECL, baseline HR, and HRV were not collected during regulation games which did not allow us to fully quantify the physiological load endured by the athletes during a given in-season training week. As such, it is unclear as to whether the physiological load of the game influenced the ECL of the subsequent week's training sessions and vice versa. However, the game-day physiological load was indirectly measured as the data were collected during "in-season" training. Third, the small sample size precluded our ability to analyze the correlations between ECL, HR recovery, and maximum speed by football position. However, the inter-position variability in movement patterns was reduced as only positions with "heavy running" were included in the analyses. Lastly, other factors potentially affecting ANS activity were not accounted for such as sleep, ergogenic aids, and psychological stress.

4.2. Practical Implications

This study highlights the importance of coaches appropriately designing exercise training programs during the in-season. Because the in-season includes many regulation games, athletes endure significantly greater physiological loads nearly every week. As such, strength, and conditioning coaches, as recommended by sports performance experts, must dramatically modify their training programs to provide sufficient rest following games, yet simultaneously provide sufficient physiological stimulus to maintain fitness levels. By optimizing training programs throughout the year, sports performance outcomes, such as maximum running speed, can be improved.

5. Conclusions

In conclusion, the current study demonstrated that exposure to both high acute, and more importantly, cumulative ECLs, may negatively influence sports performance, specifically maximum running speed. Additionally, the observed decrement in running speed may be a manifestation of a deteriorating ANS, an early warning sign of overtraining. As such, it is imperative that coaches account for the increased physiological load of games thus, optimizing in-season training programs that improve sports performance. Further research is needed to continue identifying optimal training: recovery ratios during off-, pre-, and in-season phases for many sports. We recommend that future investigations monitor, year-round, the physiological loads of training programs to inform coaches of the best practices for preparing for off-, pre-, and in-season training, and providing adequate recovery. Importantly, researchers should also identify ineffective sports training programs that lead to declines in performance.

Author Contributions: Conceptualization, S.H.W., E.R., H.L.W., M.J.W., S.L., K.B., J.G., T.V. and L.A.F.; methodology, S.C., E.D.W., S.H., K.B., J.G. and D.H.; software, S.H.W., H.L.W. and M.J.W.; validation, S.H.W., H.L.W. and M.J.W.; formal analysis, M.J.W., H.L.W. and S.M.M.; investigation, S.C., E.D.W., S.H., K.B., J.G. and D.H.; resources, S.H.W., H.L.W., K.B., J.G. and E.R.; data curation, M.J.W.; writing—original draft preparation, S.M.M.; writing—review and editing, S.M.M., H.L.W. and M.J.W.; visualization, S.M.M., H.L.W. and M.J.W.; supervision, S.H.W., H.L.W. and M.J.W.; project administration, H.L.W., S.C., K.B., J.G. and L.A.F.; funding acquisition, S.H.W and H.L.W. All authors have read and agreed to the published version of the manuscript.

Funding: This research received no external funding.

Institutional Review Board Statement: The study was conducted in accordance with the Declaration of Helsinki and approved by the Institutional Review Board of University of Miami (IRB# 20191223 and 22 June 2020) for studies involving humans.

Informed Consent Statement: Informed consent was obtained from all subjects involved in the study.

Data Availability Statement: Data presented in the current paper are available upon request.

Acknowledgments: The authors would like to thank Army Applications Laboratory and Thomas M. Mead for their support in the research and development of the WarFighter Monitor^{TM}, a device aimed to improve the safety and performance of our service members.

Conflicts of Interest: The following authors are paid employees of Tiger Tech Solutions Inc., owner of the Warfighter Monitor (WFM) used in this study: S.H.W., H.L.W., M.J.W., S.C., E.D.W., S.H., D.H. and S.M.M. Authors K.B., S.L., L.A.F. and E.R. have no conflict of interest to disclose.

References

1. Kellmann, M.; Bertollo, M.; Bosquet, L.; Brink, M.; Coutts, A.J.; Duffield, R.; Erlacher, D.; Halson, S.L.; Hecksteden, A.; Heidari, J.; et al. Recovery and Performance in Sport: Consensus Statement. *Int. J. Sports Physiol. Perform.* **2018**, *13*, 240–245. [CrossRef]
2. Freeman, J.V.; Dewey, F.E.; Hadley, D.M.; Myers, J.; Froelicher, V.F. Autonomic Nervous System Interaction with the Cardiovascular System During Exercise. *Prog. Cardiovasc. Dis.* **2006**, *48*, 342–362. [CrossRef]
3. Jensen, J.L.; Marstrand, P.C.D.; Nielsen, J.B. Motor Skill Training and Strength Training Are Associated with Different Plastic Changes in the Central Nervous System. *J. Appl. Physiol.* **2005**, *99*, 1558–1568. [CrossRef]
4. Pincivero, D.M.; Lephart, S.M.; Karunakara, R.G. Effects of Rest Interval on Isokinetic Strength and Functional Performance after Short-Term High Intensity Training. *Br. J. Sports Med.* **1997**, *31*, 229. [CrossRef]
5. Pincivero, D.M.; Bompa, T.O. A Physiological Review of American Football. *Sports Med.* **1997**, *23*, 247–260. [CrossRef]
6. Edwards, T.; Spiteri, T.; Piggott, B.; Haff, G.G.; Joyce, C. A Narrative Review of the Physical Demands and Injury Incidence in American Football: Application of Current Knowledge and Practices in Workload Management. *Sports Med.* **2018**, *48*, 45–55. [CrossRef]
7. Kreher, J.B.; Schwartz, J.B. Overtraining Syndrome: A Practical Guide. *Sports Health* **2012**, *4*, 128–138. [CrossRef]
8. Lehmann, M.; Foster, C.; Gastmann, U.; Keizer, H.; Steinacker, J.M. Definition, Types, Symptoms, Findings, Underlying Mechanisms, and Frequency of Overtraining and Overtraining Syndrome. In *Overload, Performance Incompetence, and Regeneration in Sport*; Lehmann, M., Foster, C., Gastmann, U., Keizer, H., Steinacker, J.M., Eds.; Springer: Boston, MA, USA, 1999; pp. 1–6. [CrossRef]
9. Tiidus, P.M. (Ed.) *Skeletal Muscle Damage and Repair*; Human Kinetics: Champaign, IL, USA, 2008. [CrossRef]
10. O'Reilly, K.P.; Warhol, M.J.; Fielding, R.A.; Frontera, W.R.; Meredith, C.N.; Evans, W.J. Eccentric Exercise-Induced Muscle Damage Impairs Muscle Glycogen Repletion. *J. Appl. Physiol.* **1987**, *63*, 252–256. [CrossRef]
11. Howatson, G.; Milak, A. Exercise-Induced Muscle Damage Following a Bout of Sport Specific Repeated Sprints. *J. Strength Cond. Res.* **2009**, *23*, 2419–2424. [CrossRef]
12. Pearce, A.J.; Sacco, P.; Byrnes, M.L.; Thickbroom, G.W.; Mastaglia, F.L. The Effects of Eccentric Exercise on Neuromuscular Function of the Biceps Brachii. *J. Sci. Med. Sport* **1998**, *1*, 236–244. [CrossRef]
13. Flockhart, M.; Nilsson, L.C.; Tais, S.; Ekblom, B.; Apró, W.; Larsen, F.J. Excessive Exercise Training Causes Mitochondrial Functional Impairment and Decreases Glucose Tolerance in Healthy Volunteers. *Cell Metab.* **2021**, *33*, 957–970.e6. [CrossRef]
14. Halson, S.L. Monitoring Training Load to Understand Fatigue in Athletes. *Sports Med.* **2014**, *44*, 139–147. [CrossRef]
15. Gabbett, T.J. The Training—Injury Prevention Paradox: Should Athletes Be Training Smarter and Harder? *Br. J. Sports Med.* **2016**, *50*, 273. [CrossRef]

16. National Collegiate Athletics Association. *NCAA Sports Sponsorship and Participation Rates Report (1956–57 through 2021–22)*; NCAA/06071983; National Collegiate Athletics Association: Indianapolis, IN, USA, 2022; p. 135.
17. Cross, M.J.; Williams, S.; Trewartha, G.; Kemp, S.P.; Stokes, K.A. The Influence of In-Season Training Loads on Injury Risk in Professional Rugby Union. *Int. J. Sports Physiol. Perform.* **2016**, *11*, 350–355. [CrossRef]
18. Rogalski, B.; Dawson, B.; Heasman, J.; Gabbett, T.J. Training and Game Loads and Injury Risk in Elite Australian Footballers. *J. Sci. Med. Sport* **2013**, *16*, 499–503. [CrossRef]
19. Peck, J.; Wishon, M.J.; Wittels, H.; Lee, S.J.; Hendricks, S.; Davila, H.; Wittels, S.H. Single Limb Electrocardiogram Using Vector Mapping: Evaluation and Validation of a Novel Medical Device. *J. Electrocardiol.* **2021**, *67*, 136–141. [CrossRef]
20. Speed, C.; Arneil, T.; Harle, R.; Wilson, A.; Karthikesalingam, A.; McConnell, M.; Phillips, J. Measure by Measure: Resting Heart Rate across the 24-Hour Cycle. *PLoS Digit. Health* **2023**, *2*, e0000236. [CrossRef]
21. Bourdillon, N.; Yazdani, S.; Vesin, J.-M.; Schmitt, L.; Millet, G.P. RMSSD Is More Sensitive to Artifacts Than Frequency-Domain Parameters: Implication in Athletes' Monitoring. *J. Sports Sci. Med.* **2022**, *21*, 260–266. [CrossRef]
22. Yuan, Q.; Chen, I.-M. Simultaneous Localization and Capture with Velocity Information. In Proceedings of the 2011 IEEE/RSJ International Conference on Intelligent Robots and Systems, San Francisco, CA, USA, 25–30 September 2011; pp. 2935–2940. [CrossRef]
23. Li, Q.; Young, M.; Naing, V.; Donelan, J.M. Walking Speed Estimation Using a Shank-Mounted Inertial Measurement Unit. *J. Biomech.* **2010**, *43*, 1640–1643. [CrossRef]
24. Sampson, J.A.; Murray, A.; Williams, S.; Halseth, T.; Hanisch, J.; Golden, G.; Fullagar, H.H.K. Injury Risk-Workload Associations in NCAA American College Football. *J. Sci. Med. Sport* **2018**, *21*, 1215–1220. [CrossRef]
25. Jalilvand, F.; Chapman, D.; Lockie, R. Strength and Conditioning Considerations for Collegiate American Football. *J. Aust. Strength Cond.* **2019**, *27*, 72–85.
26. Manresa-Rocamora, A.; Flatt, A.A.; Casanova-Lizón, A.; Ballester-Ferrer, J.A.; Sarabia, J.M.; Vera-Garcia, F.J.; Moya-Ramón, M. Heart Rate-Based Indices to Detect Parasympathetic Hyperactivity in Functionally Overreached Athletes. A Meta-Analysis. *Scand. J. Med. Sci. Sports* **2021**, *31*, 1164–1182. [CrossRef]
27. Mourot, L.; Bouhaddi, M.; Perrey, S.; Cappelle, S.; Henriet, M.T.; Wolf, J.P.; Rouillon, J.D.; Regnard, J. Decrease in Heart Rate Variability with Overtraining: Assessment by the Poincaré Plot Analysis. *Clin. Physiol. Funct. Imaging* **2004**, *24*, 10–18. [CrossRef]
28. Burma, J.S.; Copeland, P.V.; Macaulay, A.; Khatra, O.; Smirl, J.D. Effects of High-Intensity Intervals and Moderate-Intensity Exercise on Baroreceptor Sensitivity and Heart Rate Variability during Recovery. *Appl. Physiol. Nutr. Metab.* **2020**, *45*, 1156–1164. [CrossRef]
29. Sacha, J. Interaction between Heart Rate and Heart Rate Variability. *Ann. Noninvasive Electrocardiol.* **2014**, *19*, 207–216. [CrossRef]
30. Dong, J.-G. The Role of Heart Rate Variability in Sports Physiology. *Exp. Ther. Med.* **2016**, *11*, 1531–1536. [CrossRef]
31. Meyler, S.; Bottoms, L.; Wellsted, D.; Muniz-Pumares, D. Variability in Exercise Tolerance and Physiological Responses to Exercise Prescribed Relative to Physiological Thresholds and to Maximum Oxygen Uptake. *Exp. Physiol.* **2023**, *108*, 581–594. [CrossRef]

Disclaimer/Publisher's Note: The statements, opinions and data contained in all publications are solely those of the individual author(s) and contributor(s) and not of MDPI and/or the editor(s). MDPI and/or the editor(s) disclaim responsibility for any injury to people or property resulting from any ideas, methods, instructions or products referred to in the content.

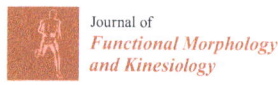

Article

Running-Related Overuse Injuries and Their Relationship with Run and Resistance Training Characteristics in Adult Recreational Runners: A Cross-Sectional Study

Lea R. Stenerson [1,2,*], Bridget F. Melton [1,3], Helen W. Bland [4] and Greg A. Ryan [5,*]

1. Department of Health and Human Performance, Concordia University of Chicago, River Forest, IL 60305, USA; bmelton@georgiasouthern.edu
2. Department of Biology, Regis University, Denver, CO 80221, USA
3. Department of Health Sciences and Kinesiology, Georgia Southern University, Statesboro, GA 30458, USA
4. Department of Health Policy and Community Health, Georgia Southern University, Statesboro, GA 30458, USA; hwbland@georgiasouthern.edu
5. Department of Health Sciences, Piedmont University, Demorest, GA 30535, USA
* Correspondence: lstenerson@regis.edu (L.R.S.); gryan@piedmont.edu (G.A.R.)

Abstract: This study aimed to characterize running-related injuries (RRIs), explore their relationship with run and resistance training (RT) parameters, and identify perceived prevention measures among adult recreational runners. An anonymous online survey was designed and distributed via social media and email. Data were analyzed with chi-square, t-test, or analysis of variance (ANOVA), with significance accepted at $p \leq 0.05$. Data from 616 participants (76.8% female, age: 42.3 ± 10.5 y) were analyzed. Most runners (84.4%) had an injury history, with 44.6% experiencing one in the past year. The most common RRI sites included the foot/ankle (30.9%) and knee (22.2%). RRI prevalence was higher in those running >19 miles weekly (48.4%, $p = 0.05$), but there were no differences based on RT participation status. Among those using RT, relatively more RRIs were observed in runners who trained the hip musculature (50.3%, $p = 0.005$) and did not include the upper body (61.6%, $p < 0.001$). A disproportionately high RRI prevalence was found for several of the other risk-reduction strategies. RRIs remain a substantial problem, particularly around the ankle/foot and knee. Higher run volume and performance motives were positively associated with RRIs. Most runners incorporated RRI risk-reduction techniques, with over half using RT. The current study did not determine whether preventative strategies were implemented before or after injury; therefore, prospective studies controlling for previous injuries are required to evaluate the effectiveness of RT in preventing future RRIs.

Keywords: running-related injury prevalence; recreational runners; resistance training; injury prevention

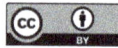

1. Introduction

Practical, efficient, and accessible, running is one of the most popular exercise modes worldwide, with involvement continuing to rise [1,2]. Along with higher participation rates, runner characteristics have evolved over the decades to include more female participants, a slower average pace, a higher average age [1], and those with health versus performance motives [1,3]. The current runner demographics exemplify the more casual, social, or recreational runner [4], who falls between novice and sub-elite or elite and ostensibly represents most of the running populace.

Recreational athletes may indeed reap the countless health benefits associated with running, including weight loss, cardiorespiratory fitness, lipoprotein profiles, mental health, and increased lifespan [5–7], but these rewards are concomitant with a high running-related injury (RRI) risk—defined herein as "running-related (training or competition) musculoskeletal pain in the lower limbs that causes a restriction or stoppage of running (distance, speed, duration, or training) for at least 7 days or 3 consecutive scheduled training sessions, or that requires the runners to consult a physician or other health professional" [8] (p. 375). RRIs are associated with direct and indirect costs (i.e., healthcare, time away from work) and represent a considerable economic burden [9,10]. Additionally, a history of an RRI is the main determinant of future RRIs and the primary reason people quit running [11,12]. Due to heterogeneous reporting methods and inconsistent definitions [8,13], RRI prevalence varies widely from 10 to 90%, with an average of 42.7% of runners experiencing an RRI annually [14,15]. Notably, these prevalence data were an amalgamation of novice to elite runners, triathletes, and orienteers and did not provide a unifying definition of RRI or delineate between the different athlete types, sex, age, or run distance.

The popularity of running, its indisputable benefits, and the high likelihood of nefarious outcomes highlight the necessity of incorporating RRI risk-reduction strategies. Efforts to reduce RRIs are not novel, but evidence of effective strategies remains elusive, likely due to the complexity of RRIs' etiologies. Nonetheless, RRIs are universally characterized as a load–capacity imbalance [16], and while reducing RRIs requires a multifaceted approach, focusing on modifiable factors to improve runners' capacity is imperative. Salient modifiable factors include strength and neuromuscular insufficiencies [17–21] and posture control or balance deficits [19,22,23]. Resistance training (RT), sometimes referred to as "weight" or "strength" training and described herein as requiring the body to resist an external force or load, can elicit positive neuromusculoskeletal adaptations, improving intrinsic capacity. For example, various RT modalities, from body weight to heavy load exercises, can correct strength imbalances; increase bone density; and improve overall strength, speed, power, balance, coordination, and posture control [24,25].

RT is posited to reduce injury prevalence in team sports [26]; however, the relationship between RT participation status and RRIs is equivocal among recreational runners. Two studies aimed to investigate the relationship between RT participation and RRIs in recreational runners [27,28], both reporting no benefit or association. However, Toresdahl et al. [27] did not account for RT participation in their observational group and reported poor compliance in the RT group. Voight et al. [28] found no association between RRIs and cross-training, but cycling was the most common cross-training modality, with RT representing only a small percentage. Moreover, no studies have investigated the specific RT programming parameters as they relate to RRIs, and little is known about the proportion of recreational runners who use RT to reduce RRIs or what other measures are perceived to achieve this goal. Thus, this study aimed to characterize overuse running-related injuries (RRIs), explore their relationship with specific run and resistance training (RT) parameters, and identify perceived prevention strategies among adult recreational runners. Uniquely, the current study: (a) used Yamato et al.'s [8] consensus definition of RRIs to assess overuse injuries, which are the most common RRI among distance runners [15]; (b) explicitly targeted recreational runners, defined as running an average of at least 2 times per week for at least a year, and considering running their primary exercise mode; (c) examined RRI's association with RT participation and specific program parameters for all participants and by sex, age, and run distance; and (d) identified perceived prevention strategies currently in use.

2. Materials and Methods

2.1. Participants

Following institutional review board (IRB) approval, volunteers were recruited using a combination of non-probability purposeful convenience and snowball sampling. Inclusion criteria included recreational runners aged 18–65 who considered running their primary exercise mode and averaged at least 2 weekly runs for at least 1 year. Familiarity with the English language and internet access were requisite for study participation.

2.2. Procedures

This study used a quantitative, cross-sectional, online survey design. A 4-part survey was created with influence from related surveys [29–38] to reduce bias in question creation and promote consistency within the field. Each section (running history, RT characteristics, injury history, and standard demographics) had 2–11 questions, depending on the answers selected. The running-specific questions asked about years of experience, frequency, weekly distance, duration, and reasons for running. RT questions addressed participation status, experience, frequency, duration, workout parameters (i.e., sets, repetitions, effort level, type of RT, and targeted muscles), and reasons for participation. The RRI segment began with a definition of an overuse RRI that was adapted from other researchers [8]. Questions were asked about RRI history, the RRI prevalence in the past year, and the RRI location and severity if one was present. This section also assessed the use of perceived injury-prevention strategies.

The survey underwent unbiased peer review and was piloted with a small subset of the population for feedback and readability. A web-based Flesch–Kincaid readability test indicated a 7th–8th grade reading level, which is considered adequate for those 18 years and older. A brief study overview, an invitation to participate, and the Qualtrics (Provo, UT, USA) survey link were distributed broadly via Facebook (Menlo Park, CA, USA) and email lists with encouragement to share among other recreational runners. Survey questions were available only after agreeing to informed consent and eligibility criteria.

2.3. Statistical Analysis

All data were analyzed with IMB SPSS Statistics version 28 (Chicago, IL, USA). G*power's (Aichach, Germany) minimum sample size for chi-square with a medium effect (Cohen's W = 0.3), powered at 80%, and 5 degrees of freedom, was 143. Descriptive statistics are presented as mean and standard deviation (continuous variables) or frequency with percentage (categorical data). The survey questions yielded predominantly ordinal and nominal data. Cross-tabulation with chi-square analysis determined associations between the categorical variables. Independent t-tests or analysis of variance (ANOVA) were used for continuous data (e.g., years of experience). Significance was accepted at $p \leq 0.05$ for all, and a post hoc Bonferroni correction was applied when omnibus significance was determined from the cross-tabulated chi-square analyses. Missing values were excluded from the analysis.

3. Results

3.1. Participants

Data from 616 eligible volunteers (76.8% female, M ± SD, age: 42.3 ± 10.5 y, body mass index (BMI) = 23.6 ± 3.6 kg·m^{-2}) were included in the analyses. On average, participants had about 13 years of experience and ran approximately four times per week, totaling 3–6 h. There were slight but statistically significant sex differences: men had a higher BMI and ran more frequently, while women had more running experience (Table 1).

Table 1. Participant characteristics.

Variable	All	Female	Male
Total	616 (100%)	473 (76.8%)	143 (23.2%)
Age (y)	42.3 ± 10.5	42.3 ± 10.1	42.3 ± 11.8
BMI (kg·m^{-2})	23.6 ± 3.6	23.3 ± 3.7	24.9 ± 3.2 ***
Education			
High school or equivalent	29 (4.7%)	14 (3%)	15 (10.5%) **
Trade/technical	20 (3.2%)	15 (3.2%)	5 (3.5%)
Associates	22 (3.6%)	14 (3%)	8 (5.6%)
Bachelors	202 (32.8%)	155 (32.8%)	47 (32.9%)
Masters/doctorate	342 (55.5%)	275 (58.1%)	67 (46.9%)

Table 1. Cont.

Variable	All	Female	Male
Community			
Urban	130 (21.1%)	97 (20.5%)	33 (23.1%)
Suburban	374 (60.7%)	295 (62.4%)	79 (55.2%)
Rural	111 (18%)	81 (17.1%)	30 (21%)
Race			
Asian/Pacific Islander	12 (1.9%)	7 (1.5%)	5 (3.5%)
Black/African American	5 (0.8%)	5 (1.1%)	-
Native American/Alaskan	1 (0.2%)	-	1 (0.7%)
White/Caucasian	565 (91.7%)	436 (92.2%)	129 (90.2%)
Bi- or multi-racial	13 (2.1%)	10 (2.1%)	3 (2.1%)
Other	19 (3.1%)	14 (3.0%)	5 (3.5%)
Run experience (y)	12.8 ± 9.6	13.3 ± 9.6 *	11.3 ± 9.7
Frequency (d/wk)	3.95 ± 1.3	3.9 ± 1.2	4.3 ± 1.4 **
Weekly distance (miles)			
≤19	298 (48.4%)	242 (51.2%)	56 (39.2%)
>19	318 (51.6%)	231 (48.8%)	87 (60.8%) *
Weekly duration (h)			
1–2	79 (12.8%)	60 (12.7%)	19 (13.3%)
3–4	228 (37%)	186 (39.3%)	42 (29.4%)
5–6	181 (29.4%)	136 (28.8%)	45 (31.5%)
7+	128 (20.8%)	91 (19.2%)	37 (25.9%)

Note. Continuous data are presented as $M \pm SD$. Categorical data are presented as frequency (n) and percentage. BMI = body mass index. * $p < 0.05$, ** $p < 0.01$, *** $p < 0.001$.

3.2. Injury Prevalence and Characteristics

RRI prevalence for all runners and by sex, age, and run-distance categories are presented in Table 2. Nearly 85% of participants had a history of RRI, and about 45% reported one in the past year, with similar proportions across sex and age categories. RRI prevalence in the past year was higher than expected among those who ran >19 miles per week (48.4%), $\chi^2(1) = 3.81$, $p = 0.05$, and for those that selected "performance" as a dominant reason for running (51.3%), $\chi^2(1) = 4.87$, $p = 0.03$. Runners in the 51–65 age category were more likely than expected to experience an injury requiring moderate (vs. mild or major) training modifications (50%), $\chi^2(1) = 10.86$, $p = 0.03$.

Table 2. Injury characteristics by frequency and percentage.

Variable	Category (n)	History of RRI	RRI in the Past Year
	Total (n = 616)	520 (84.4%)	275 (44.6%)
Sex	F (n = 473)	398 (84.1%)	202 (42.7%)
	M (n = 143)	122 (85.3%)	73 (51.0%)
p		0.74	0.08
Age	18–34 (n = 144)	120 (83.3%)	71 (49.3%)
	35–50 (n = 327)	277 (84.7%)	140 (42.8%)
	51–65 (n = 145)	123 (84.8%)	64 (44.1%)
p		0.92	0.42
Run (miles/wk)	<19 (n = 298)	250 (83.9%)	121 (40.6%)
	19+ (n = 318)	270 (84.9%)	154 (48.4%) *
p		0.73	0.05

Note. RRI = running-related injury. F = female, M = male. * $p \leq 0.05$.

RRIs occurred most frequently at the foot/ankle (30.9%), knee (22.2%), hip/groin (17.5%), and calf/Achilles (16.4%), as presented in Figure 1. The proportion of RRIs at the calf/Achilles was higher than expected for men versus women (26.0% and 12.9%, respectively), $\chi^2(6) = 14.32$, $p = 0.03$. No other significant differences in injury location were determined across sex, age, and run-distance categories.

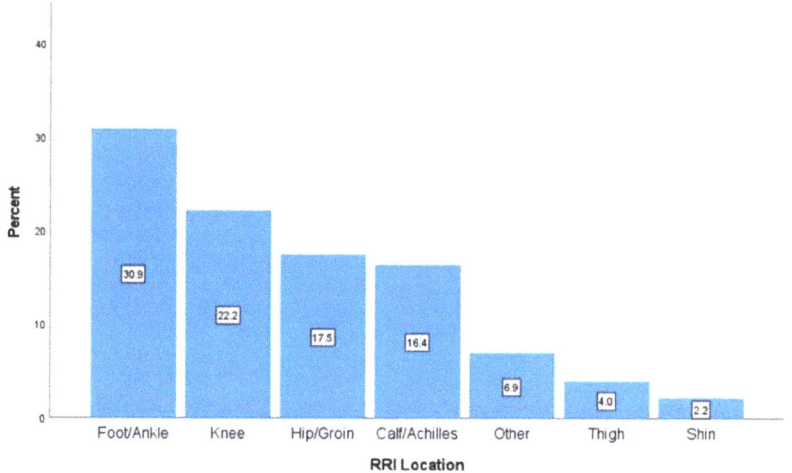

Figure 1. Percentage of injuries by anatomical location.

3.3. Relationships with Resistance Training Characteristics

No differences ($p > 0.05$) in RRI prevalence were observed between those who used RT and those who did not, which was consistent across sex, age, and run-distance categories (Table 3). Regarding RRI severity, sub-analysis showed that among those in the 35–50 age category who did not participate in RT, there was a lower proportion (14.3%) than expected of moderate RRI-related training modifications ($p = 0.03$).

Table 3. Running-related injuries and resistance-training status across sex, age, and run-distance categories.

	RRI in Past Year		p	RRI Severity			p
	Yes	No		Mild	Moderate	Major	
All			0.49				0.13
Yes	195 (45.6%)	233 (54.4%)		57 (29.2%)	73 (37.4%)	65 (33.3%)	
No	80 (42.6%)	108 (57.4%)		30 (37.5%)	20 (25.0%)	30 (37.5%)	
Sex							
Female			0.08				0.37
Yes	156 (45.1%)	190 (54.9%)		47 (30.1%)	61 (39.1%)	48 (30.8%)	
No	46 (36.2%)	81 (63.8%)		15 (32.6%)	13 (28.3%)	18 (39.1%)	
Male			0.33				0.24
Yes	39 (47.6%)	43 (52.4%)		10 (25.6%)	12 (30.8%)	17 (43.6%)	
No	34 (55.7%)	27 (44.3%)		15 (44.1%)	7 (20.6%)	12 (35.3%)	
Age							
18–34							
Yes	51 (50.0%)	51 (50.0%)	0.80	14 (27.5%)	14 (27.5%)	23 (45.1%)	0.33
No	20 (47.6%)	22 (52.4%)		9 (45.0%)	5 (25.0%)	6 (30.0%)	
35–50							
Yes	98 (43.2%)	129 (56.8%)	0.84	32 (32.7%)	36 (36.7%)	30 (30.6%)	0.03
No	42 (42.0%)	58 (58.0%)		18 (42.9%)	6 (14.3%) *	18 (42.9%)	
51–65							
Yes	46 (46.5%)	53 (53.5%)	0.41	11 (23.9%)	23 (50.0%)	12 (26.1%)	0.76
No	18 (39.1%)	28 (60.9%)		3 (16.7%)	9 (50.0%)	6 (33.3%)	

Table 3. Cont.

	RRI in Past Year		p	RRI Severity			p
	Yes	No		Mild	Moderate	Major	
			Run Distance (miles)				
≤19							
Yes	89 (41.8%)	124 (58.2%)	0.51	31 (34.8%)	36 (40.4%)	22 (24.7%)	0.06
No	32 (37.6%)	53 (62.4%)		9 (28.1%)	8 (25.0%)	15 (46.9%)	
>19 miles							
Yes	106 (57.3%)	79 (42.7%)	0.65	26 (24.5%)	37 (34.9%)	43 (40.6%)	0.06
No	48 (49.3%)	55 (53.4%)		21 (43.8%)	12 (25.0%)	15 (31.3%)	

Note. RT = resistance training. RRI = running-related injury. RRI severity reflects the extent to which training was altered. Data are presented as frequency (n) and percentage. In the case of omnibus significance, a post hoc Bonferroni adjustment was applied. * $p < 0.001$ after Bonferroni adjustment.

A disproportionately high number of RRIs was observed in runners that included hip musculature in their RT (50.3%), $\chi^2(1) = 7.97$, $p = 0.005$, and in those that did not include the upper body musculature in their RT (61.6%), $\chi^2(1) = 13.25$, $p < 0.001$. Runners who selected "general health" as a reason for using RT were less likely than expected to have an RRI (42.1%), $\chi^2(1) = 8.98$, $p = 0.003$, while those using RT for performance gains were more likely to have an RRI (50.2%), $\chi^2(1) = 4.23$, $p = 0.04$. The 40.4% of runners following a personalized RT program—developed by an exercise professional such as a personal trainer, strength coach, or physical therapist—had a relatively higher RRI prevalence (52%), $\chi^2(1) = 4.89$, $p = 0.03$. Significant differences in RRI prevalence and severity were not observed ($p > 0.05$) across RT years of experience, duration of sessions, sets, repetitions, effort, and type of modality used (Table 4).

Table 4. Resistance-training characteristics by running-related injury status.

Characteristics	RRI in Past Year		p
	Yes (n = 195)	No (n = 233)	
RT experience (y)	8.6 ± 9.1	9.5 ± 9.0	0.32
RT frequency (d/wk)	2.6 ± 1.2	2.5 ± 1.1	0.44
RT min/session	30–44 (72, 44.7%)	30–44 (89, 55.3%)	0.62
Repetition range	7–12 (128, 46.4%)	7–12 (148, 53.6%)	0.99
Effort level (0–10)	6.2 ± 1.4	6.2 ± 1.4	0.66

Note. RT = resistance training. RRI = running-related injury. Data are presented as $M \pm SD$ or as mode with frequency (n) and percentage.

3.4. Strategies for Reducing Injury Risk

Runners identified various strategies for injury prevention, with the most frequently reported methods including resistance training, passive stretching, foam rolling, and dynamic stretching (Figure 2). About 90% of all runners engaged with one or more strategies they perceived to help reduce injury risk. Runners using no risk-reduction measures had a disproportionately low RRI prevalence (21.2%), $\chi^2(1) = 12.68$, $p < 0.001$. There was a higher proportion of RRIs than expected among runners that used percussive devices (56.1%), $\chi^2(1) = 9.56$, $p = 0.002$, massage (51.3%), $\chi^2(1) = 6.39$, $p = 0.01$, dynamics (48.4%), $\chi^2(1) = 3.95$, $p = 0.047$, and who altered their run training (59.5%), $\chi^2(1) = 24.45$, $p < 0.001$. Sub-analyses revealed that those running >19 miles per week were more likely to use percussive devices (29.2%), $\chi^2(1) = 16.79$, $p < 0.001$, while those running fewer miles were more likely to include passive stretching (64.8%), $\chi^2(1) = 13.13$, $p < 0.001$. Males were also more likely to include passive stretching (67.8%), $\chi^2(1) = 8.44$, $p = 0.004$, and used run-training modifications more than expected (37.8%), $\chi^2(1) = 4.18$, $p = 0.04$. Whereas a higher proportion of females than males indicated using RT to reduce RRIs (60.7%), $\chi^2(1) = 4.19$, $p = 0.04$.

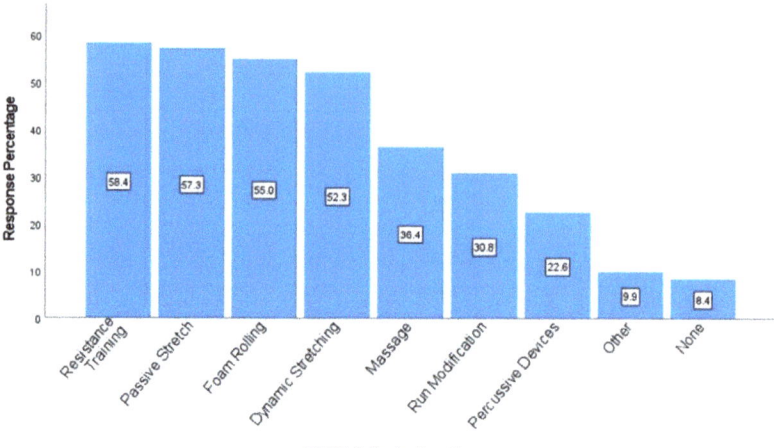

Figure 2. Percentage of runners using each strategy for reducing injuries (multi-response question).

4. Discussion

The purpose of the current study was to characterize overuse RRIs, explore their relationship with specific run and RT parameters, and identify the perceived prevention strategies used by adult recreational runners. The investigation incorporated a consensus definition of RRIs with a focus on overuse injuries and is the first study to delineate RRI characteristics and the use of prevention methods, including RT and the specific RT parameters, across sex, age, and run-distance categories.

4.1. Injury Prevalence and Location

A major finding of our study is the alarmingly high likelihood of sustaining an RRI, with 85% of runners reporting a history of injury. Moreover, nearly half (44.6%) of the participants had incurred an injury within the past year. These results are consistent with other research with mixed populations that identified broad RRI prevalence ranges from about 19 to 80% [39] or 10 to 90%, averaging about 43% [14]. There were no differences in injury prevalence by sex, despite the finding that proportionally more males ran >19 miles per week, and there was a higher injury prevalence among those averaging greater distances (48.4%) versus those running ≤19 weekly miles (40.6%). This finding suggests that weekly running distance may be a more salient factor in RRIs than sex. Injury proportion by sex is somewhat mixed in the literature, with some reporting that females have a higher RRI risk relative to males [40] and others reporting the opposite [41,42]. There is supporting evidence that higher mileage is positively associated with RRIs [30,43]. Concomitantly, our results showed a higher proportion of RRIs than expected (51.3%) among recreational runners with event-performance motives, which aligns with studies reporting a high injury rate (67.4%) among competitive runners [30] and a positive relationship between running mileage and competition level [44].

The most common anatomical locations of RRIs were the foot/ankle and knee, which is consistent with findings from a recent systematic review [14], with the exception that in our study, foot/ankle injuries (30.9%) were more common than knee injuries (22.2%), rather than the reverse, as shown in the review. Earlier studies have also reported higher injury incidence at the knee (30.7%) compared to the ankle (8.3%) or foot (14.6%) [42]. As exemplified in our study, it is plausible that foot injuries may be on the rise, which, while still speculative, may be related to the growing popularity of carbon-plated super shoes [45].

4.2. Injury Associations with Resistance Training

No associations were found between RT participation status (yes or no) and RRI prevalence among all participants and within sex, age, and run-distance categories, nor were differences determined for RRI prevalence and severity across RT experience, session duration, sets, repetitions, effort, and type of modality used. Our overall prevalence results agree with other research also depicting no relationships between RT status and injuries [27,28]. Somewhat counterintuitively, a recent study of competitive runners determined that only a small percentage of those without RRIs had participated in RT activities [30], which aligns with the disproportionately high RRI prevalence revealed in the current study among those using hip muscles during RT. However, given the numerous beneficial neuromusculoskeletal adaptations that RT can stimulate [24,25,46] and the strong evidence of its efficacy in reducing injury risk in team sports [26,47,48], it is very likely that our and other's [28] findings of no association or a positive association [30] between RT and RRI are the product of study design. Importantly, the current study design did not allow for a temporal determination of RT relative to sustaining an RRI; thus, it is unclear if RT use was preemptive or rehabilitative.

4.3. Strategies for Reducing Injury Risk

About 10% of runners in this study do not use RRI-prevention strategies, while other studies have found that nearly 20% do not use injury-reduction strategies [31]. RT, passive stretching, foam rolling, and dynamic stretching were most frequently used to reduce injury risk, with each selected by just over 50% of runners. Many competitive runners also use RT, stretching, and foam rolling (62.5%, 86.2%, and 54.7%, respectively) [30]. Interestingly, the current study found that several of the perceived prevention strategies were associated with a high proportion of RRIs. However, as with RT participation, the time frame for commencing injury-prevention measures was not determined, and sustaining an injury is likely to facilitate the incorporation of risk-reducing strategies [31]. Nonetheless, understanding prevention preferences for the sub-populations (sex, age, and distance categories) can inform exercise and healthcare professionals about preferences among these runners—with the caveat that conclusive evidence about the efficacy of each strategy for reducing RRIs is scarce.

4.4. Limitations

Important limitations exist for this study aside from the design not allowing for the elucidation of the timeline for RRIs and RT use or other prevention measures, thus precluding causal inferences. The study results were subject to recall bias as the survey was self-administered and self-reported. Survey questions were predominantly closed-ended, and more nuanced responses may have been generated by including open-ended questions. Though inclusion criteria were intentionally broad to approximate the larger population of recreational runners, convenience sampling led to a disproportionally high percentage of female, well-educated, and Caucasian runners, thus reducing external validity and limiting applicability to the current study population. However, considering the traditionally male-dominated nature of research, the high representation of females in this study is simultaneously a strength.

5. Conclusions

Recreational runners' risk of RRI is high, with an overall prevalence of about 85% and an annual prevalence of nearly 50%. While completely eradicating RRIs is unrealistic, coaches and practitioners should educate recreational runners about the high RRI prevalence and encourage proactive risk-reducing measures, particularly for those running higher distances and with performance motives. Injury-prevention measures, including RT, were not associated with lower RRIs in this study, but these results were substantially confounded by participation timing considerations, which were not determined herein. Nonetheless, RT can improve runners' capacity to tolerate training load and, thus, should be recommended. Lastly, cross-sectional retrospective studies are not adequate to elucidate the effect of RT on reducing future RRIs—prospective studies that control for previous injuries while tracking the use and timing of RT and other prevention measures relative to the RRI are necessary.

Author Contributions: All authors made substantial intellectual contributions to this study. L.R.S. developed the protocol, conducted data collection and analyses, and drafted the manuscript with guidance and review from B.F.M., H.W.B. and G.A.R. All authors have read and agreed to the published version of the manuscript.

Funding: This research received no external funding.

Institutional Review Board Statement: The study protocol was approved by Concordia University of Chicago's Institutional Review Board (2013040-1).

Informed Consent Statement: Informed consent was obtained from all subjects involved in the study.

Data Availability Statement: Data available upon reasonable request.

Acknowledgments: The authors would like to thank all the recreational runners who answered our survey and made this study possible.

Conflicts of Interest: The authors declare no conflict of interest.

References

1. Andersen, J.; RunRepeat. The State of Running 2019. 2021. Available online: https://runrepeat.com/state-of-running (accessed on 8 July 2022).
2. Lange, D.; Statistica. Running & Jogging—Statistics & Facts. 2020. Available online: https://www.statista.com/topics/1743/running-and-jogging/ (accessed on 8 July 2022).
3. Malchrowicz, J.; Malchrowicz-Mośko, E.; Fadigas, A. Age-related motives in mass running events participation. *Olimp. J. Olymp. Stud.* **2018**, *2*, 257–273. [CrossRef]
4. Janssen, M.; Walravens, R.; Thibaut, E.; Scheerder, J.; Brombacher, A.; Vos, S. Understanding different types of recreational runners and how they use running-related technology. *Int. J. Environ. Res. Public Health* **2020**, *17*, 2276. [CrossRef] [PubMed]
5. Hespanhol, L.C., Jr.; Pillay, J.D.; van Mechelen, W.; Verhagen, E. Meta-analyses of the effects of habitual running on indices of health in physically inactive adults. *Sports Med.* **2015**, *45*, 1455–1468. [CrossRef] [PubMed]
6. Quirk, H.; Bullas, A.; Haake, S.; Goyder, E.; Graney, M.; Wellington, C.; Copeland, R.; Reece, L.; Stevinson, C. Exploring the benefits of participation in community-based running and walking events: A cross-sectional survey of parkrun participants. *BMC Public Health* **2021**, *21*, 1978. [CrossRef]
7. Lee, D.; Brellenthin, A.G.; Thompson, P.D.; Sui, X.; Lee, I.M.; Lavie, C.J. Running as a key lifestyle medicine for longevity. *Prog. Cardiovasc. Dis.* **2017**, *60*, 45–55. [CrossRef] [PubMed]
8. Yamato, T.P.; Saragiotto, B.T.; Lopes, A.D. A consensus definition of running-related injury in recreational runners: A modified Delphi approach. *J. Orthop. Sports Phys. Ther.* **2015**, *45*, 375–380. Available online: http://www.jospt.org/doi/10.2519/jospt.2015.5741 (accessed on 5 May 2020). [CrossRef] [PubMed]
9. Centers for Disease Control and Prevention [CDC]. *Trends in Meeting the 2008 Physical Activity Guidelines, 2008–2018*; CDC: Atlanta, GA, USA, 2018.
10. Hespanhol, L.C., Jr.; van Mechelen, W.; Postuma, E.; Verhagen, E. Health and economic burden of running-related injuries in runners training for an event: A prospective cohort study. *Scand. J. Med. Sci. Sports* **2016**, *26*, 1091–1099. [CrossRef]
11. Fokkema, T.; Hartgens, F.; Kluitenberg, B.; Verhagen, E.; Backx, F.J.G.; van der Worp, H.; Bierma-Zeinstra, S.M.; Koes, B.W.; van Middelkoop, M. Reasons and predictors of discontinuation of running after a running program for novice runners. *J. Sci. Med. Sport* **2019**, *22*, 106–111. [CrossRef]
12. Desai, P.; Jungmalm, J.; Borjesson, M.; Karlsson, J.; Grau, S. Recreational runners with a history of injury are twice as likely to sustain a running-related injury as runners with no history of injury: A 1-year prospective cohort study. *J. Orthop. Sports Phys. Ther.* **2021**, *51*, 144–150. [CrossRef]
13. Kluitenberg, B.; van Middelkoop, M.; Verhagen, E.; Hartgens, F.; Huisstede, B.; Diercks, R.; van der Worp, H. The impact of injury definition on injury surveillance in novice runners. *J. Sci. Med. Sport* **2016**, *19*, 470–475. [CrossRef]
14. Francis, P.; Whatman, C.; Sheerin, K.; Hume, P.; Johnson, M.I. The proportion of lower limb running injuries by gender, anatomical location and specific pathology: A systematic review. *J. Sports Sci. Med.* **2019**, *18*, 21–31. [PubMed]
15. Hollander, K.; Baumann, A.; Zech, A.; Verhagen, E. Prospective monitoring of health problems among recreational runners preparing for a half marathon. *BMJ Open Sport Exerc. Med.* **2018**, *4*, 308. [CrossRef] [PubMed]

16. Soligard, T.; Schwellnus, M.; Alonso, J.M.; Bahr, R.; Clarsen, B.; Dijkstra, H.P.; Gabbett, T.; Gleeson, M.; Hägglund, M.; Hutchinson, M.R.; et al. How much is too much? (Part 1) International Olympic Committee consensus statement on load in sport and risk of injury. *Br. J. Sports Med.* **2016**, *50*, 1030–1041. [CrossRef]
17. Brund, R.B.K.; Rasmussen, S.; Nielsen, R.O.; Kersting, U.G.; Laessoe, U.; Voigt, M. The association between eccentric hip abduction strength and hip and knee angular movements in recreational male runners: An explorative study. *Scand. J. Med. Sci. Sports* **2018**, *28*, 473–478. [CrossRef] [PubMed]
18. Ferreira, A.S.; de Oliveira Silva, D.; Barton, C.J.; Briani, R.V.; Taborda, B.; Pazzinatto, M.F.; de Azevedo, F.M. Impaired isometric, concentric, and eccentric rate of torque development at the hip and knee in patellofemoral pain. *J. Strength Cond. Res.* **2019**, *35*, 2492–2497. [CrossRef] [PubMed]
19. Palmer, K.; Hebron, C.; Williams, J.M. A randomised trial into the effect of an isolated hip abductor strengthening programme and a functional motor control programme on knee kinematics and hip muscle strength. *BMC Musculoskelet. Disord.* **2015**, *16*, 105. [CrossRef] [PubMed]
20. Radzak, K.N.; Stickley, C.D. Fatigue-induced hip-abductor weakness and changes in biomechanical risk factors for running-related injuries. *J. Athl. Train.* **2020**, *55*, 1270–1276. [CrossRef] [PubMed]
21. Ramskov, D.; Barton, C.; Nielsen, R.O.; Rasmussen, S. High eccentric hip abduction strength reduces the risk of developing patellofemoral pain among novice runners initiating a self-structured running program: A 1-year observational study. *J. Orthop. Sports Phys. Ther.* **2015**, *45*, 153–161. [CrossRef]
22. Brachman, A.; Kamieniarz, A.; Michalska, J.; Pawłowski, M.; Słomka, K.J.; Juras, G. Balance training programs in athletes-A systematic review. *J. Hum. Kinet.* **2017**, *58*, 45–64. [CrossRef]
23. Sudhakar, S.; Veena Kirthika, S.; Padmanabhan, K.; Senthil Nathan, C.V.; Ramachandran, S.; Rajalaxmi, V.; Sowmiya, S.; Selvam, P.S. Which is efficient in improving postural control among the novice runners? Isolated ankle strengthening or functional balance training programme: A randomized controlled trial. *Res. J. Pharm. Technol.* **2018**, *11*, 1461–1466. [CrossRef]
24. McGill, E.A.; Montel, I. (Eds.) *NASM Essentials of Sports Performance Training*, 2nd ed.; Jones & Bartlett Learning: Burlington, MA, USA, 2019.
25. Haff, G.G.; Triplett, N.T. (Eds.) *Essentials of Strength Training and Conditioning*, 4th ed.; Human Kinetics: Champaign, IL, USA, 2016.
26. Lauersen, J.B.; Andersen, T.E.; Andersen, L.B. Strength training as superior, dose-dependent and safe prevention of acute and overuse sports injuries: A systematic review, qualitative analysis and meta-analysis. *Br. J. Sports Med.* **2018**, *52*, 1557–1563. [CrossRef] [PubMed]
27. Toresdahl, B.G.; McElheny, K.; Metzl, J.; Ammerman, B.; Chang, B.; Kinderknecht, J. A randomized study of a strength training program to prevent injuries in runners of the New York City Marathon. *Sports Health* **2020**, *12*, 74–79. [CrossRef]
28. Voight, A.M.; Roberts, B.; Lunos, S.; Chow, L. Pre- and postmarathon training habits of nonelite runners. *Open Access J. Sports Med.* **2011**, *2*, 13. Available online: www.dovepress.com (accessed on 21 June 2022). [PubMed]
29. Bampton, E.A.; Johnson, S.T.; Vallance, J.K. Correlates and preferences of resistance training among older adults in Alberta, Canada. *Can. J. Public Health* **2016**, *107*, e272–e277. [CrossRef] [PubMed]
30. Blagrove, R.C.; Brown, N.; Howatson, G.; Hayes, P.R. Strength and conditioning habits of competitive distance runners. *J. Strength Cond. Res.* **2020**, *34*, 1392–1399. [CrossRef] [PubMed]
31. Fokkema, T.; De Vos, R.J.; Bierma-Zeinstra, S.M.A.; Van Middelkoop, M. Opinions, barriers, and facilitators of injury prevention in recreational runners. *J. Orthop. Sports Phys. Ther.* **2019**, *49*, 736–745. [CrossRef]
32. García-Pinillos, F.; Lago-Fuentes, C.; Jaén-Carrillo, D.; Bujalance-Moreno, P.; Latorre-Román, P.Á.; Roche-Seruendo, L.E.; Ramirez-Campillo, R. Strength training habits in amateur endurance runners in Spain: Influence of athletic level. *Int. J. Environ. Res. Public Health* **2020**, *17*, 8184. [CrossRef]
33. Hespanhol Junior, L.C.; Costa, L.O.P.; Carvalho, A.C.A.; Lopes, A.D. A description of training characteristics and its association with previous musculoskeletal injuries in recreational runners: A cross-sectional study. *Braz. J. Phys. Ther.* **2012**, *16*, 46–53. [CrossRef]
34. Hespanhol Junior, L.C.; Pena Costa, L.O.; Lopes, A.D. Previous injuries and some training characteristics predict running-related injuries in recreational runners: A prospective cohort study. *J. Physiother.* **2013**, *59*, 263–269. [CrossRef]
35. Linton, L.; Valentin, S. Running with injury: A study of UK novice and recreational runners and factors associated with running related injury. *J. Sci. Med. Sport* **2018**, *21*, 1221–1225. [CrossRef]
36. Luckin, K.; Badenhorst, C.; Hoyne, G.; Cripps, A.; Landers, G.; Merrells, R. Strength training in long-distance triathletes: Barriers and characteristics. *J. Strength Cond. Res.* **2018**, *21*, S30. [CrossRef]
37. Shakespear-Druery, J.; De Cocker, K.; Biddle, S.J.H.; Bennie, J. Muscle-Strengthening Exercise Questionnaire (MSEQ): An assessment of concurrent validity and test-retest reliability. *BMJ Open Sport Exerc. Med.* **2022**, *8*, e001375. [CrossRef] [PubMed]
38. Taunton, J.E.; Ryan, M.B.; Clement, D.B.; McKenzie, D.C.; Lloyd-Smith, D.R.; Zumbo, B.D. A prospective study of running injuries: The Vancouver Sun Run "In Training" clinics. *Br. J. Sports Med.* **2003**, *37*, 239–244. [CrossRef] [PubMed]
39. Van Gent, R.N.; Siem, D.; Van Middelkoop, M.; Van Os, A.G.; Bierma-Zeinstra, S.M.A.; Koes, B.W. Incidence and determinants of lower extremity running injuries in long distance runners: A systematic review. *Br. J. Sports Med.* **2007**, *41*, 469–480. [CrossRef] [PubMed]
40. Dempster, J.; Dutheil, F.; Ugbolue, U.C. The prevalence of lower extremity injuries in running and associated risk factors: A systematic review. *Phys. Act. Health* **2021**, *5*, 133–145. [CrossRef]

41. van Poppel, D.; van der Worp, M.; Slabbekoorn, A.; van den Heuvel, S.S.P.; van Middelkoop, M.; Koes, B.W.; Verhagen, A.P.; Scholten-Peeters, G.G. Risk factors for overuse injuries in short- and long-distance running: A systematic review. *J. Sport Health Sci.* **2021**, *10*, 14–28. [CrossRef]
42. Van Middelkoop, M.; Kolkman, J.; Van Ochten, J.; Bierma-Zeinstra, S.M.A.; Koes, B. Prevalence and incidence of lower extremity injuries in male marathon runners. *Scand. J. Med. Sci. Sports* **2008**, *18*, 140–144. [CrossRef]
43. van Poppel, D.; Scholten-Peeters, G.G.M.; van Middelkoop, M.; Verhagen, A.P. Prevalence, incidence and course of lower extremity injuries in runners during a 12-month follow-up period. *Scand. J. Med. Sci. Sports* **2014**, *24*, 943–949. [CrossRef]
44. Karp, J.R. Training characteristics of qualifiers for the U.S. Olympic Marathon Trials. *Int. J. Sports Physiol. Perform.* **2007**, *2*, 72–92. [CrossRef]
45. Tenforde, A.; Hoenig, T.; Saxena, A.; Hollander, K. Bone stress injuries in runners using carbon fiber plate footwear. *Sports Med.* **2023**, *53*, 1499–1505. [CrossRef]
46. Clark, M.; Lucett, S.; Sutton, B. (Eds.) *NASM Essentials of Corrective Exercise Training*; Jones & Bartlett Learning: Burlington, MA, USA, 2014.
47. Lauersen, J.B.; Bertelsen, D.M.; Andersen, L.B. The effectiveness of exercise interventions to prevent sports injuries: A systematic review and meta-analysis of randomised controlled trials. *Br. J. Sports Med.* **2014**, *48*, 871–877. [CrossRef] [PubMed]
48. Leppänen, M.; Aaltonen, S.; Parkkari, J.; Heinonen, A.; Kujala, U.M. Interventions to prevent sports related injuries: A systematic review and meta-analysis of randomised controlled trials. *Sports Med.* **2014**, *44*, 473–486. [CrossRef] [PubMed]

Disclaimer/Publisher's Note: The statements, opinions and data contained in all publications are solely those of the individual author(s) and contributor(s) and not of MDPI and/or the editor(s). MDPI and/or the editor(s) disclaim responsibility for any injury to people or property resulting from any ideas, methods, instructions or products referred to in the content.

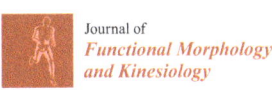

Article

Analysis of Individual $\dot{V}O_{2max}$ Responses during a Cardiopulmonary Exercise Test and the Verification Phase in Physically Active Women

Pasquale J. Succi, Brian Benitez, Minyoung Kwak and Haley C. Bergstrom *

Department of Kinesiology and Health Promotion, University of Kentucky, Lexington, KY 40536, USA; pj.succi@uky.edu (P.J.S.); bbe241@uky.edu (B.B.); mkw223@uky.edu (M.K.)
* Correspondence: hbergstrom@uky.edu

Abstract: This study aimed to investigate the test–retest reliability, mean, and individual responses in the measurement of maximal oxygen consumption ($\dot{V}O_{2max}$) during a cardiopulmonary exercise test (CPET) and the verification phase during cycle ergometry in women. Nine women (22 ± 2 yrs, 166.0 ± 4.5 cm, 58.6 ± 7.7 kg) completed a CPET, passively rested for 5 min, and then completed a verification phase at 90% of peak power output to determine the highest $\dot{V}O_2$ from the CPET ($\dot{V}O_{2CPET}$) and verification phase ($\dot{V}O_{2verification}$) on 2 separate days. Analyses included a two-way repeated measures ANOVA, intraclass correlation coefficients ($ICC_{2,1}$), standard errors of the measurement (SEM), minimal differences (MD), and coefficients of variation (CoV). There was no test (test 1 versus test 2) × method (CPET vs. verification phase) interaction ($p = 0.896$) and no main effect for method ($p = 0.459$). However, test 1 (39.2 mL·kg^{-1}·min^{-1}) was significantly higher than test 2 (38.3 mL·kg^{-1}·min^{-1}) ($p = 0.043$). The $\dot{V}O_{2CPET}$ (ICC = 0.984; CoV = 1.98%; SEM = 0.77 mL·kg^{-1}·min^{-1}; MD = 2.14 mL·kg^{-1}·min^{-1}) and $\dot{V}O_{2verification}$ (ICC = 0.964; CoV = 3.30%; SEM = 1.27 mL·kg^{-1}·min^{-1}; MD = 3.52 mL·kg^{-1}·min^{-1}) demonstrated "excellent" reliability. Two subjects demonstrated a test 1 $\dot{V}O_{2CPET}$ that exceeded the test 2 $\dot{V}O_{2CPET}$, and one subject demonstrated a test 1 $\dot{V}O_{2verification}$ that exceeded the test 2 $\dot{V}O_{2verification}$ by more than the respective CPET and verification phase MD. One subject demonstrated a $\dot{V}O_{2CPET}$ that exceeded the $\dot{V}O_{2verification}$, and one subject demonstrated a $\dot{V}O_{2verification}$ that exceeded the $\dot{V}O_{2CPET}$ by more than the MD. These results demonstrate the importance of examining the individual responses in the measurement of the $\dot{V}O_{2max}$ and suggest that the MD may be a useful threshold to quantify real individual changes in $\dot{V}O_2$.

Keywords: exercise test; women; verification phase; oxygen consumption

1. Introduction

The examination of individual responses to an exercise or nutritional intervention has gained increasing interest with the development of individualized exercise prescription, medicine, and genetic testing [1–4]. Despite this increased focus on individual responses, most primary research continues to base conclusions on group or mean effects. For example, training interventions that have examined changes in the volume of maximal oxygen consumption ($\dot{V}O_{2max}$) utilized the mean response alone as justification for or against the efficacy of the given training protocol, despite high variability in the individual responses [4]. Therefore, the main effect and overall conclusion about the efficacy of the intervention may be driven by a few individuals that demonstrated exaggerated responses [5]. The misstep of drawing conclusions based primarily on the mean responses has also been observed in the examination of the methodologies used for the determination of the primary outcomes such as the $\dot{V}O_{2max}$. Specifically, the call to perform a verification phase upon completion of an initial cardiopulmonary exercise test (CPET) to verify that the $\dot{V}O_{2max}$ was achieved

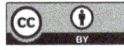

has been made primarily based on the mean responses [6–11]. However, the determination of the $\dot{V}O_{2max}$ should be made using individual thresholds, since the mean responses do not identify those who have or have not attained a 'true' $\dot{V}O_{2max}$. The few studies that have examined the individual responses have used a threshold based solely on the measurement error of the respective metabolic analyzer used, corresponding to a 2–3% difference, to determine significance among the individual responses [4,7,12–14]. Thus, there is a need for a method to compare individual responses that is based on the combined biological variability in addition to the error of the measurement being examined.

Previous work [15–17] has called for a test–retest approach to the quantification of individual responses. In particular, Weir [17] advocated for the use of the minimal difference (MD) to be considered real, which represents a 95% confidence interval around the standard error of the measurement (SEM), as a more statistically grounded threshold to determine 'real' individual differences test–retest. The MD is derived from test and subsequent retest values of the measure of interest, each with a true component and an error component [17]. By using the test and retest values, the MD thereby contains the error from the biological variability in addition to the measurement error of the given test [17]. Thus, the MD can be used to examine whether an individual difference from one test to another is the result of a 'real' difference, or if it is just the result of the day-to-day variability associated with the measure [17]. By quantifying the MD in a given population for the measurement of a primary outcome, such as the $\dot{V}O_{2max}$, future researchers may be able to use the MD as a threshold to examine individual differences during a training or interventional study.

The measurement of the $\dot{V}O_{2max}$ is a prevalent primary outcome in the examination of endurance exercise; yet, debate exists surrounding its measurement [18]. Traditional definitions of the $\dot{V}O_{2max}$ use the presence of a plateau in the $\dot{V}O_2$ (<150 mL·min^{-1}) with increasing work rate as the primary criterion or secondary criteria, such as the attainment of a percentage of the age-predicted maximal heart rate (HR), a respiratory exchange ratio (RER) of 1.1 or greater, and a rating of perceived exertion (RPE) greater than or equal to 17 [18–21]. These criteria have come under criticism [18] due to the low incidence of a plateau in $\dot{V}O_2$, and the inability of the secondary criteria to distinguish between the individual variation in responses for those who truly did attain a $\dot{V}O_2$ and those who did not [18,21,22]. To address these criticisms, there has been an increased call to perform a verification phase upon the completion of a CPET to verify the attainment of the $\dot{V}O_{2max}$ [18]. However, there is no consensus for a universal methodology for the administration of a verification phase to confirm the attainment of $\dot{V}O_{2max}$. A recent review and meta-analysis with 54 studies found no difference between the highest $\dot{V}O_{2max}$ attained in the CPET and that from the verification phase [23]. While the authors concluded the verification phase appears to be a robust procedure to confirm a 'true' $\dot{V}O_{2max}$ has been attained, they also questioned its necessity in all populations based on the lack of mean differences between the $\dot{V}O_{2max}$ from the CPET ($\dot{V}O_{2CPET}$) and the verification phase ($\dot{V}O_{2verification}$). The purpose of a verification phase is to, on an individual basis, examine the $\dot{V}O_2$ responses to verify the individual attainment of the $\dot{V}O_{2max}$ [24]. Thus, to fully examine the necessity of the verification phase in the measurement of $\dot{V}O_{2max}$, the individual $\dot{V}O_2$ responses should be examined during the CPET and verification phase.

Similar to the lack of consensus on the verification phase methodology, there is a lack of consensus on the specific magnitude of the difference between the $\dot{V}O_{2CPET}$ and $\dot{V}O_{2verification}$ needed to detect a real change or indicate whether the result is a consequence of measurement error or biological variability [17]. To compound this issue, the specific number of subjects in a given sample that demonstrate a difference in the $\dot{V}O_2$ responses is often not reported [10,11]. Previous works that have attempted to examine individual differences have used a 2–3% threshold to define an individual difference as real [4,7,12,14]. Using this threshold, Weatherwax et al. [4] demonstrated 2.6% of subjects

(4 out of 156 tests) demonstrated a 3% difference between the $\dot{V}O_{2CPET}$ and $\dot{V}O_{2verification}$. Other more recent work [25] has extrapolated the $\dot{V}O_2$ versus work rate relationship to predict the $\dot{V}O_{2verification}$ and used the predicted value as a method to confirm the individual attainment of the $\dot{V}O_{2max}$ following the recommendation of Midgley et al. [26]. These authors [25] demonstrated that the $\dot{V}O_{2verification}$ was on average 5% lower than the $\dot{V}O_{2CPET}$, but that on an individual basis, the $\dot{V}O_{2max}$ was 'confirmed' in all participants since the difference between the predicted and actual $\dot{V}O_{2max}$ was less than half the regression slope [25,26]. While this method represents an improvement upon the 3% threshold, this may not serve as a threshold for future studies to use to examine individual responses. Thus, the need still exists for a threshold that encapsulates the biological variability and the error associated with the measurement that can be potentially used as a threshold for future studies.

Previous work [27–29] has used the MD to examine the individual differences in the $\dot{V}O_{2CPET}$ and $\dot{V}O_{2verification}$ in treadmill running in men and women and in cycle ergometry in men. These works, in addition to others [4,25,30], demonstrated that young healthy subjects accustomed to exhaustive exercise seldom demonstrate differences between the $\dot{V}O_{2CPET}$ and $\dot{V}O_{2verification}$, and in some cases, they demonstrate no differences at all. The lack of individual subjects who demonstrate $\dot{V}O_{2verification}$ values that are either equivalent or are significantly less than the $\dot{V}O_{2CPET}$ [4,25,27–29] support previous work [23] that has questioned the need for the verification phase in measuring the $\dot{V}O_{2max}$ in all populations and settings. The additional benefit of the quantification of the MD in specific populations and in different modalities is that future works, such as training or nutritional interventions, are able to use the MD as a threshold by which individual responses can be examined without the need to perform verification phases. However, no study has quantified the MD during cycle ergometry in women. Thus, the purpose of this study was to use a test–retest approach to examine the reliability, mean, and individual differences between the $\dot{V}O_{2CPET}$ and $\dot{V}O_{2verification}$ in healthy, recreationally trained, and well-motivated women during cycle ergometry. Based on previous examinations of the verification phase using similar methodologies [27–29], it was hypothesized that (1) both the $\dot{V}O_{2CPET}$ and $\dot{V}O_{2verification}$ would have 'excellent' test–retest reliabilities; (2) there would be no mean differences between the $\dot{V}O_{2CPET}$ and $\dot{V}O_{2verification}$; (3) no individual would exceed the MD between the test and retest difference for the $\dot{V}O_{2CPET}$ or $\dot{V}O_{2verification}$; and (4) based on the previously reported incidence of individual differences [4,13], two or fewer subjects would exhibit a difference between the $\dot{V}O_{2CPET}$ and $\dot{V}O_{2verification}$ that exceeded the MD.

2. Materials and Methods

2.1. Experimental Approach

This study used a test–retest design to determine the reliability and validity of the determination of $\dot{V}O_{2max}$ with a verification phase. The study consisted of 3 visits total with each visit being separated by at least 48 h. The first visit consisted of a familiarization trial where subjects performed a cardiopulmonary exercise test (CPET) followed by a verification phase on an electronically braked cycle ergometer to familiarize themselves with the protocol and the effort required to determine the $\dot{V}O_{2CPET}$ and $\dot{V}O_{2verification}$. The second and third visits followed the same procedures as the familiarization visit and were used to determine the mean and individual differences in the measurement of the $\dot{V}O_{2CPET}$ and the $\dot{V}O_{2verification}$.

2.2. Subjects

Ten moderately trained recreationally active women were recruited from university students and from the general public in the surrounding area. One subject withdrew due to scheduling conflicts. Therefore, 9 women were included in the analyses (mean ± SD,

22 ± 2 years, 166.0 ± 4.5 cm, 58.6 ± 7.7 kg). The subjects' physical activities included a combination of running (n = 7), cycling (n = 2), resistance training (n = 5), and yoga (n = 2). Individuals were eligible for inclusion if they had been endurance training 30 min a day, 5 days a week, for the past 6 months and had no known cardiovascular, metabolic, or musculoskeletal diseases or disorders. The subjects were asked to maintain their current level of physical activity, but to abstain from high intensity exercise at least 24 h prior to their testing session and abstain from caffeine consumption 4 h before their testing session. All subjects completed a health history form and signed a written informed consent document approved by the University Institutional Review Board for Human Subjects (IRB#64999) prior to beginning the study.

2.3. Graded Exercise Test with Verification Phase

Each subject performed 3 CPET's on a calibrated cycle ergometer (Lode, Corival, Groningen, The Netherlands) on different days each separated by at least 48 h. The first visit served as a familiarization trial so that subjects understood the effort required for each visit. The second and third trials were used for the test–retest determination of the $\dot{V}O_{2CPET}$ and $\dot{V}O_{2verification}$. Each subject was fitted with a nose clip, mouthpiece mounted to a headset (Hans Rudolph 2700 breathing valve, Kansas City, MO, USA), and heart rate monitor (Polar Heart Watch system, Polar Electro Inc., Lake Success, NY, USA) during all visits. Expired gas samples were collected and analyzed using a calibrated TrueMax 2400 metabolic cart (Parvo Medics, Sandy, UT, USA). Prior to testing, the gas analyzers were calibrated to room air and gases of known concentrations, and the flow meter was calibrated using a 3L syringe. The oxygen ($\dot{V}O_2$) and carbon dioxide ($\dot{V}CO_2$) parameters were expressed as 20 s averages [31]. Each subject performed a 4-min warmup at 50 W at 70 rev·min^{-1} cadence, followed by one minute of passive rest. The CPET started at 50 W, and the power output was increased 30 W every two minutes until the subjects could no longer maintain the 70 rev·min^{-1} cadence despite strong verbal encouragement. After the subject signaled for exhaustion, the subject was given 5 min of passive recovery, then the power output was increased to 90% of their peak power from the CPET. This intensity was maintained until the subject could no longer maintain the 70 rev·min^{-1} cadence despite strong verbal encouragement. The protocol for the current study was based on the work of Sawyer et al. [11], which indicated that a 90% verification phase was the ideal intensity to elicit the highest $\dot{V}O_{2verification}$ values compared to 80, 100, and 105% of peak power in moderately trained individuals. The greater $\dot{V}O_2$ response at 90% peak power, relative to the other submaximal, maximal, or supramaximal intensities, likely resulted because there was sufficient time for the development of the $\dot{V}O_2$ slow component phenomenon causing the $\dot{V}O_2$ to increase to the $\dot{V}O_{2max}$ [32]. The $\dot{V}O_{2CPET}$ and $\dot{V}O_{2verificaiton}$ were defined as the highest 20 s $\dot{V}O_2$ value obtained from the step protocol and the verification phase, respectively. The rating of perceived exertion (RPE) was recorded using the Borg 6–20 scale at the end of each stage during the CPET and after each minute during the verification phase [33]. The respiratory exchange ratio (RER) was defined as the highest 20 s value obtained from the step protocol and verification phase, respectively.

2.4. Statistical Analyses

Separate, 2 (Test [Test 1 vs. Test 2]) × 2 (Method [CPET vs Verification]) repeated measures analyses of variance (ANOVA) were used to examine the interaction and main effects for the mean responses for the highest $\dot{V}O_2$ demonstrated from the CPET and verification phase ($\dot{V}O_{2CPET}$ and $\dot{V}O_{2verification}$), as well as for the time to exhaustion (T_{Lim}), heart rate (HR), respiratory exchange ratio (RER), rating of perceived exertion (RPE), and power output for the CPET and the verification phase with appropriate follow-up pairwise comparisons. The test–retest reliability of each variable was calculated using an intraclass correlation coefficient (ICC, relative reliability) (2,1) model [17,34–36] using the equation:

$$ICC_{2,1} = \frac{MS_S - MS_E}{MS_S + (k-1)MS_E + \left(\frac{k(MS_T - MS_E)}{n}\right)}, \quad (1)$$

where the MS_S is the mean square error of the between-subjects effects, MS_E is the mean square error of the within-subjects effects, and MS_T is the mean square factor of the within-subjects effects from separate one-way repeated measures ANOVA for each method (CPET, verification phase). Additionally, k is the number of tests (k = 2), and n represents the sample size. A 2,1 ICC model was selected so that the ICC values could be generalized to outside testers [17,34–36]. The ICC values were classified as "excellent" (0.80–1.0), "good" (0.60–0.80), or "poor" (<0.60) [37]. A 95% confidence interval (CI) was calculated around each ICC value to confirm the rejection of the null hypothesis that each ICC was statistically different from zero. The standard error of the measurement (SEM, absolute reliability) was calculated using the equation:

$$SEM = \sqrt{MS_E}. \quad (2)$$

Additionally, the minimal difference to be considered real (MD) was calculated using the equation:

$$MD = SEM * 1.96 * \sqrt{2} \quad (3)$$

to examine the individual differences for each variable from test 1 to test 2. The coefficient of variation (CoV) was also calculated to display a normalized measure of the SEM using the equation:

$$CoV = \frac{SEM}{GrandMean} * 100. \quad (4)$$

Based on previous recommendations [38], a CoV of <10% was used as an indication of sufficient absolute reliability. However, the overall reliability of the measures was characterized by taking into account the ICC value, in conjunction with the CoV, SEM, and the MD. The effect size for each variable of the ANOVAs was expressed as the partial eta squared ($p\eta^2$). An a priori alpha level was set at 0.05, and all of the data were analyzed using IBM SPSS Statistical Software Version 28 (IBM SPSS Inc., Chicago, IL, USA).

3. Results

The individual responses and the mean ± SD for each variable (test 1 $\dot{V}O_{2CPET}$, test 2 $\dot{V}O_{2CPET}$, test 1 $\dot{V}O_{2verification}$, and test 2 $\dot{V}O_{2verification}$) are listed in Table 1 and shown in Figures 1 and 2. The results of the two-way repeated measures ANOVA for peak $\dot{V}O_2$ demonstrated no significant test x method interaction ($F = 0.018$, $p = 0.896$, $p\eta^2 = 0.002$) and no main effect for the method ($F = 0.605$, $p = 0.459$, $p\eta^2 = 0.070$), but there was a significant main effect for the test ($F = 8.465$, $p = 0.043$, $p\eta^2 = 0.419$). Followup comparisons indicated that collapsed across the method (i.e., the average of both the CPET and verification phase), test 1 (39.2 ± 7.2 mL·kg^{-1}·min^{-1}) was significantly higher than test 2 (38.3 ± 7.7 mL·kg^{-1}·min^{-1}). The mean ± SD T_{Lim} for test 1 and test 2 for the CPET and verification phase, as well as the peak power output (PPO) from the CPET, the verification phase power output, and the maximal HR, RER, and RPE for the CPET and verification phase are listed in Table 2. There were no significant interactions, but there was a main effect for the method that indicated the T_{Lim} for the CPET was longer than the verification phase ($p < 0.001$), and the peak power output ($p < 0.001$) and RER ($p < 0.001$) during the CPET were greater than the verification phase. There were no interactions or main effects for the test or method for the maximal HR or RPE ($p = 0.062$–0.512).

Table 1. Mean ± SD and individual responses for the highest $\dot{V}O_2$ values from the cardiopulmonary exercise test ($\dot{V}O_{2CPET}$) and the verification phase ($\dot{V}O_{2verification}$) for test 1 (T1) and test 2 (T2).

Subject	T1 $\dot{V}O_{2CPET}$	T2 $\dot{V}O_{2CPET}$	T1 $\dot{V}O_{2verification}$	T2 $\dot{V}O_{2verification}$
1	45.5 *	43.1	44.1	43.9
2	31.0	30.5	31.9	30.6
3	40.6	39.5 ‡	41.7 †	36.8
4	40.8	40.1	41.1	41.9
5	35.1 *	32.8	35.4	34.0
6	35.6	34.0	38.0 ‡	35.4
7	56.4	57.3	55.5	56.2
8	33.6	33.6	34.6	34.3
9	39.5	38.8	38.4	38.5
Mean	39.8	38.9	40.1	39.1
SD	7.6	8.1	6.9	7.6

* indicates test 1 versus test 2 for the CPET exceeded the minimal difference to be considered real (MD) (2.14 mL·kg^{-1}·min^{-1}). † indicates test 1 versus test 2 for the verification phase exceeded the MD (3.52 mL·kg^{-1}·min^{-1}). ‡ indicates the CPET versus the verification phase exceeded the MD (2.14 mL·kg^{-1}·min^{-1}).

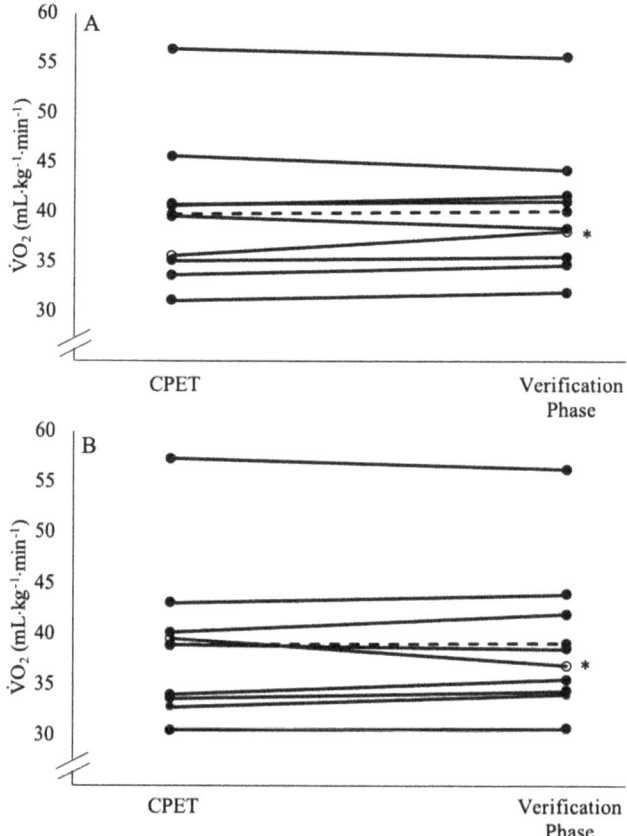

Figure 1. Individual (solid line and closed circles) and mean (dashed line) $\dot{V}O_2$ responses from the cardiopulmonary exercise test (CPET) and the verification phase for test 1 (**A**) and test 2 (**B**). * indicates an individual (solid line open circles) exceeded the minimal difference to be considered real (2.14 mL·kg^{-1}·min^{-1}) between the CPET and verification phase.

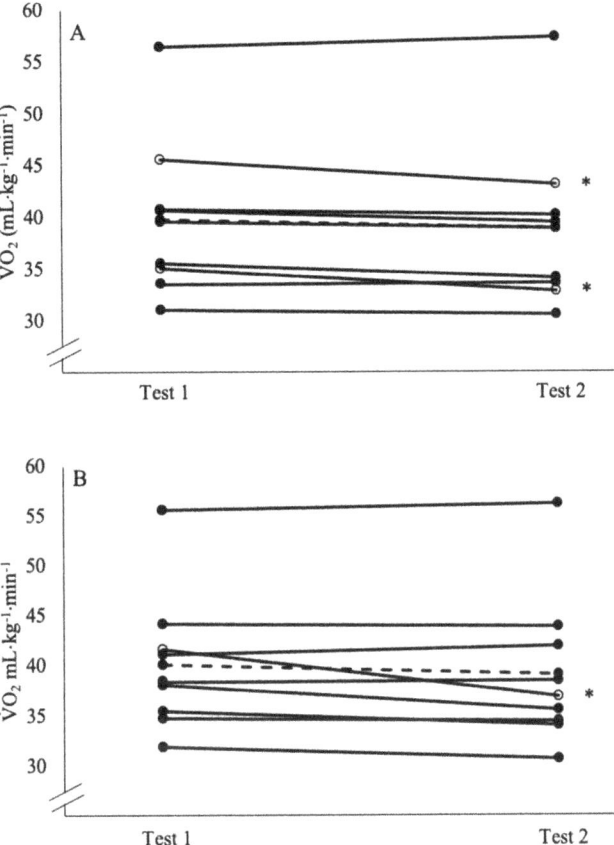

Figure 2. Individual (solid line and closed circles) and mean (dashed line) $\dot{V}O_2$ responses from the cardiopulmonary exercise test (CPET) 1 compared to test 2 (**A**), and the verification phase test 1 compared to test 2 (**B**). * indicates an individual (solid line and open circles) exceeded the minimal difference to be considered real for the CPET (2.14 mL·kg^{-1}·min^{-1}) or the verification phase (3.52 mL·kg^{-1}·min^{-1}).

Table 2. Mean ± SD for time to exhaustion (T$_{Lim}$), peak power output, heart rate (HR), respiratory exchange ratio (RER), and rating of perceived exertion (RPE) for test 1 (T1) and test 2 (T2) cardiopulmonary exercise test (CPET) and verification phase.

	T1 CPET	T2 CPET	T1 Verification	T2 Verification
T$_{Lim}$ (min) *	11.25 ± 1.27	11.43 ± 1.23	3.01 ± 0.98	3.14 ± 0.88
Power Output (W) *	203 ± 23	203 ± 23	183 ± 21	183 ± 21
HR (b·min^{-1})	182 ± 6	180 ± 8	181 ± 8	180 ± 8
RER *	1.18 ± 0.05	1.20 ± 0.06	1.08 ± 0.07	1.11 ± 0.05
RPE	19 ± 1	19 ± 1	19 ± 1	19 ± 1

Power output for the CPET represents the peak power output (PPO), and for the verification phase represents 90% of the peak power output from the CPET. * T$_{Lim}$, power output, and RER during the CPET was greater than verification phase, collapsed across test ($p < 0.001$).

The reliability statistics are presented in Table 3. The test 1 $\dot{V}O_{2CPET}$ was significantly higher than the test 2 $\dot{V}O_{2CPET}$ ($F = 6.563$, $p = 0.034$, $p\eta^2 = 0.451$), but there was no difference between the test 1 $\dot{V}O_{2verification}$ and the test 2 ($F = 2.833$, $p = 0.131$, $p\eta^2 = 0.261$).

The ICC values of the $\dot{V}O_{2CPET}$ (R = 0.984) and the $\dot{V}O_{2verification}$ (R = 0.964) indicated both methods demonstrated 'excellent' test–retest reliabilities [37]. The CoV for the $\dot{V}O_{2CPET}$ (1.98%) and $\dot{V}O_{2verification}$ (3.30%) were both below the 10% threshold used to be considered reliable [38]. Two subjects exceeded the MD (2.14 mL·kg^{-1}·min^{-1}; 0.12 L·min^{-1}) for the $\dot{V}O_{2CPET}$ test–retest. In addition, one subject exceeded the MD (3.30 mL·kg^{-1}·min^{-1}; 0.22 L·min^{-1}) for the $\dot{V}O_{2verification}$ test–retest. Lastly, one subject demonstrated a $\dot{V}O_{2CPET}$ that was greater than the $\dot{V}O_{2verification}$ by a value that exceeded the MD (2.14 mL·kg^{-1}·min^{-1}), and one subject demonstrated a $\dot{V}O_{2verification}$ that was greater than the $\dot{V}O_{2CPET}$ by a value that was greater than the MD (Table 1).

Table 3. Reliability analyses including the mean ± SD, intraclass correlation coefficient (ICC), standard error of the measure (SEM), minimal difference (MD) to be considered real, and the coefficient of variation (CoV) for the $\dot{V}O_2$ from the cardiopulmonary exercise test ($\dot{V}O_{2CPET}$) and the verification phase ($\dot{V}O_{2verification}$).

$\dot{V}O_2$ (Mean ± SD)	Test 1	Test 2	p	ICC (95% CI)	SEM (mL·kg^{-1}·min^{-1})	MD (mL·kg^{-1}·min^{-1})	CoV (%)
$\dot{V}O_{2CPET}$	39.8 ± 7.6	38.9 ± 8.1	0.034	0.984 (0.879–0.997)	0.77	2.14	1.98
$\dot{V}O_{2verification}$	40.1 ± 6.9	39.1 ± 7.6	0.131	0.964 (0.841–0.992)	1.27	3.53	3.30

4. Discussion

The purpose of this study was to use a test–retest approach to examine the reliability, mean, and individual differences between the $\dot{V}O_{2CPET}$ and $\dot{V}O_{2verification}$ in healthy, recreationally trained, and well-motivated women during cycle ergometry. The recommendation for researchers to perform verification phase testing when determining the $\dot{V}O_{2max}$ in all populations has become more prevalent [18]. It is of note that the verification phase may be necessary in novice, unmotivated, older, or especially diseased populations [39]. However, it has been suggested that the verification phase may not be necessary in young healthy subjects that are accustomed to exhaustive exercise [18]. In addition, previous studies in this population have demonstrated highly reproducible $\dot{V}O_{2max}$ values based on the group mean responses [18,23,27–29]. The findings of the current study provide additional support to this notion as both the $\dot{V}O_{2CPET}$ and $\dot{V}O_{2verification}$ demonstrated "excellent" reliabilities based on the ICC along with the MD, SEM, and CoV (Table 3). Although the test–retest mean responses for the $\dot{V}O_{2CPET}$ indicated systematic variability (test 1 > test 2), this mean difference reflected a real difference, based on the MD, for only two of the nine subjects. The use of several indices of reliability allows for the determination of the absolute and relative reliability, which enables an individual to compare across studies [17,40]. The ICC, MD, SEM, and CoV for the $\dot{V}O_{2CPET}$ and $\dot{V}O_{2verification}$ in this study were consistent with previous work examining the CPET and verification phase protocols (ICCs = 0.89–0.99, MDs = 0.17–0.21 L·min^{-1}, SEMs = 0.06–0.16 L·min^{-1}, and CoVs = 2.1–3.8%) [6,11,12,27–29]. Thus, the current findings further supported that the $\dot{V}O_{2CPET}$ and $\dot{V}O_{2verification}$ can be reliably determined in younger, healthy, and well-motivated subjects.

Previous work investigating the need for a verification phase in the determination of the $\dot{V}O_{2max}$ has examined the mean responses of the $\dot{V}O_2$ determined from the CPET compared to the $\dot{V}O_2$ determined from the verification phase. Other works have demonstrated no mean difference in the $\dot{V}O_{2max}$ between the CPET and verification phase, yet still recommend its use in all populations [8,25]. However, as has been previously pointed out [23,24], the examination of the individual responses is more important than the mean responses in regard to the attainment of the highest $\dot{V}O_2$ ($\dot{V}O_{2max}$). In the current study, there was no main effect for method (i.e., no difference for the $\dot{V}O_2$ determined from the

CPET vs. the verification phase). This lack of difference between the CPET and the verification phase is consistent with previous studies [4,6–8,11] but is also in contrast to other works [27–29,41] that demonstrated that the CPET $\dot{V}O_{2max}$ was significantly greater than the verification phase. However, in contrast to other works [4,6–8,11,12,27–29], the $\dot{V}O_2$ from test 1 in this study was significantly greater than test 2, collapsed across the CPET and verification phase. It is important to note that the mean difference between test 1 (39.2 ± 7.2 mL·kg^{-1}·min^{-1}) and test 2 (38.3 ± 7.7 mL·kg^{-1}·min^{-1}) was 0.9 ± 1.2 mL·kg^{-1}·min^{-1} (~2.2%), and there were no differences in the time to exhaustion, power output, or maximal HR between test 1 and test 2. On an individual basis, only two of the nine subjects for the CPET and one of the nine subjects for the verification phase test–retest exceeded the MD for the test–retest responses. These findings demonstrate a potential pitfall of using the mean responses alone to evaluate the changes in the $\dot{V}O_{2max}$ across time or as the result of a training or dietary intervention. That is, evaluation of the mean response alone would suggest a significant change across time; however, this reflected a real difference for only three out eighteen total test–retest responses. Thus, these findings illustrate that using the mean responses may not be sufficient to fully examine the proper methodology for the measurement of the $\dot{V}O_{2max}$ and highlight the potential usefulness in examining changes across time and the need for the examination of individual responses.

The utility of the verification phase is to determine on an individual basis whether the $\dot{V}O_2$ obtained from the CPET is truly the maximal $\dot{V}O_2$ that an individual is capable of producing. However, in past works, the threshold that has been used to determine whether there were individual differences was set at 2–3% between measures [4,7,12,14]. Using this threshold presents a flawed approach as it does not consider the standard error of the measurement of the $\dot{V}O_2$ in addition to the biological variability associated with the measurement. The use of the minimal difference (MD) to be considered real provides a threshold with increased statistical backing to determine whether the differences between the CPET and the verification phase are real differences or are just due to the error of the measure [17]. The MD for the measurement of the $\dot{V}O_2$ from the CPET and verification phase has previously been quantified in men and women during treadmill running [27,28] and in men during cycle ergometry [29], but it has yet to be determined for women during cycle ergometry. Therefore, the quantification of the MD in women during cycle ergometry (2.14 mL·kg^{-1}·min^{-1}) may allow future researchers to examine the individual responses in the $\dot{V}O_{2max}$ to potential changes in interventional studies. Using this approach, one individual demonstrated a $\dot{V}O_{2verification}$ that exceeded the $\dot{V}O_{2CPET}$ by more than the MD, while one individual demonstrated a $\dot{V}O_{2CPET}$ that was greater than the $\dot{V}O_{2verification}$ by more than the MD. These data suggest that a verification phase is not necessary in the measurement of the $\dot{V}O_{2max}$ in healthy well-motivated women on a cycle ergometer. In addition, the MD may provide a valuable tool to examine individual differences in the $\dot{V}O_{2max}$ across time or as the result of an intervention.

Limitations

The variation in the $\dot{V}O_{2max}$ for those subjects who exceeded the MD for the test–retest responses may be a result of the increased variation in the $\dot{V}O_2$ due to biological factors and may highlight 'responders' vs. 'non-responders' [42] due to factors that may influence the maximal performance, such as the time of day [43] or the menstrual cycle phase [44], in addition to other factors such as diet, hydration, or sleep [42]. However, additional work is needed to explore the magnitude of the effect that these factors may have on individual performance measures. While the time of day of testing was kept consistent in the current study (±2 h), Knaier et al. [43] demonstrated that individual $\dot{V}O_2$ values can vary even when there are minor variations (<3 h) in the time of day that the testing is repeated. Furthermore, Lebrun et al. [44] demonstrated that the $\dot{V}O_{2max}$ can vary across the menstrual cycle phases. The individual menstrual cycle phase was not tracked in the current study; however, all test–retest responses were recorded within 48–72 h. Although it is possible that menstrual cycle phase transitions introduced sufficient variability to alter the $\dot{V}O_{2max}$, based on the timing of the testing protocol and the lack of effect for these same subjects on the verification phase $\dot{V}O_2$ responses, this seems unlikely to be the primary driver of the variations in the $\dot{V}O_{2max}$. Future researchers should examine factors that may impact maximal day-to-day performance to determine the possible magnitude of these effects. In addition, future studies should quantify the MD using a larger sample size.

5. Conclusions

The results of the current study suggested that its use in healthy well-motivated women who are accustomed to maximal exhaustive exercise may not be necessary. The performance of additional maximal tests increases the demand on subjects to push themselves to their limit more than may be necessary and increases the burden on researchers to perform these additional tests. Day et al. [30], and more recently Poole and Jones [18] have previously made this claim; however, there were no specific data as support. The current study has shown that there were no mean differences between the $\dot{V}O_{2CPET}$ and $\dot{V}O_{2verification}$, and both measures demonstrated 'excellent' test–retest reliabilities. Therefore, these data support the claims made in previous work [18,30], which suggested young, healthy, and well-motivated subjects may not need to perform additional tests in the measurement of the $\dot{V}O_{2max}$. In addition, this study has added to the quantification of the MD that has previously been determined for men in running and cycling and in women in running but had not been derived for women in cycling. There were two individuals who demonstrated differences in the $\dot{V}O_{2CPET}$ test–retest and one individual who demonstrated differences in the $\dot{V}O_{2verification}$ test–retest. Thus, the few individual differences in combination with the lack of mean difference between the CPET and verification phase responses, suggested that the verification phase may not be necessary in healthy motivated women. The MD allows for the examination of individual responses with a threshold that is based on the standard error of the measure and presents an improvement on the 2–3% threshold, which has previously been used. Thus, the MD may prove useful for other researchers to examine the individual $\dot{V}O_{2max}$ responses to potential training or nutritional intervention studies.

Author Contributions: P.J.S. and H.C.B. conceived and designed the study. P.J.S., B.B. and M.K. conducted the experiments and collected the data. P.J.S. and H.C.B. analyzed the data. P.J.S., B.B., M.K. and H.C.B. all contributed to the interpretation of the findings and the manuscript preparation. All authors have read and agreed to the published version of the manuscript.

Funding: This research received no external funding.

Institutional Review Board Statement: This study was approved by the University of Kentucky Institutional Review Board for Human Subjects (IRB#64999, approved 5 May 2021) meeting the ethical standards of the Declaration of Helsinki.

Informed Consent Statement: Informed consent was obtained from all subjects involved in the study.

Data Availability Statement: The data presented in this study are available upon request to the corresponding author.

Conflicts of Interest: The authors declare no conflict of interest.

References

1. Dionne, F.T.; Turcotte, L.; Thibault, M.C.; Boulay, M.R.; Skinner, J.S.; Bouchard, C. Mitochondrial DNA Sequence Polymorphism, VO$_{2max}$, and Response to Endurance Training. *Med. Sci. Sports Exerc.* **1991**, *23*, 177–185. [CrossRef] [PubMed]
2. Dipla, K. The FITT Principle in Individuals with Type 2 Diabetes: From Cellular Adaptations to Individualized Exercise Prescription. *J. Adv. Med. Med. Res.* **2017**, *22*, 1–18. [CrossRef]

3. Marks, P.; Witten, C. Toward a New Framework for the Development of Individualized Therapies. *Gene Ther.* **2021**, *28*, 615–617. [CrossRef]
4. Weatherwax, R.M.; Harris, N.K.; Kilding, A.E.; Dalleck, L.C. Incidence of VO_{2max} Responders to Personalized versus Standardized Exercise Prescription. *Med. Sci. Sports Exerc.* **2019**, *51*, 681–691. [CrossRef] [PubMed]
5. Pollet, T.V.; Stulp, G.; Henzi, S.P.; Barrett, L. Taking the Aggravation out of Data Aggregation: A Conceptual Guide to Dealing with Statistical Issues Related to the Pooling of Individual-Level Observational Data. *Am. J. Primatol.* **2015**, *77*, 727–740. [CrossRef] [PubMed]
6. Kirkeberg, J.M.; Dalleck, L.C.; Kamphoff, C.S.; Pettitt, R.W. Validity of 3 Protocols for Verifying VO_{2max}. *Int. J. Sports Med.* **2011**, *32*, 266–270. [CrossRef]
7. Midgley, A.W.; McNaughton, L.R.; Carroll, S. Verification Phase as a Useful Tool in the Determination of the Maximal Oxygen Uptake of Distance Runners. *Appl. Physiol. Nutr. Metab.* **2006**, *31*, 541–548. [CrossRef]
8. Midgley, A.W.; Carroll, S. Emergence of the Verification Phase Procedure for Confirming "true" VO(2max). *Scand. J. Med. Sci. Sports* **2009**, *19*, 313–322. [CrossRef]
9. Murias, J.M.; Pogliaghi, S.; Paterson, D.H. Measurement of a True VO_{2max} during a Ramp Incremental Test Is not Confirmed by a Verification Phase. *Front. Physiol.* **2018**, *9*, 143. [CrossRef]
10. Rossiter, H.B.; Kowalchuk, J.M.; Whipp, B.J. A Test to Establish Maximum O_2 Uptake despite No Plateau in the O_2 Uptake Response to Ramp Incremental Exercise. *J. Appl. Physiol.* **2006**, *100*, 764–770. [CrossRef]
11. Sawyer, B.J.; McMahon, N.; Thornhill, K.L.; Baughman, B.R.; Mahoney, J.M.; Pattison, K.L.; Freeberg, K.A.; Botts, R.T. Supra-Versus Submaximal Cycle Ergometer Verification of VO_{2max} in Males and Females. *Sports* **2020**, *8*, 163. [CrossRef] [PubMed]
12. Astorino, T.A.; DE LA Rosa, A.B.; Clark, A.; DE Revere, J.L. Verification Testing to Confirm VO_{2max} Attainment in Inactive Women with Obesity. *Int. J. Exerc. Sci.* **2020**, *13*, 1448–1458. [PubMed]
13. Iannetta, D.; de Almeida Azevedo, R.; Ingram, C.P.; Keir, D.A.; Murias, J.M. Evaluating the Suitability of Supra-POpeak Verification Trials after Ramp-Incremental Exercise to Confirm the Attainment of Maximum O_2 Uptake. *Am. J. Physiol. Regul. Integr. Comp. Physiol.* **2020**, *319*, R315–R322. [CrossRef] [PubMed]
14. Dalleck, L.C.; Astorino, T.A.; Erickson, R.M.; McCarthy, C.M.; Beadell, A.A.; Botten, B.H. Suitability of Verification Testing to Confirm Attainment of VO_{2max} in Middle-Aged and Older Adults. *Res. Sports Med.* **2012**, *20*, 118–128. [CrossRef] [PubMed]
15. Hecksteden, A.; Kraushaar, J.; Scharhag-Rosenberger, F.; Theisen, D.; Senn, S.; Meyer, T. Individual Response to Exercise Training—A Statistical Perspective. *J. Appl. Physiol.* **2015**, *118*, 1450–1459. [CrossRef]
16. Hopkins, W.G. Individual Responses Made Easy. *J. Appl. Physiol.* **2015**, *118*, 1444–1446. [CrossRef]
17. Weir, J.P. Quantifying Test-Retest Reliability Using the Intraclass Correlation Coefficient and the SEM. *J. Strength Cond. Res.* **2005**, *19*, 231–240. [CrossRef]
18. Poole, D.C.; Jones, A.M. Measurement of the Maximum Oxygen Uptake VO_{2max}: VO_{2peak} Is No Longer Acceptable. *J. Appl. Physiol.* **2017**, *122*, 997–1002. [CrossRef]
19. Taylor, H.L.; Buskirk, E.; Henschel, A. Maximal Oxygen Intake as an Objective Measure of Cardio-Respiratory Performance. *J. Appl. Physiol.* **1955**, *8*, 73–80. [CrossRef]
20. Howley, E.T.; Bassett, D.R.; Welch, H.G. Criteria for Maximal Oxygen Uptake: Review and Commentary. *Med. Sci. Sports Exerc.* **1995**, *27*, 1292–1301. [CrossRef]
21. Poole, D.C.; Wilkerson, D.P.; Jones, A.M. Validity of Criteria for Establishing Maximal O_2 Uptake during Ramp Exercise Tests. *Eur. J. Appl. Physiol.* **2008**, *102*, 403–410. [CrossRef] [PubMed]
22. Robergs, R.A.; Landwehr, R. The Surprising History of the "HRmax=220-Age" Equation. *J. Exerc. Physiol.* **2002**, *5*, 1–10.
23. Costa, V.A.B.; Midgley, A.W.; Carroll, S.; Astorino, T.A.; de Paula, T.; Farinatti, P.; Cunha, F.A. Is a Verification Phase Useful for Confirming Maximal Oxygen Uptake in Apparently Healthy Adults? A Systematic Review and Meta-Analysis. *PLoS ONE* **2021**, *16*, e0247057. [CrossRef]
24. Noakes, T.D. Maximal Oxygen Uptake as a Parametric Measure of Cardiorespiratory Capacity: Comment. *Med. Sci. Sports Exerc.* **2008**, *40*, 585. [CrossRef] [PubMed]
25. Pryor, J.L.; Lao, P.; Leija, R.G.; Perez, S.; Morales, J.; Looney, D.P.; Cochrane-Snyman, K.C. Verification Phase Confirms VO_{2max} in a Hot Environment in Sedentary Untrained Males. *Med. Sci. Sports Exerc.* **2023**, *55*, 1069–1075. [CrossRef] [PubMed]
26. Midgley, A.W.; Carroll, S.; Marchant, D.; McNaughton, L.R.; Siegler, J. Evaluation of True Maximal Oxygen Uptake Based on a Novel Set of Standardized Criteria. *Appl. Physiol. Nutr. Metab.* **2009**, *34*, 115–123. [CrossRef]
27. Succi, P.J.; Benitez, B.; Kwak, M.; Bergstrom, H.C. VO_{2max} Is Reliably Measured from a Stand-Alone Graded Exercise Test in Healthy Women. *J. Exerc. Physiol. Online* **2022**, *25*, 14–25.
28. Succi, P.J.; Benitez, B.; Kwak, M.; Bergstrom, H.C. Methodological Considerations for the Determination of VO_{2max} in Healthy Men. *Eur. J. Appl. Physiol.* **2023**, *123*, 191–199. [CrossRef]
29. Succi, P.J.; Benitez, B.; Kwak, M.; Bergstrom, H.C. The Minimal Difference as an Individual Threshold to Examine the Utility of a Verification Bout in Determining VO_{2max}. *Med. Sci. Sports Exerc.* **2023**, *55*, 1063–1068. [CrossRef]
30. Day, J.R.; Rossiter, H.B.; Coats, E.M.; Skasick, A.; Whipp, B.J. The Maximally Attainable VO_2 during Exercise in Humans: The Peak vs. Maximum Issue. *J. Appl. Physiol.* **2003**, *95*, 1901–1907. [CrossRef]
31. Robergs, R.A.; Dwyer, D.; Astorino, T. Recommendations for Improved Data Processing from Expired Gas Analysis Indirect Calorimetry. *Sports Med.* **2010**, *40*, 95–111. [CrossRef] [PubMed]

32. Jones, A.M.; Grassi, B.; Christensen, P.M.; Krustrup, P.; Bangsbo, J.; Poole, D.C. Slow Component of VO$_2$ Kinetics: Mechanistic Bases and Practical Applications. *Med. Sci. Sports Exerc.* **2011**, *43*, 2046–2062. [CrossRef] [PubMed]
33. Borg, G. Perceived Exertion as an Indicator of Somatic Stress. *Scand. J. Rehabil. Med.* **1970**, *2*, 92–98. [CrossRef] [PubMed]
34. Hopkins, W.G. Measures of Reliability in Sports Medicine and Science. *Sports Med.* **2000**, *30*, 1–15. [CrossRef] [PubMed]
35. Shrout, P.E.; Fleiss, J.L. Intraclass Correlations: Uses in Assessing Rater Reliability. *Psychol. Bull.* **1979**, *86*, 420–428. [CrossRef]
36. Vincent, W.J.; Weir, J.P. *Statistics in Kinesiology*, 4th ed.; Human Kinetics: Champaign, IL, USA, 2012.
37. Buckthorpe, M.W.; Hannah, R.; Pain, T.G.; Folland, J.P. Reliability of Neuromuscular Measurements during Explosive Isometric Contractions, with Special Reference to Electromyography Normalization Techniques. *Muscle Nerve* **2012**, *46*, 566–576. [CrossRef]
38. Atkinson, G.; Nevill, A.M. Statistical Methods for Assessing Measurement Error (Reliability) in Variables Relevant to Sports Medicine. *Sports Med.* **1998**, *26*, 217–238. [CrossRef]
39. Rose, G.A.; Davies, R.G.; Appadurai, I.R.; Williams, I.M.; Bashir, M.; Berg, R.M.G.; Poole, D.C.; Bailey, D.M. "Fit for Surgery": The Relationship between Cardiorespiratory Fitness and Postoperative Outcomes. *Exp. Physiol.* **2022**, *107*, 787–799. [CrossRef]
40. Succi, P.J.; Dinyer, T.K.; Byrd, M.T.; Soucie, E.P.; Voskuil, C.C.; Bergstrom, H.C. Test-Retest Reliability of Critical Power, Critical Heart Rate, Time to Exhaustion, and Average Heart Rate during Cycle Ergometry. *J. Exerc. Physiol. Online* **2021**, *24*, 33–52.
41. Astorino, T.A.; DeRevere, J. Efficacy of Constant Load Verification Testing to Confirm VO$_{2max}$ Attainment. *Clin. Physiol. Funct. Imaging* **2018**, *38*, 703–709. [CrossRef]
42. Pickering, C.; Kiely, J. Do Non-Responders to Exercise Exist-and If So, What Should We Do about Them? *Sports Med.* **2019**, *49*, 1–7. [CrossRef] [PubMed]
43. Knaier, R.; Infanger, D.; Niemeyer, M.; Cajochen, C.; Schmidt-Trucksäss, A. In Athletes, the Diurnal Variations in Maximum Oxygen Uptake Are More than Twice as Large as the Day-to-Day Variations. *Front. Physiol.* **2019**, *10*, 219. [CrossRef] [PubMed]
44. Lebrun, C.M.; McKenzie, D.C.; Prior, J.C.; Taunton, J.E. Effects of Menstrual Cycle Phase on Athletic Performance. *Med. Sci. Sports Exerc.* **1995**, *27*, 437–444. [CrossRef] [PubMed]

Disclaimer/Publisher's Note: The statements, opinions and data contained in all publications are solely those of the individual author(s) and contributor(s) and not of MDPI and/or the editor(s). MDPI and/or the editor(s) disclaim responsibility for any injury to people or property resulting from any ideas, methods, instructions or products referred to in the content.

Article

Vertical Jump Kinetic Parameters on Sand and Rigid Surfaces in Young Female Volleyball Players with a Combined Background in Indoor and Beach Volleyball

George Giatsis [1,*], Vassilios Panoutsakopoulos [1], Christina Frese [2] and Iraklis A. Kollias [1]

[1] Biomechanics Laboratory, School of Physical Education and Sport Science at Thessaloniki, Aristotle University of Thessaloniki, 54124 Thessaloniki, Greece; bpanouts@phed.auth.gr (V.P.); hkollias@phed.auth.gr (I.A.K.)

[2] Department for Biomechanics and Sportbiology, Institute of Sport and Movement Science, University Stuttgart, Allmandring 28 A, Vaihingen, 70569 Stuttgart, Germany; christina.frese@inspo.uni-stuttgart.de

* Correspondence: ggiatsis@phed.auth.gr; Tel.: +30-231-099-2208

Abstract: Little is known about the differences in vertical jump biomechanics executed on rigid (RJS) and sand (SJS) surfaces in female indoor and beach volleyball players. Eleven young female beach volleyball players with a combined indoor and beach volleyball sport background performed squat jumps, countermovement jumps with and without an arm swing, and drop jumps from 40 cm on a RJS (force plate) and SJS (sand pit attached to the force plate). The results of the 2 (surface) × 4 (vertical jump test) repeated-measure ANOVA revealed a significant ($p < 0.05$) main effect of the surface and the vertical jump test on the jump height and time to achieve peak vertical body center of mass velocity. A significant ($p < 0.05$) main effect of the test, but not of the surface ($p > 0.05$), was observed for the other examined biomechanical parameters. The only significant ($p < 0.05$) jump height gain difference between RJS and SJS was observed for the utilization of the stretch-shortening cycle, which was higher in SJS (15.4%) compared to RJS (7.5%). In conclusion, as the testing was conducted during the beach volleyball competitive season, the examined female players showed adaptations relating the effective utilization of the pre-stretch and enhanced stability during the execution of the vertical jump tests on a SJS compared to RJS.

Keywords: biomechanical analysis; kinetics; kinematics; stretch-shortening cycle; vertical jumping; surface stability; gender differences; drop jump

1. Introduction

Vertical jump tests are widely considered diagnostic conditioning tests for volleyball and beach volleyball (BV) players [1–5] since most jumps performed in both sports are executed with countermovement and an arm swing [6]. In specific, the countermovement jump (CMJ) is observed during the execution of blocks, standing jump float serve and special counterattack actions [7].

The most common diagnostic vertical jump tests are the squat jump (SQJ), CMJ and drop jump (DJ), providing different information about physical fitness. Kinetic parameters, such as force, power and work, among others, as well as their respective time curves in each jump test, evaluate specific strength and conditioning capabilities. For example, a SQJ is considered an appropriate evaluation tool of the concentric muscular strength application capability [8]. As for the CMJ without an arm swing (CMJA), the effectiveness of the pre-stretch that occurs during the stretch-shortening cycle (SCC) is evaluated [9], while a CMJ with an arm swing (CMJF) tests the ability to utilize the proximal-to-distal energy flow generated from the work produced at the shoulders [10]. Finally, a DJ is used to check the ability to effectively use the SSC in a pre-stretch of great extent [11].

In addition, the difference in jump height (h_{JUMP}) between a SQJ and CMJA is widely considered to represent the gain resulted from the SSC [9], and the respective gain between CMJA and CMJF is suggested to represent the upper and lower limb intra-segmental neuromuscular coordination [10,12,13]. Finally, the gain in h_{JUMP} between SQJ and DJ evaluates the effect of a greater pre-stretch on jumping ability [14]. The examination of the kinetic and temporal parameters among the different vertical jump tests is considered to provide useful insight into the neuromuscular mechanisms responsible for the optimization of jumping performance [10,12–14].

A vast amount of information on the decreased h_{JUMP} on sand (SJS) compared to a rigid (RJS) jumping surface exists in the literature for BV players [2,15–21]. The decreased h_{JUMP} on a SJS compared to RJS is associated with a lower force and power outputs [2,17–19] due to the less stiff surface and larger friction compared to indoor sport surfaces [15]. This deprives practitioners of applying force fast during the jumping tests, resulting in a lower power output and eventually poor jumping performance [17–19]. However, volleyball-specific training on a SJS during the indoor volleyball off-season resulted in higher physical fitness, such as higher endurance of quadriceps and calf muscles [22], as well as in higher jump height in SQJ and CMJ on both surfaces [22], and in the spike jump on a RJS [23]. Furthermore, there is evidence that CMJs on a RJS are not only useful to gain information regarding performance on a SJS, but also in relation to diagnosing neuromuscular imbalances in players with a mixed indoor volleyball and BV sport background for the spike jump on a SJS [16].

Previous literature has shown that game patterns [24] are gender-specific, whereby female players have slower attack tempos, but use more placed attacks and play longer rallies. Furthermore, men jump higher than women in the spike jump [25], which probably results from a combination of higher strength and power generation capabilities [26–28]. Furthermore, it can be also a result of different movement characteristics such as approach speed, torso incline, use of arm swing [25,28], plant angle of the dominant limb and neuromuscular activation in spike [25]. Differences in power generation capabilities could be the reason for higher kinetic parameters in CMJ despite the fact that the maximal rate of force development was even for both genders [29,30]; however, it does not explain the higher loss of jump height on a SJS compared to a RJS for women (-13%) compared to men (-9.4%) [31]. As such, it is worth noting that, although vertical jump biomechanics on a SJS have been extensively reported for male BV players, such information is missing for female BV players. With respect to the SJS, to the best of our knowledge, the only available information is that vertical jump performance in female BV players is rather constant, regardless of the sand surface [32,33], but the h_{JUMP} of the spike jump on a SJS was lower compared to a RJS [33,34].

To conclude, the respective literature lacks evidence about the modification of the jumping kinetics of female BV players when executing diagnostic vertical jump tests on a SJS, since they might have different movement characteristics than male players. The aim of the study was to investigate the possible differences in the performance and biomechanical parameters of common diagnostic vertical jump tests executed on a RJS and SJS in young female volleyball players. It was hypothesized that vertical jumps on a SJS will result in a decreased h_{JUMP} and performance gains, as well as a lower force and power outputs compared to those on a RJS.

2. Materials and Methods
2.1. Participants

The research was conducted following the requirements of the Declaration of Helsinki and the Research Ethics Code of the Aristotle University of Thessaloniki after obtaining ethical approval from the Institutional Ethics Committee (approval no.: 87/2021). A convenience sample comprising 13 young female BV players (20.2 ± 3.2 years, 1.72 ± 0.05 m, 62.9 ± 3.9 kg) was selected for examination. The participants needed to have experience on both the RJS and SJS. Participation was voluntary and was granted after obtaining a signed consent form. Of the recruited players, seven were members of the national team, with four of them having participated in major international competitions, four being national-level players and two varsity-level players.

At the time of testing, all players were participating in the competitive BV season. The inclusion criteria were participation in official BV tournaments within the previous five years, systematic participation in their training and competition BV schedule, and having been systematically (>10 h/wk) trained in indoor volleyball during the past winter. The exclusion criterion was having sustained an injury that prevented them from competition within the 6 months before the study.

2.2. Procedure

Basic anthropometric measures (body height, body mass) were acquired using a SECA 220 (Seca Deutschland, Hamburg, Germany) stadiometer and a Delmac PS400L (Delmac Instrumetns S.A., Athens, Greece) electronic scale. An 817E Monark Exercise Cycle (Monark-Crescent AB, Varberg, Sweden) was used for warm up, followed by dynamic stretching exercises and six sub-maximal vertical jumps, with a progressive increase in countermovement and intensity.

The examined vertical jump tests included an SQJ, CMJA, CMJF and a DJ from 40 cm (DJ40). Three trials were allowed for each jumping test. The intra- and inter-test resting period was 1 min and 4 min, respectively. All jumps were executed barefooted, employing procedures implemented in previous studies [17–19]. The surface of the force plate was considered a RJS. The vertical jump tests on a SJS were conducted on sand weighing 112.12 kg, that was contained in a wooden sand pit (Figure 1) and the depth of the sand was 0.31 m. The top-side dimensions of the wooden pit were 0.59 × 0.63 m. The bottom-side dimensions of the wooden pit were 0.46 × 0.50 m. This size was selected so that the sand pit was firmly attached to the force plate. In terms of safety, soft materials covered the edges of the wooden pit. In addition, a safety platform (1.16 × 1.50 × 0.31 m, length, width and height, respectively) surrounded the wooden pit. According to the results of a series of tests performed following the American Society for Testing and Materials (ASTM) [18], it was established that the physical properties of the sand and its grain size distribution satisfied the Federation International de Volleyball (FIVB) requirements. To avoid the compaction of sand particles during the vertical jump tests on a SJS, a tool with a 0.31 m length was used to mix and spread the sand in its entire volume within the sand pit before each trial. During data acquisition, the equality of participants' body masses between the force plate recordings with and without the sand pit was checked.

The order of the jumping tests and the jumping surface was randomized using Matlab R2021 (The MathWorks Inc., Natick, MA, USA) scripts. In all tests, the instruction was to "jump as high as you can with the shortest push-off time". The SQJ test initiated from a knee angle of 90° and with full foot contact on the jumping surface. If the force recordings indicated a downward movement, the trial was cancelled [17]. For the CMJ test, no restrictions were set concerning the depth of the countermovement [18]. A one-dimensional force plate (1-Dynami, ©: Biomechanics Lab AUTh, Thessaloniki, Greece) was used as the drop platform [19]. In the case of the DJ40 on the SJS, the drop force plate was fixed and adjusted within the safety platform at a height of 0.71 m. The instruction was to execute the drop with a "roll-off", while no specific requirements were set about the depth of the countermovement during the ground contact [19].

The foot–SJS interaction was recorded with a Redlake Motionscope PCI 1S camera (Redlake Imaging Corporation, Morgan Hill, CA, USA; sampling frequency: 250 fps) to ensure that no excessive plunging into the sand occurred. This was established after the visual review of the recorded contact phase by an experienced researcher.

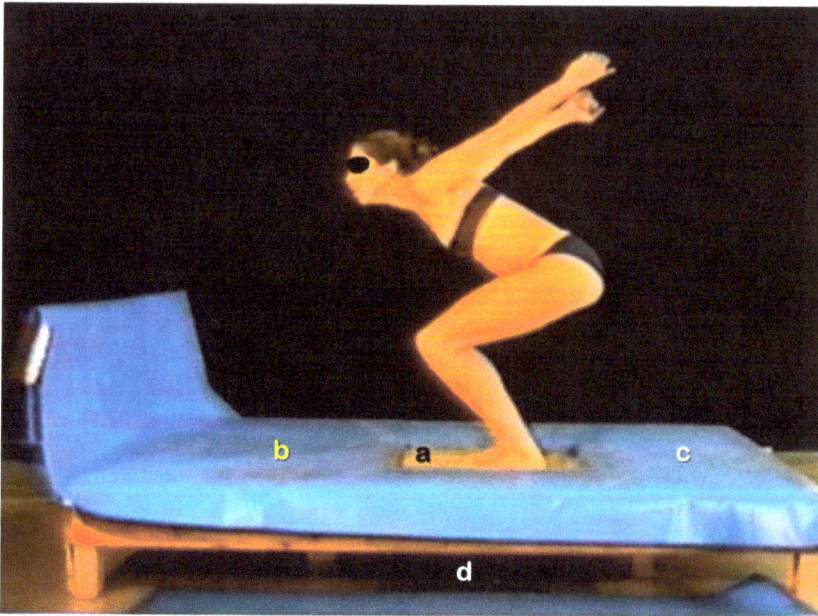

Figure 1. Representational depiction of the experimental set-up and execution of the countermovement jump with an arm swing on the sand jumping surface: (a) sand surface; (b) safety platform; (c) fixation points for the drop force plate; (d) force plate.

2.3. Data Acquisition and Analysis

Only the best jump in each test using the h_{JUMP} as a criterion was selected for further analysis. The criterion parameter was calculated from the vertical body center of mass (CoM) take-off velocity, which was extracted as the first-time integral of the net vertical ground reaction force (GRF) using the trapezoid rule [18]. The vertical GRF was acquired with an AMTI OR6-5-1 force plate (AMTI, Newton, MA, USA; sampling frequency: 500 Hz). GRF data recording and analysis were completed with the modules of the K-Dynami 2018 (©: Iraklis A. Kollias, Biomechanics Laboratory, Aristotle University of Thessaloniki, Thessaloniki, Greece) software. The following vertical jump biomechanical parameters were calculated using the procedures described previously [17–19]:

1. Temporal parameters: total push-off time (tC), time to achieve a maximum vertical GRF (tFz), time to achieve peak vertical CoM velocity (tUz) and time to achieve peak power (tP$_{Max}$);
2. Spatial/kinematic parameters: h_{JUMP}, actual drop take-off height (h_{DROP}), peak CoM vertical velocity (Uz$_{MAX}$) and maximum downward vertical CoM displacement (S$_{DOWN}$);
3. Kinetic parameters: peak vertical GRF (Fz$_{MAX}$), peak rate of force development (RFD) and peak power (P$_{MAX}$).

The temporal parameters were extracted from the time curves of the respective kinetic parameters. As for h_{DROP}, it was calculated with an integration of the vertical CoM velocity that was recorded from the drop force plate [19]. In turn, S$_{DOWN}$ was extracted after integration of the vertical CoM velocity [18]. The first-time derivative of the recorded vertical GRF defined RFD, while P$_{MAX}$ was the peak value of the multiplication product of the vertical GRF by the vertical CoM velocity during the propulsive phase [17]. Based on h_{JUMP}, the following vertical jump performance parameters were also calculated [35,36]:

1. SSC gain (Equation (1)):

$$\text{SSC gain} = \left(\frac{h_{\text{JUMP(CMJA)}} - h_{\text{JUMP(SQJ)}}}{h_{\text{JUMP(SQJ)}}}\right) \times 100 \quad (1)$$

2. Arm swing gain (Equation (2)):

$$\text{Arm Swing gain} = \left(\frac{h_{\text{JUMP(CMJF)}} - h_{\text{JUMP(CMJA)}}}{h_{\text{JUMP(CMJA)}}}\right) \times 100 \quad (2)$$

3. Drop jump gain (Equation (3)):

$$\text{Drop Jump gain} = \left(\frac{h_{\text{JUMP(DJ40)}} - h_{\text{JUMP(SQJ)}}}{h_{\text{JUMP(SQJ)}}}\right) \times 100 \quad (3)$$

2.4. Statistical Analyses

The Shapiro–Wilk ($p > 0.05$) and the Levene tests ($p < 0.05$) were used to establish the existence of a normal distribution and equality of variance of the data, respectively. Based on the results of the above-mentioned tests, a 2 (surface: RJS vs. SJS) × 4 (jump tests: SQJ, CMJA, CMJF, DJ40) repeated-measure ANOVA with the Bonferroni adjustment was run to investigate the main effects and interaction of surface and jump modality on the biomechanical parameters of the examined vertical jumps. Significant differences were followed up with pairwise comparisons. The partial eta-squared (η_p^2) statistic was used for the determination of the effect sizes as follows: small (>0.01), medium (>0.06), and large (>0.14).

The paired sample t-test was used for the search of possible significant differences between the RJS and SJS relating the h_{DROP} and h_{JUMP} gain due to the SSC, the arm swing and the drop. Effect sizes were estimated based on Cohen's d (≤ 0.49 = small, 0.50–0.79 = medium, and ≥ 0.80 = large effect sizes, respectively).

All statistical analyses were conducted with the level of significance set at $a = 0.05$. The IBM SPSS Statistics v.29 software (International Business Machines Corp., Armonk, NY, USA) was used for the execution of the statistical analyses.

3. Results

Due to the imposed inclusion and exclusion criteria, only 11 players (21.2 ± 2.3 years, 1.74 ± 0.04 m, 64.1 ± 3.5 kg) were examined. In order to reach a power of 0.8 at $a = 0.05$ with a sample size of 11 participants and 2 (surfaces) × 4 (jump types) testing, high effect sizes (0.75) are required to obtain a statistically relevant result according to the estimation made using the G*power v.3.1.9.6 software (©Franz Faul, University of Kiel, Kiel, Germany).

The results for the vertical jump biomechanical parameters are presented in Table 1. Significant ($p < 0.05$) main effects for h_{JUMP} and tUz were found between the surfaces. For both parameters, the values for the SJS condition were lower than the RJS.

In most spatio-temporal and kinetic parameters, significant ($p < 0.05$) differences among jumps, but not between surfaces, were observed. The DJ40 test was significantly different ($p < 0.05$) from the no-arm swing vertical jump tests relating the examined force parameters and power output.

Finally, no significant surface × jumping test interaction was revealed ($p > 0.05$).

No significant differences ($p > 0.05$) were revealed concerning the examined vertical jump performance parameters, except for the SSC utilization ratio, which was significantly ($p < 0.05$) higher (two-fold) on a SJS compared to RJS (Table 2). Finally, h_{DROP} was not different ($t = 2.043$, $p = 0.068$, $d = 0.60$) between the examined surfaces (34.5 ± 4.5 cm and 37.0 ± 3.8 cm for the RJS and SJS, respectively).

Table 1. Mean (standard deviation) of the biomechanical vertical jump parameters on rigid (RJS) and sand (SJS) jumping surfaces (n = 11).

Surface	RJS				SJS				F	p	η_p^2
Parameter	SQJ	CMJA	CMJF	DJ40	SQJ	CMJA	CMJF	DJ40	Test Surface	Test Surface	Test Surface
Body center of mass displacement											
h_{JUMP} (cm)	17.8 (2.2)	18.8 (2.6)	21.5 [a] (3.2)	13.3 [abc] (2.9)	15.1 * (1.2)	17.5 (2.6)	20.8 [ab] (3.2)	11.8 [abc] (2.7)	40.292 7.566	<0.001 0.007	0.599 0.085
S_{DOWN} (cm)	-	−30.9 (4.2)	−30.8 (4.6)	−36.3 (7.0)	-	−31.2 (2.7)	−30.4 (4.1)	−39.6 [bc] (7.7)	369.864 0.615	<0.001 0.436	0.302 0.010
Temporal parameters											
tC (ms)	492.3 (63.9)	504.7 (57.4)	550.1 (100.2)	425.3 [c] (80.4)	451.9 (78.8)	505.8 (39.8)	533.7 (53.1)	470.9 (92.5)	6.843 0.026	<0.001 0.872	0.202 0.000
tFz (%tC)	62.2 (17.2)	65.7 (4.7)	62.4 (17.7)	73.1 (11.5)	57.9 (17.3)	66.7 (6.5)	62.5 (17.8)	74.5 [a] (15.4)	3.964 0.023	0.011 0.881	0.128 0.000
tUz (%tC)	75.5 (1.7)	75.9 (1.9)	76.6 (2.5)	71.9 [abc] (3.2)	72.8 (1.2)	74.9 (2.0)	75.9 [a] (3.4)	68.9 [abc] (4.3)	20.608 10.720	<0.001 0.002	0.433 0.117
tP_{MAX} (%tC)	74.4 (3.6)	75.3 (3.0)	76.0 (4.9)	71.1 (15.2)	71.6 (4.4)	75.4 (2.1)	78.0 (8.6)	70.5 (8.7)	2.896 0.052	0.040 0.821	0.097 0.001
Kinematic parameters											
Uz_{MAX} (m/s)	2.46 (0.12)	2.52 (0.12)	2.67 [a] (0.14)	2.23 [abc] (0.18)	2.36 (0.09)	2.46 (0.13)	2.65 [ab] (0.14)	2.19 [abc] (0.16)	40.550 3.840	<0.001 0.053	0.600 0.045
Kinetic parameters											
Fz_{MAX} (N/kg)	2.06 (0.12)	2.27 (0.16)	2.28 (0.14)	3.27 [abc] (0.75)	2.06 (0.16)	2.26 (0.13)	2.30 (0.18)	2.97 [abc] (0.64)	34.827 0.820	<0.001 0.368	0.566 0.010
RFD (kN/s)	5.1 (1.5)	8.5 (5.6)	7.3 (4.1)	31.5 [abc] (9.8)	5.9 (1.7)	9.0 (4.2)	7.0 (3.0)	38.1 *[abc] (12.0)	108.053 2.033	<0.001 0.158	0.800 0.158
P_{MAX} (W/kg)	21.4 (2.7)	21.5 (3.2)	25.6 (4.3)	28.7 [b] (8.1)	20.2 (3.2)	20.7 (3.7)	26.7 [ab] (4.3)	26.9 [ab] (3.4)	14.564 0.530	<0.001 0.469	0.350 0.006

*: $p < 0.05$ vs. RJS surface; [a]: $p < 0.05$ vs. SQJ; [b]: $p < 0.05$ vs. CMJA; [c]: $p < 0.05$ vs. CMJF. Abbreviations: h_{JUMP}: jump height; S_{DOWN}: maximum vertical downward body center of mass (CoM) displacement; tC: total push-off time; tFz: time to achieve maximum vertical ground reaction force (GRF); tUz: time to achieve maximum vertical CoM velocity; tP_{MAX}: time to achieve maximum power during the upward phase; Uz_{MAX}: peak vertical CoM velocity; Fz_{MAX}: peak vertical GRF; RFD: peak rate of force development; P_{MAX}: peak power.

Table 2. Mean (standard deviation) of the vertical jump performance ratios on rigid (RJS) and sand (SJS) jumping surfaces (n = 11).

Parameter	RJS	SJS	MD	SE	t	p	d
SSC gain (%)	7.5 (8.4)	15.4 (8.6)	7.9	3.6	2.516	0.031 *	0.93
Arm swing gain (%)	14.9 (9.2)	18.9 (10.7)	4.0	4.3	0.748	0.471	0.40
Drop jump gain (%)	−23.7 (12.9)	−22.3 (15.2)	1.4	6.0	0.260	0.800	0.10

*: $p < 0.05$; Abbreviations: SSC: stretch-shortening cycle: MD: mean difference; SE: standard error of the mean; d: Cohen's d.

4. Discussion

The purpose of the present research was to examine the possible differences in vertical jump tests executed on RJS and SJS surfaces in young female volleyball players. The results revealed that jumping performance was lower on a SJS than RJS, but there was no difference in the examined kinetic parameters. In addition, tUz values were reached faster on a SJS compared to RJS. Furthermore, SSC gain was higher on a SJS than RJS.

In agreement with past reports [2,15–21,37,38], h_{JUMP} was higher on a RJS compared to SJS. Although this is not statistically relevant for all jump results yet, it is attributed to the low sample size, since only large effect sizes and not small or moderate effect sizes in a small population lead to a statically relevant result. In respect to the vertical jump tests, only h_{JUMP} on an SQJ was significantly different between the tested surfaces. This might be explained by the reported differences in the SSC gain, which could be the result of regular CMJF variation use in BV [6], such as block jumps, standing jump float serve and special counterattack actions [7], leading to better inter-segmental coordination. These adaptations have already been reported [22,39–41]. Since the participants were at the peak of the BV competitive period, such adaptations were most likely to occur. Biomechanical variables, such as power output, confirm the h_{JUMP} height, because no differences were observed. Similar results were reported in the past [18], but are contradictory to other previous findings [2,17].

The SJS also influenced tUz (η_p^2 = 0.433), as participants reached their peak vertical CoM velocity earlier compared to the vertical jump tests executed on a RJS. It has been suggested [14] that the generation of vertical CoM velocity is the result of the capacity of neural recruitment. A possible mechanism for this finding could be the effect of plyometric activities conducted by the players on sand that has been shown to increase the motor unit recruitment [42]. Other possible factors are the instability of the SJS, which increases the need to maintain balance. This eventually results in increased work expenditure due to the larger amount of energy absorbed [2,15,18,20,21,43,44] and decreased ability to reuse stored elastic energy during the SCC [45].

Another finding was that there was no difference in Uz_{MAX} between a SJS and RJS (p = 0.053). It is suggested that the Uz_{MAX} is a determinant factor for the performance differences between men and women [46]. Even though it shall not be connected with the eccentric phase of vertical jump tests [47], it is proposed that it is beneficial to achieve a higher CoM velocity during the eccentric phase [48]. This is related to increased force and power outputs at the initiation and through the entire concentric phase [49,50] that eventually result in a higher h_{JUMP} [51].

The only difference revealed for the vertical jump performance parameters was the SSC gain. The SCC gain in the present study was in reasonable agreement with past research reports [30,52]. However, our findings derived from the examined young female BV players is not in agreement with past research, suggesting that the effectiveness of SSC movements on sand rely more on the concentric rather than eccentric muscle action. This can be a result of the degradation of elastic energy resulting from the sand instability [45,53], since tC was not changed between RJS and SJS, indicating an efficient SSC function [23]. The larger SSC gain can be attributed to the fact that, as training on sand improves postural control [54], the examined young female players might have been more stable on a SJS and, thus, they optimized their jumping mechanics. This can be further supported by the fact that jump training on a SJS results in an increased CMJ jump height compared to jump training on a RJS [39].

Regarding DJ40, no drop jump gain was obtained, but rather an approximate 23% reduction in h_{JUMP}. This can be attributed to a possible reduced capacity of the participants to efficiently use the SSC, since previous research on male athletes on a RJS and SJS has shown that peak angular velocity in the ankle joint when landing in a SJS is significantly lower, thus reducing the stretch mechanism [19,55]. The results for h_{DROP} confirm the above rationale, as h_{DROP} was almost two-fold from the h_{JUMP} achieved, with recommendation for the optimum h_{DROP} being in the range of 50–100% of the h_{JUMP} in CMJA for male volleyball players [56]. In contrast to previous studies on elite male BV players [19] and despite the larger RFD compared to RJS, there were no indications that the SJS led to an unstable execution of DJ40, since tFz was not different between the examined jumping surfaces. Nevertheless, it is worth noting that increased differences between a RJS and SJS compared to the other jumps were observed in DJ40 in regard to the h_{JUMP}, tUz, and force parameters, especially in the RFD (+18% on SJS).

As depicted in Figure 1, the examined female BV players performed the CMJ with a full-arm swing, which is typical for volleyball players [57]. Nevertheless, a lower h_{JUMP} arm swing gain was observed in the present study when compared to professional male BV players [18], confirming previous evidence that the arm swing provides a larger h_{JUMP} gain to males than females [28]. Contrarily to the previously mentioned research, no surface effect was revealed. Past research revealed a larger range of motion in the ankle and hip joints in the CMJF compared to the CMJA on a SJS than RJS [18]. In the same study, the arm swing on a SJS was associated with a larger forward inclination of the body at the lowest position of the CoM. In general, the arm swing generates mechanical work from the musculature of the shoulder that is transferred to the lower limb muscles and eventually results in an augmented energy production for the propulsion for the jump [10,12,13]. It has been suggested that the greater upper body strength production capability in men enhances the effectiveness of this mechanism more than in women [28].

Regarding the inter-test comparison, the present study reveals that an excessive pre-stretch tension imposed by the DJ resulted in a higher force, RFD and power outcomes compared to the other jumping tests, especially those without the use of an arm swing. It has been suggested that the reflex potentiation provides additional enhancement in jumping performance [14]. This can also be attributed to the fact that SSC exercises executed on a SJS increase motor unit recruitment [42]. The comparison of the examined biomechanical parameters in vertical jump tests led to the conclusion that plyometric training aiming for a fast force application seem to improve explosiveness more effectively. However, the largest Uz_{MAX} was observed in the CMJF compared to the other jumping tests. This can be attributed to the fact that most sport-specific jumps are conducted with counter-movements and arm swings [6]. This also seems to be related to the higher P_{MAX} in the CMJF on a SJS. Nevertheless, the absence of an inter-test difference regarding tP_{MAX} can be attributed to the fact that young female volleyball players were found to rely less on fast time-depended parameters in order to maximize vertical squat jump performance [51].

We want to acknowledge some limitations of this study. First, the small sample size and homogeneity of the playing level might prevent a broad generalization of the present findings, since there are contradictory findings regarding playing level and vertical jump test performance [58–60], which might also be jump-specific [61]. There are some findings [60], particularly in DJ40, which show that performance is not associated with a sport-specific background rather than the ability to execute the jumping task with an optimized utilization of its kinetic factors. Second, we assumed that kinematical differences might be present between the surfaces, since the subjects did not get any instructions on the depth of the countermovement; therefore, they could self-select their movement strategy to enhance CMJ performance. Thus, a kinematical analysis would have been useful to detect such changes [50].

Future research should not only emphasize on the kinetic, but also on kinematic and electromyographic differences when jumping on rigid and sand surfaces, to examine the loading imposed on the lower limb joints and the possible modifications in the function of the neuromuscular system. The retrieved information from such studies could be applied to both performance enhancement and injury prevention. This is because in contrast to current beliefs, sand training does not necessarily involve lower kinetic parameters such as the Fz_{MAX} and P_{MAX}, at least for double-legged jumps in young female players. This information might be especially important for physiotherapists working with athletes and chronic knee pain, since it likely leads to similar tendon loading compared to jumps on a RJS.

5. Conclusions

Young female players with a combined indoor and beach volleyball sport background performed the common diagnostic vertical jump tests on rigid and sand surfaces with no between-surface differences concerning the examined kinetic parameters. Jumping on sand resulted in: (1) a decreased jump height, especially on an SQJ; (2) a shorter time to achieve peak vertical body center of mass vertical velocity; and (3) a higher jump height gain when the countermovement was applied on the sand compared to application on a rigid surface.

The observed alterations when jumping on sand may lead to an enhanced utilization of the pre-stretch and therefore might enhance stability during the execution of the vertical jump tests. Also, the inclusion of plyometric jump training on a sand surface could stimulate the neuromuscular mechanisms that enhance jumping performance. In conclusion, the jumps performed on sand with a countermovement and arm swing or excessive pre-stretch loads imposed by drop jumps comprise jumping activities that involve favorable patterns for greater power outputs.

Author Contributions: Conceptualization, G.G. and I.A.K.; methodology, G.G., V.P. and I.A.K.; software, I.A.K.; validation, G.G., V.P. and I.A.K.; formal analysis, G.G.; investigation, G.G. and V.P.; resources, I.A.K.; data curation, G.G.; writing—original draft preparation, G.G. and C.F.; writing—review and editing, V.P. and C.F.; visualization, G.G. and V.P.; supervision, I.A.K.; project administration, G.G. All authors have read and agreed to the published version of the manuscript.

Funding: This research received no external funding.

Institutional Review Board Statement: The study was conducted in accordance with the Declaration of Helsinki, and approved by the Institutional Ethics Committee of the School of Physical Education and Sport Science at Thessaloniki, Aristotle University of Thessaloniki, Greece (approval no: 87/2021-04.11.2021).

Informed Consent Statement: Informed consent was obtained from all subjects involved in the study.

Data Availability Statement: The data that were acquired and analyzed in the present study are available from the corresponding author upon reasonable request.

Conflicts of Interest: The authors declare no conflict of interest.

References

1. Aouadi, R.; Jlid, M.C.; Khalifa, R.; Hermassi, S.; Chelly, M.S.; van den Tillaar, R.; Gabbett, T. Association of anthropometric qualities with vertical jump performance in elite male volleyball players. *J. Sports Med. Phys. Fit.* **2012**, *52*, 11–17.
2. Bishop, D.A. Comparison between land and sand-based tests for beach volleyball assessment. *J. Sports Med. Phys. Fit.* **2003**, *43*, 418–423.
3. Ricarte Batista, G.; Freire De Araujo, R.; Oliveira Guerra, R. Comparison between vertical jumps of high performance athletes on the Brazilian men's beach volleyball team. *J. Sports Med. Phys. Fit.* **2008**, *48*, 172–176.
4. Sheppard, J.M.; Newton, R.U. Long-term training adaptations in elite male volleyball players. *J. Strength Cond. Res.* **2012**, *26*, 2180–2184. [CrossRef] [PubMed]
5. Ziv, G.; Lidor, R. Vertical jump in female and male volleyball players: A review of observational and experimental studies. *Scand. J. Med. Sci. Sports* **2010**, *20*, 556–567. [CrossRef] [PubMed]
6. Turpin, J.P.; Cortell, J.M.; Chinchilla, J.J.; Cejuera, R.; Suarez, C. Analysis of jump patterns in competition for elite male Beach Volleyball players. *Int. J. Perform. Anal. Sport* **2008**, *8*, 94–101. [CrossRef]
7. Giatsis, G. Jumping quality and quantitative analysis of beach volleyball game. *Exerc. Soc. J. Sports Sci.* **2001**, *28* (Suppl. 1), 95.
8. Bosco, C. *La Valutazione Della Forza con il Test di Bosco*; 3S-Societa Stampa Sportiva: Rome, Italy, 1992.
9. Tufano, J.J.; Walker, S.; Seitz, L.B.; Newton, R.U.; Häkkinen, K.; Blazevich, A.J.; Haff, G.G. Reliability of the reactive strength index, eccentric utilisation ratio, and pre-stretch augmentation in untrained, novice jumpers. *J. Aus. Strength Cond.* **2013**, *21*, 31–33.
10. Lees, A.; Vanrenterghem, J.; De Clercq, D. Understanding how an arm swing enhances performance in the vertical jump. *J. Biomech.* **2004**, *37*, 1929–1940. [CrossRef]
11. Komi, P.V.; Nicol, C. Stretch-Shortening Cycle of muscle function. In *Neuromuscular Aspects of Sport Performance*; Komi, P.V., Ed.; Blackwell Publishing Ltd.: West Sussex, UK, 2011; pp. 15–31.
12. Feltner, M.E.; Fraschetti, D.J.; Crisp, R.J. Upper extremity augmentation of lower extremity kinetics during countermovement vertical jumps. *J. Sports Sci.* **1999**, *17*, 449–466. [CrossRef]
13. Hara, M.; Shibayama, A.; Takeshita, D.; Hay, D.C.; Fukashiro, S. A comparison of the mechanical effect of arm swing and countermovement on the lower extremities in vertical jumping. *Hum. Mov. Sci.* **2008**, *27*, 636–648. [CrossRef] [PubMed]
14. Bosco, C.; Komi, P.V.; Ito, A. Prestretch potentiation of human skeletal muscle during ballistic movement. *Acta Physiol. Scand.* **1981**, *111*, 135–140. [CrossRef]
15. Bisciotti, G.N.; Ruby, A.; Jaquemod, C. Biomechanics of jumps in the volleyball and in the beach-volley. *Riv. Cult. Sport.* **2001**, *20*, 29–34.
16. Frese, C.; Bubeck, D.; Alt, W. Reduced Vastus Medialis/Lateralis EMG ratio in volleyballers with chronic knee pain on sports-specific surfaces: A pilot study. *Int. J. Environ. Res. Public Health* **2022**, *19*, 9920. [CrossRef]
17. Giatsis, G.; Kollias, I.; Panoutsakopoulos, V.; Papaiakovou, G. Biomechanical differences in elite beach-volleyball players in vertical squat jump on rigid and sand surface. *Sports Biomech.* **2004**, *3*, 145–158. [CrossRef]
18. Giatsis, G.; Panoutsakopoulos, V.; Kollias, I.A. Biomechanical differences of arm swing countermovement jumps on sand and rigid surface performed by elite beach volleyball players. *J. Sports Sci.* **2018**, *36*, 997–1008. [CrossRef]
19. Giatsis, G.; Panoutsakopoulos, V.; Kollias, I.A. Drop jumping on sand is characterized by lower power, higher rate of force development and larger knee joint range of motion. *J. Funct. Morphol. Kinesiol.* **2022**, *7*, 17. [CrossRef] [PubMed]

20. Miyama, M.; Nosaka, K. Influence of surface on muscle damage and soreness induced by consecutive drop jumps. *J. Strength Cond. Res.* **2004**, *18*, 206–211. [CrossRef] [PubMed]
21. Muramatsu, S.; Fukudome, A.; Miyama, M.; Arimoto, M.; Kijima, A. Energy expenditure in maximal jumps on sand. *J. Physiol. Anthropol.* **2006**, *25*, 59–61. [CrossRef]
22. Balasas, D.G.; Christoulas, K.; Stefanidis, P.; Vamvakoudis, E.; Bampouras, T. The effect of beach volleyball training on muscle performance of indoor volleyball players. *J. Sports Med. Phys. Fit.* **2018**, *58*, 1240–1246. [CrossRef]
23. Trajkovic, N.; Sporis, G.; Kristicevic, T. Does training on sand during off-season improves physical performance in indoor volleyball players? *Acta Kinesiol.* **2016**, *10*, 107–111.
24. Costa, G.; Brand, E.; Mesquita, I. Differences in game patterns between male and female youth volleyball. *Kinesiology* **2009**, *44*, 60–66.
25. Fuchs, P.X.; Menzel, H.-J.K.; Guidotti, F.; Bell, J.; von Duvillard, S.P.; Wagner, H. Spike jump biomechanics in male versus female elite volleyball players. *J. Sports Sci.* **2019**, *37*, 2411–2419. [CrossRef] [PubMed]
26. Johnson, D.L.; Bahamonde, R. Power output estimate in university athletes. *J. Strength Cond. Res.* **1996**, *10*, 161–166.
27. Mayhew, J.L.; Salm, P.C. Gender differences in anaerobic power tests. *Eur. J. Appl. Physiol. Occup. Physiol.* **1990**, *60*, 133–138. [CrossRef]
28. Walsh, M.S.; Boehm, H.; Butterfield, M.M.; Santhosam, J. Gender bias in the effects of arms and countermovement on jumping performance. *J. Strength Cond. Res.* **2007**, *21*, 362–366. [CrossRef]
29. Ebben, W.; Flanagan, E.; Jensen, R. Gender similarities in rate of force development and time to takeoff during the countermovement jump. *J. Exer. Physiol. Online* **2007**, *10*, 10–17.
30. Riggs, M.P.; Sheppard, J.M. The relative importance of strength and power qualities to vertical jump height of elite beach volleyball players during the counter-movement and squat jump. *J. Hum. Sport Exerc.* **2009**, *4*, 221–236. [CrossRef]
31. Lames, D.L.M. Sprungtechniken im Beachvolleyball: Zum einfluss der closing-time und des fußaufsatzes auf die sprunghöhe im sand. *Leistungssport* **2006**, *36*, 35–38.
32. Pastore, J.; Ferreira, C.A.; Costa, F.C.; João, P. Evaluation of variables according to agility, speed, and power to the type of sand of different beaches for the practice of beach volleyball. *Int. J. Sports Phys. Educ.* **2017**, *3*, 1–8. [CrossRef]
33. Frese, C. Biomechanical differences of general jumps and volleyball specific jumps on hard floor and two sand types. In *Book of Abstracts of the 27th Annual Congress of the European College of Sport Science*; Dela, F., Piacentini, M.F., Helge, J.W., Calvo Lluch, Á., Sáez, E., Pareja Blanco, F., Tsolakidis, E., Eds.; European College of Sport Science: Sevilla, Spain, 2022; pp. 291–292.
34. Tilp, M.; Wagner, H.; Müller, E. Differences in 3D kinematics between volleyball and beach volleyball spike movements. *Sports Biomech.* **2008**, *7*, 386–397. [CrossRef] [PubMed]
35. Panoutsakopoulos, V.; Kotzamanidou, M.C.; Giannakos, A.K.; Kollias, I.A. Relationship of vertical jump performance and ankle joint range of motion: Effect of knee joint angle and handedness in young adult handball players. *Sports* **2022**, *10*, 86. [CrossRef]
36. Bassa, E.; Adamopoulos, I.; Panoutsakopoulos, V.; Xenofondos, A.; Yannakos, A.; Galazoulas, C.; Patikas, D.A. Optimal drop height in prepubertal boys is revealed by the performance in the squat jump. *Sports* **2022**, *11*, 1. [CrossRef] [PubMed]
37. Arianasab, H.; Mohammadipour, F.; Amiri-Khorasani, M. Comparison of knee joint kinematics during a countermovement jump among different sports surfaces in male soccer players. *Sci. Med. Footb.* **2017**, *1*, 74–79. [CrossRef]
38. Buscà, B.; Alique, D.; Salas, C.; Hileno, R.; Pena, J.; Morales, J.; Bantulà, J. Relationship between agility and jump ability in amateur beach volleyball male players. *Int. J. Perform. Anal. Sport* **2015**, *15*, 1102–1113. [CrossRef]
39. Ahmadi, M.; Nobari, H.; Ramirez-Campillo, R.; Pérez-Gómez, J.; Ribeiro, A.L.d.A.; Martínez-Rodríguez, A. Effects of plyometric jump training in sand or rigid surface on jump-related biomechanical variables and physical fitness in female volleyball players. *Int. J. Environ. Res. Public Health* **2021**, *18*, 13093. [CrossRef]
40. Gortsila, E.; Theos, A.; Nesic, G.; Maridaki, M. Effect of training surface on agility and passing skills of prepubescent female volleyball players. *J. Sports Med. Doping Stud.* **2013**, *3*, 1000128. [CrossRef]
41. Mirzaei, B.; Asghar Norasteh, A.; Saez de Villarreal, E.; Asadi, A. Effects of six weeks of depth jump vs. countermovement jump training on sand on muscle soreness and performance. *Kinesiology* **2014**, *46*, 97–108.
42. Mirzaei, B.; Norasteh, A.A.; Asadi, A. Neuromuscular adaptations to plyometric training: Depth jump vs. countermovement jump on sand. *Sport Sci. Health* **2013**, *9*, 145–149. [CrossRef]
43. Pinnington, H.; Dawson, B. Running economy of elite surf iron men and male runners, on soft dry beach sand and grass. *Eur. J. Appl. Physiol.* **2001**, *86*, 62–70. [CrossRef]
44. Smith, R. Movement in the sand: Training implications for beach volleyball. *Strength Cond. J.* **2006**, *28*, 19–21. [CrossRef]
45. Impellizzeri, F.M.; Rampinini, E.; Castagna, C.; Martino, F.; Fiorini, S.; Wisloff, U. Effect of plyometric training on sand versus grass on muscle soreness and jumping and sprinting ability in soccer players. *Br. J. Sports Med.* **2008**, *42*, 42–46. [CrossRef] [PubMed]
46. McMahon, J.J.; Rej, S.J.E.; Comfort, P. Sex differences in countermovement jump phase characteristics. *Sports* **2017**, *5*, 8. [CrossRef]
47. Jidovtseff, B.; Quievre, J.; Nigel, H.; Cronin, J. Influence of jumping strategy on kinetic parameters. *J. Sports Med. Phys. Fit.* **2014**, *54*, 129–138.
48. Sánchez-Sixto, A.; Harrison, A.J.; Floría, P. Larger Countermovement Increases the Jump Height of Countermovement Jump. *Sports* **2018**, *6*, 131. [CrossRef] [PubMed]

49. Cormie, P.; McBride, J.M.; McCaulley, G.O. Power-Time, Force-Time, and Velocity-Time Curve Analysis of the Countermovement Jump: Impact of Training. *J. Strength Cond. Res.* **2009**, *23*, 177–186. [CrossRef]
50. Kirby, T.J.; McBride, J.M.; Haines, T.L.; Dayne, A.M. Relative net vertical impulse determines jumping performance. *J. Appl. Biomech.* **2011**, *27*, 207–214. [CrossRef]
51. Panoutsakopoulos, V.; Papachatzis, N.; Kollias, I.A. Sport specificity background affects the principal component structure of vertical squat jump performance of young adult female athletes. *J. Sport Health Sci.* **2014**, *3*, 239–247. [CrossRef]
52. Freire, R.; Hausen, M.; Pereira, G.; Itaborahy, A. Body composition, aerobic fitness, isokinetic profile, and vertical jump ability in elite male and female Volleyball and Beach Volleyball players. *J. Sci. Sport Exerc.* **2022**, 1–11. [CrossRef]
53. Binnie, M.J.; Dawson, B.; Pinnington, H.; Landers, G.; Peeling, P. Sand training: A review of current research and practical applications. *J. Sports Sci.* **2014**, *32*, 8–15. [CrossRef]
54. Sebastia-Amat, S.; Ardigò, L.P.; Jimenez-Olmedo, J.M.; Pueo, B.; Penichet-Tomas, A. The effect of balance and sand training on postural control in elite Beach Volleyball players. *Int. J. Environ. Res. Public Health* **2020**, *17*, 8981. [CrossRef]
55. Gillen, Z.M.; Jahn, L.E.; Shoemaker, M.E.; McKay, B.D.; Mendez, A.I.; Bohannon, N.A.; Cramer, J.T. Effects of eccentric pre-loading on concentric vertical jump performance in young female athletes. *J. Sci. Sport Exerc.* **2021**, *3*, 98–106. [CrossRef]
56. Peng, H.T.; Song, C.Y.; Wallace, B.J.; Kernozek, T.W.; Wang, M.H.; Wang, Y.H. Effects of relative drop heights of drop jump biomechanics in male volleyball players. *Int. J. Sports Med.* **2019**, *40*, 863–870. [CrossRef] [PubMed]
57. Vaverka, F.; Jandačka, D.; Zahradník, D.; Uchytil, J.; Farana, R.; Supej, M.; Vodičar, J. Effect of an arm swing on countermovement vertical jump performance in elite volleyball players. *J. Hum. Kinet.* **2016**, *53*, 41–50. [CrossRef]
58. Barnes, J.L.; Schilling, B.K.; Falvo, M.J.; Weiss, L.W.; Creasy, A.K.; Fry, A.C. Relationship of jumping and agility performance in female volleyball athletes. *J. Strength Cond. Res.* **2007**, *21*, 1192–1196. [CrossRef]
59. Sattler, T.; Hadžic, V.; Derviševic, E.; Markovic, G. Vertical jump performance of professional male and female volleyball players: Effects of playing position and competition level. *J. Strength Cond. Res.* **2015**, *29*, 1486–1493. [CrossRef] [PubMed]
60. Panoutsakopoulos, V.; Chalitsios, C.; Nikodelis, T.; Kollias, I.A. Kinetic time-curves can classify individuals in distinct levels of drop jump performance. *J. Sports Sci.* **2022**, *40*, 2143–2152. [CrossRef] [PubMed]
61. Carvalho, A.; Roriz, P.; Duarte, D. Comparison of morphological profiles and performance variables between female volleyball players of the First and Second Division in Portugal. *J. Hum. Kinet.* **2020**, *71*, 109–117. [CrossRef]

Disclaimer/Publisher's Note: The statements, opinions and data contained in all publications are solely those of the individual author(s) and contributor(s) and not of MDPI and/or the editor(s). MDPI and/or the editor(s) disclaim responsibility for any injury to people or property resulting from any ideas, methods, instructions or products referred to in the content.

MDPI AG
Grosspeteranlage 5
4052 Basel
Switzerland
Tel.: +41 61 683 77 34
www.mdpi.com

Journal of Functional Morphology and Kinesiology Editorial Office
E-mail: jfmk@mdpi.com
www.mdpi.com/journal/jfmk

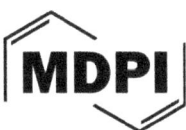

Disclaimer/Publisher's Note: The statements, opinions and data contained in all publications are solely those of the individual author(s) and contributor(s) and not of MDPI and/or the editor(s). MDPI and/or the editor(s) disclaim responsibility for any injury to people or property resulting from any ideas, methods, instructions or products referred to in the content.

www.ingramcontent.com/pod-product-compliance
Lightning Source LLC
LaVergne TN
LVHW070658100526
838202LV00013B/994